Royal Statistical Society Lecture Note Series

Royal Statistical Society Lecture Note Series

---

1. Monica A. Walker (ed.): *Interpreting crime statistics*
2. Wojtek J. Krzanowski (ed.): *Recent advances in descriptive multivariate analysis*
3. Byron J. T. Morgan (ed.): *Statistics in toxicology*

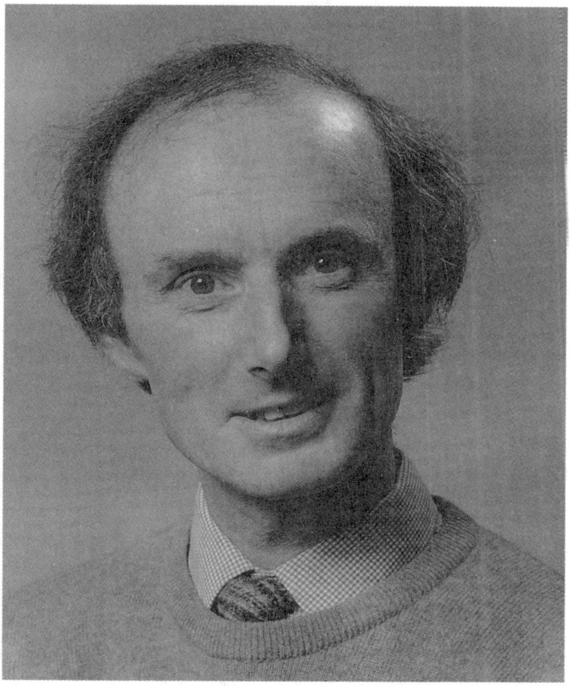

David A. Williams

Statistics in Toxicology

A Volume in Memory of David A. Williams

Edited by

B. J. T. MORGAN

Institute of Mathematics and Statistics
University of Kent

CLARENDON PRESS • OXFORD

1996

Oxford University Press, Walton Street, Oxford OX2 6DP
Oxford New York
Athens Auckland Bangkok Bombay
Calcutta Cape Town Dar es Salaam Delhi
Florence Hong Kong Istanbul Karachi
Kuala Lumpur Madras Madrid Melbourne
Mexico City Nairobi Paris Singapore
Taipei Tokyo Toronto
and associated companies in
Berlin Ibadan

Oxford is a trade mark of Oxford University Press

Published in the United States
by Oxford University Press Inc., New York

A catalogue record for this book is available from the British Library

Library of Congress Cataloging in Publication Data
(Data available)

ISBN 0 19 852329 7

Typeset by Technical Typesetting Ireland
Printed in Great Britain by
Redwood Books, Trowbridge, Wiltshire

Preface

This volume celebrates the life and work of David A. Williams who, at the time of his death, was one of the foremost statisticians in the world working in the area of toxicology. This can be appreciated from the many references to his work in this volume.

In May 1992, the British Region of the international Biometric Society held a meeting in Edinburgh in memory of David. Several of the contributors to this volume (Eryl Shirley, Barry Margolin, Andy Grieve, Anne Whitehead, and Louise Ryan) spoke at that meeting. It was introduced by Professor David Finney, and an edited version of his comments is included in this volume.

Found by Margaret Shotter amongst David's papers was the written version of an invited talk he gave in Vienna, in 1988, to the Third International Workshop on Statistical Modelling. As it has previously only been given limited circulation, we are pleased to be able to include this paper here, as Chapter 7. Special thanks are due to Anne Miller, David's wife, who agreed to this, and supplied the photograph used as the frontispiece.

B.J.T.M

Contents

Contributors

M. Becka, Universitat Dortmund, Fachbereich Statistik, Statistische Methoden in der Genetik, Campus Nord/Gebaude Mathematik, Vogelpothsweg 87, D-44227 Dortmund, Germany

R. N. Curnow, Department of Applied Statistics, University of Reading, Whiteknights, PO Box 217, Reading RG6 2AN, UK

Michael F. W. Festing, MRC Toxicology Unit, Hodgkin Building, University of Leicester, PO Box 138, Lancaster Road, Leicester LE1 9HN, UK

D. J. Finney, 13 Oswald Court, South Oswald Road, Edinburgh EH9 2HY, UK

Karen Fung, Department of Mathematics and Statistics, University of Windsor, Windsor, Ontario, Canada N9B 3P4

Andrew P. Grieve, Pfizer Central Research, Biometrics Department, Sandwich, Kent CT13 9NJ, UK

W. G. S. Hines, Department of Mathematics and Statistics, University of Guelph, Guelph, Ontario, Canada N1G 2W1

A. Islam, Department of Mathematics and Statistics, University of Windsor, Windsor, Ontario, Canada N9B 3P4

Daniel Krewski, Health Protection Branch, Health Canada, Ottawa, Ontario, Canada K1A 0L2 *and* Department of Mathematics and Statistics, Carleton University, Ottawa, Ontario, Canada K1S 5B6

Myrto Lefkopoulou, Department of Biostatistics, Harvard School of Public Health and Division of Biostatistics, DFCI, 44 Binney Street, Boston, MA 02115, USA

D. P. Lovell, BIBRA International, Woodmansterne Road, Carshalton, Surrey SM5 4DS, UK

Barry H. Margolin, Department of Biostatistics, School of Public Health, University of North Carolina at Chapel Hill, Chapel Hill, North Carolina 27599, USA

B. J. T. Morgan, Institute of Mathematics and Statistics, Cornwallis Building, University of Kent at Canterbury, Canterbury, Kent CT2 7NF, UK

R. J. O'Hara Hines, Department of Statistics and Actuarial Science, University of Waterloo, Waterloo, Ontario, Canada N2L 3G1

S. R. Paul, Department of Mathematics and Statistics, University of Windsor, Windsor, Ontario, Canada N9B 3P4

Kenneth J. Risko, Northern Telecom, 200 Athens Way, Nashville, Tennessee 37228, USA

Andrea Rotnitzky, Department of Biostatistics, Harvard School of Public Health and Division of Biostatistics, DFCI, 44 Binney Street, Boston, MA 02115, USA

Louise Ryan, Department of Biostatistics, Harvard School of Public Health and Division of Biostatistics, DFCI, 44 Binney Street, Boston, MA 02115, USA

David Salsburg, Department of Clinical Research, Central Research Division, Pfizer Inc., Eastern Point Road, Groton, CT 06340, USA

Eryl Shirley, Cambridge Statistical Consultants, 61 Beaumont Road, Cambridge CB1 4PX, UK

W. Urfer, Universitat Dortmund, Fachbereich Statistik, Statistische Methoden in der Genetik, Campus Nord/Gebaude Mathematik, Vogelpothsweg 87, D-44227 Dortmund, Germany

A. Whitehead, Department of Applied Statistics, University of Reading, Whiteknights, PO Box 217, Reading RG6 2AN, UK

Yiliang Zhu, Department of Epidemiology and Biostatistics, College of Public Health, University of South Florida, Tampa, Florida 33612-3805, USA

David A. Williams

DAVID J. FINNEY

The following is a condensation of David Finney's introductory remarks to the May 1992 meeting of the British Region of the international Biometric Society.

It is my pleasant duty to welcome you all to a long and interesting programme about recent work in a wide range of biometric problems. I shall not keep you from this for long.

Our programme has been constructed to honour the memory of David Williams, and to remind us of some of the aspects of biometry to which he contributed during his too short life.

I shall not attempt to review David's whole career. I must make plain that I regarded him as a model of what a biometrician should be, knowledgeable about underlying mathematical theory, imaginative in seeing which parts of such theory are relevant to a current practical problem, and always concerned to interpret his analysis of data in terms meaningful within the scientific discipline to which those data referred. In 1966, I was immensely pleased when I persuaded this young man of great promise to join my new department here in Edinburgh. He rapidly displayed an appetite for tackling any new problem of quantitative biology that he perceived to need statistical thought and method.

His earlier association with the late Victor Rothschild, and with Frank Yates at Rothamsted, had already taught him the vital importance of talking in depth with any biologist with whom he was to collaborate, in order to gain an appreciation of the logical structure of a problem before attempting to formulate it in terms susceptible to statistical attack. This outlook became evident in his early research on synchrony of cell growth and division. His modest ease of manner enabled him to talk with biologists—some far senior to him—without manifesting the intellectual arrogance of which our profession is sometimes accused. In this way, he was able to make important contributions to the quantitative understanding of general problems that arise in drug testing, bioassay, toxicology, and even animal ecology.

Throughout this period, David was playing a vital part in the growth and development of teaching within Edinburgh's new Department of Statistics. He was a fine teacher, always clear in exposition and rigorous without undue pedantry. He showed great concern for his undergraduate and graduate students, both academically and in the personal problems that they brought to him during his long spell as a director of studies. When I look back, I am conscious of my own good fortune in all the staff who joined me in those early years, but I always think of David Williams as an outstanding tower of strength—ever willing to take on an extra task, or to produce ideas on how we might improve our teaching programme and increase our effectiveness as willing collaborators with scientists from other disciplines.

My short tribute to a fine colleague and a dear friend would be incomplete without mention of his unstinting services to our discipline, through the Biometric Society and the Royal Statistical Society, as a member of committees and especially as an editor. Those who have undertaken to clear up his correspondence and other files have told me of their amazement at discovering the enormous amount of very thorough constructively helpful editing he had undertaken for *Applied Statistics*.

Those of us who knew David Williams well are still in a state of shock at the cruel suddenness with which he was taken from us. Let me urge that any sense of mourning be replaced by a mood of rejoicing in his achievements, and in the way that they have stimulated the research of others: I am sure that we shall be made increasingly conscious of this by the excellent papers now to be presented.

Publications of David A. Williams

1965 Monozygotic twinning in mice. *Journal of Medical Genetics*, **2**, 26–31 (with M. E. Wallace).

1966 Errors of treatment comparisons when observations are missing from a randomised block experiment with additional replication of a control treatment. *Biometrics*, **22**, 632–33.

1967 The calibration of plate differences in thin-layer chromatographic determination of R_M values. *Journal of Chromatography*, **26**, 280–2.

1967 The influence of exposure time on the susceptibility of *Australorbis glabratus* to *N*-tritylmorpholine. *Annals of Tropical Medicine and Parasitology*, **61**, 15–20 (with C. B. C. Boyce).

1967 Toxicological studies with the herbicide 2,6-dichloro-thiobenzamide (Chlorthiamid, 'Prefix'). *Archiv fur Toxikologie*, **23**, 42–51 (with V. K. H. Brown, P. L. Chambers, L. W. Ferrigan, and D. E. Stevenson).

1967 Toxicity of sodium lauryl sulphate, sodium lauryl ethoxysulphate and corresponding surfactants derived from synthetic alcohols. *Food and Cosmetics Toxicology*, **5**, 763–9 (with A. I. T. Walker, V. K. H. Brown, L. W. Ferrigan, and R. G. Pickering).

1968 A re-examination of the penetration of Nitella cells by non-electrolytes. *Physiologia Plantarum*, **21**, 902–9 (with B. V. Milborrow).

1969 Quantitative measurements of osteoid in health and disease. *Clinical Orthopaedics*, **63**, 196–209 (with J. Chalmers, A. Barclay, A. M. Davidson, and D. A. D. Macleod).

1969 Linear synthesis of sucrase and phosphatases during the cell cycle of *Schizosaccharomyces pombe*. *Journal of Cell Science*, **5**, 373–91 (J. M. Mitchison and J. Creanor, with Appendix by D. A. Williams).

1969 The inhibition of human platelet 5-hydroxytryptamine uptake by tricyclic antidepressive drugs. The relation between structure and potency. *Journal of Pharmacy and Pharmacology*, **21**, 751–62 (A. Todrick and A. C. Tait, with Appendix by D. A. Williams and A. Todrick).

1970 The inhibitory effect of phosphonates on the formation of calcium phosphate crystals *in vitro* and on aortic and kidney calcification *in vivo*. *European Journal of Clinical Investigation*, **1**, 12–18 (with H. A. Fleisch, R. G. G. Russell, S. Bisaz, and R. C. Mühlbauer).

1970 Discrimination between regression models to determine the pattern of enzyme synthesis in synchronous cell cultures. *Biometrics*, **23**, 23–32.

1970 Multivariate analysis in the genetics of spermatozoan dimensions in mice. *Proceedings of the Royal Society of London B*, **175**, 313–31 (with R. A. Beatty and P. S. Burgoyne).

1970 The influence of pyrophosphate, condensed phosphates, phosphonates and other phosphate compounds on the dissolution of hydroxyapatite *in vitro* and on bone resorption induced by para-thyroid hormone in tissue culture and in thyroparathyroidectomised rats. *Calcified Tissue Research*, **6**, 183–96 (with R. G. G. Russell, R. C. Mühlbauer, S. Bisaz, and H. Fleisch).

1971 A test for differences between treatment means when several dose levels are compared with a zero dose control. *Biometrics*, **27**, 103–17.

1971 The effects of diphosphonates, polyphosphates and calcitonin on 'immobilisation osteoporosis' in rats. *European Journal of Clinical Investigation*, **1**, 336–44 (with R. C. Mühlbauer, R. G. G. Russell, and H. Fleisch).

1971 The treatment of plantar warts in the home. *The Practitioner*, **207**, 197–204 (with M. H. Bunney, J. A. A. Hunter, and M. M. Ogilvie).

1972 The comparison of several dose levels with a zero dose control. *Biometrics*, **28**, 519–31.

1973 Effect of diphosphonates and calcitonin on the chemistry and quantitative histology of rat bone. *Calcified Tissue Research*, **11**, 179–95 (with R. G. G. Russell, A. Kislig, P. A. Casey, and H. Fleisch).

1973 The estimation of relative potency from two parabolas in symmetric bioassays. *Biometrics*, **29**, 695–700.

1973 Letter to the Editor. *Applied Statistics*, **22**, 407–8.

1975 The analysis of binary responses from toxicological experiments involving reproduction and teratogenicity. *Biometrics*, **31**, 949–52.

1976 Improved likelihood ratio tests for complete contingency tables. *Biometrika*, **63**, 33–7.

1976 An assessment of methods of treating viral warts by comparative treatment trials based on a standard design. *British Journal of Dermatology*, **94**, 667–79 (with M. H. Bunney and M. W. Nolan).

1977 Some inference procedures for monotonically ordered normal means. *Biometrika*, **64**, 9–14.

1978 An exact confidence region for a relative potency estimated from combined bioassays. *Biometrics*, **34**, 659–61.

1981 The control of body size in mouse chimaeras. *Genetical Research*, **38**, 25–46 (with D. S. Falconer, I. K. Gauld, and R. C. Roberts).

1982 Extra-binomial variation in logistic linear models. *Applied Statistics*, **31**, 144–8.

1982 Patterns of protein synthesis during the cell cycle of the fission yeast *Schizosaccharomyces pombe*. *Journal of Cell Science*, **58**, 263–85 (J. Creanor and J. M. Mitchison, with Appendix by D. A. Williams).

1983 Estimation of survival from repeated sightings of tagged galahs. *Journal of Animal Ecology*, **52**, 563–73 (with S. T. Buckland and I. Rowley).

1983 The use of the deviance to test the goodness of fit of a logistic-linear model to binary data. *GLIM Newsletter*, **6**, 60–2.

1984 Residuals in generalized linear models. *Proceedings of the XIIth International Biometric Conference, Tokyo*, pp. 59–68.

1986 A note on Shirley's nonparametric test for comparing several dose levels with a zero-dose control. *Biometrics*, **42**, 183–6.

1986 A response to recent publications on multivariate bioassay. *Proceedings of the XIII International Biometric Conference, Seattle*, Session 3.

1986 Interval estimation of the median lethal dose. *Biometrics*, **42**, 641–5.

1987 Generalized linear model diagnostics using the deviance and single case deletions. *Applied Statistics*, **36**, 181–91.

1987 Dose–response models for teratological experiments. *Biometrics*, **43**, 1013–16.

1988 Estimation bias using the beta-binomial distribution in teratology. *Biometrics*, **44**, 305–9.

1988 Extrabinomial variation in toxicology. *Proceedings of the XIVth International Biometric Conference, Namur*, pp. 301–13.

1988 An exact confidence interval for the relative potency estimated from a multivariate bioassay. *Biometrics*, **44**, 861–7.

1988 Tests for differences between several small proportions. *Applied Statistics*, **37**, 421–34.

1989 Analysis of data from *in vitro* cytogenetic assays. In *Statistical evaluation of cytogenetic test data* (ed. D. J. Kirkland), pp. 141–54. Cambridge University Press, Cambridge (with C. Richardson).

1991 The reliability of tests of hypotheses when overdispersed logistic-linear models are fitted by maximum quasi-likelihood. *Biometrical Journal*, **33**(3), 259–70.

1996 Overdispersion in logistic-linear models. In this volume.

PART I

REVIEW PAPERS

1 Are animal experiments in toxicological research the 'right' size?

MICHAEL F. W. FESTING

1.1 Introduction

The use of animals in biomedical research involves complex ethical issues. Whether or not any pain and suffering experienced by the animals can be justified in terms of better future human and animal health is hotly debated. However, both scientists and those concerned with animal welfare would agree that the unnecessary or wasteful use of animals cannot be justified. This led Russell and Burch (1959) to formulate the 'three Rs' of animal experimentation:

1. *Replacement.* Those using animals should attempt to *replace* them wherever possible by non-sentient alternatives such as tissue culture, or by less highly evolved animals such as insects or nematodes.

2. *Refinement.* The methods used in animal experimentation should be *refined* so as to cause the minimum pain and suffering. Thus, surgical procedures should be carried out under anesthetic with the appropriate use of analgesics, and animals should be housed in comfortable conditions.

3. *Reduction.* The number of animals used should be *reduced* as far as consistent with good experimental practice. Experiments which are too large will lead to wastage and unnecessary suffering. Those that are too small will often fail to detect important effects, and may not be repeatable, which in the long run may be even more wasteful. The numbers of animals used can also be reduced by careful selection of experimental material so as to reduce variation, and by controlling variation using blocking and covariance analysis.

The number of animals used in a single experiment can vary enormously, from a single animal which may be used as a source of tissues, cells, or DNA to the so-called 'megamouse' experiments involving several thousand mice. Whether any given experiment is the 'right' size is not an easy question to answer. Theoretically, it is possible to estimate how large the experiment should be if the effect size of interest can be specified, acceptable type I (false positive) and type II (false negative) error rates are chosen, and there is an estimate of the variability of the material (for quantitative characters) (Cohen 1969). In practice, while this may be a reasonable approach for expensive experiments with a single dependent variable, it is quite impractical for most animal experiments designed to assess the action of toxic compounds. Such experiments usually have several or many dependent variables, and it is difficult to specify the effect size of interest for most of them. Moreover, there is often no estimate of the variability of the material for many of the dependent variables. Thus, this theoretical approach is virtually never used. Almost all experiments with laboratory animals are designed on the basis of previous experience and available facilities, and statisticians are rarely consulted.

A more practical 'resource equation' approach was suggested by Mead (1988, p. 587). He considered that most statisticians would design experiments with quantitative dependent variables so as to have about 10–20 degrees of freedom for error with about 10–50 'questions' to be answered by each experiment. The latter can be equated with the treatment degrees of freedom. The third component in the resource equation is the number of degrees of freedom associated with blocks and/or covariates.

The use of 10–20 degrees of freedom for error can be justified by the shape of the relationship between the critical values of Student's-t test (or the F-test) and the degrees of freedom (Fig. 1.1). With less than ten degrees of freedom, the

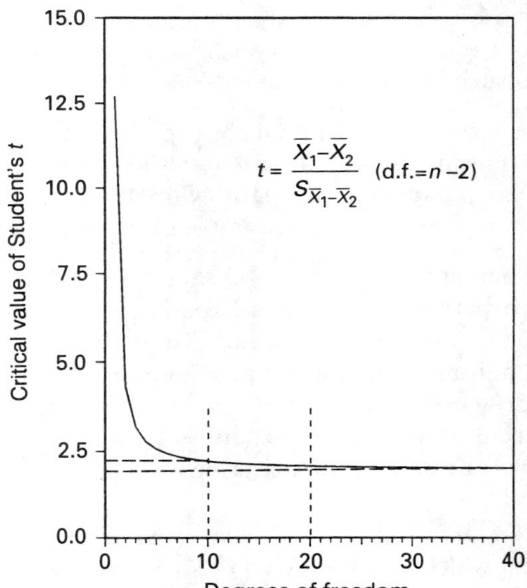

Fig. 1.1. A graph showing the 5 per cent critical values for Student's t-test against degrees of freedom (d.f. $= n - 2$, where n is the total number of observations). Mead (1988) suggested that experiments should be designed so as to have between 10 and 20 degrees of freedom for error (vertical dashed lines). With less than 10 degrees of freedom for error the chance of type II error (false negative result) increases dramatically: however, there is little benefit in having more than 20 degrees of freedom, as the effect size which can be detected only decreases slightly from that point onwards.

experiment is only capable of detecting comparatively large treatment effects. [illegible] effect size that can be detected declines rapidly as [illegible] ase from two to about ten, but it declines only [illegible] freedom exceed about 20. Mead suggests that [illegible] degrees of freedom are probably too small, and [illegible] gically important effects. In contrast, experiments [illegible] freedom for error may be unnecessarily large, as [illegible] rtance would be detected with experiments of this [illegible] d lead to a waste of resources. The exact cut-off [illegible] y. An experiment with, say, 25 to 40 or more degrees of freedom for error may well be justified in some circumstances, such as when there are many treatments and it is considered desirable to have a balanced design. However, Mead's suggestions provide a framework against which the size of actual animal experiments can be measured. The aim of this chapter is to present the results of a survey of papers published in two toxicology journals, using animals, with a view to discussing whether most experiments are well designed and correctly analysed, and appear to be of an appropriate size.

1.2 Materials and methods

All papers published in a single volume of two international toxicology journals were studied. The volumes were chosen because they were the latest bound volume in the library (dated 1989 and 1990) at the time of the survey, and the journals were chosen as being reasonably representative of the types of paper published in the discipline of toxicology. No attempt has been made to study the very large number of experiments conducted largely in the pharmaceutical industry, which do not result in a scientific paper. In many cases such studies are conducted to meet regulatory requirements, and the scientist may not have any discretion over the design. There may also be closer collaboration between research scientists and statisticians in the pharmaceutical industry than in academic departments, which are largely responsible for work published in scientific journals.

The data are expressed as percentages with approximate 95 per cent confidence intervals, even though it might be argued that the papers do not represent a true random sample of papers published in these two journals. In particular, the statistical quality of the papers may have improved since these samples were studied.

Only papers involving whole animals as the experimental unit ('animal papers') were included. Thus some papers in which animals were used as a source of cells for tissue culture were excluded, although these could legitimately be classified as animal experiments.

For each paper the number of separate experiments was noted. For each experiment the number of treatments, the total number of animals used, the experimental design (i.e. completely randomized, randomized block, etc.) and the treatment structure (i.e single factor or factorial) was recorded. The number of degrees of freedom available for estimating experimental error was calculated by subtracting the number of degrees of freedom for treatments $(T-1)$ and blocks $(B-1)$ from the total degrees of freedom $(N-1)$. The statistical methods used to analyse the data was also recorded, and a judgment was made as to whether this was an appropriate analysis. In this case, quite simple criteria were used. If there were more than two treatments, analysis by Student's t-test was considered to be inappropriate. Similarly, a one-way analysis of variance was considered to be inappropriate for analysing a factorial design. Presentation of means and standard deviations without either a statistical test or the calculation of a confidence interval was classified with 'no statistical analysis', and was regarded as inappropriate when the aim was to compare different experimental treatments. Similarly, when the method of statistical analysis was not stated, this was considered to be inappropriate, and in one case re-analysis of the data failed to support a claim of statistical significance.

1.3 Results

The number of papers studied, the number of animal papers, and the number of separate experiments are shown in Table 1.1, which also shows the approximate 95 per cent confidence intervals for any percentage quoted. In both journals animal experiments represented slightly less than half of the papers, and there was no evidence for any striking difference between the two journals either in the proportion of paper which involved animals, or in the number of experiments per paper. A large proportion of the non-animal papers used *in-vitro* methods such as tissue culture.

Somewhat surprisingly, the number of treatments per experiment was quite large (Table 1.1). The mean number of treatments per paper was 5.6 and 6.7 for the two journals. Only four papers involved only two treatments.

Among the 48 experiments, only a single one used a randomized block experimental design, and that was not statistically analysed. All other experiments presumably used a completely randomized design, although none stated explicitly the design that was used. About a third of the experiments used a factorial treatment arrangement. In most cases the factors were an experimental treatment (usually levels of a toxic compound) and a time factor, although other factors were occasionally used.

The statistical test used in each experiment is recorded in Table 1.1. Only a single paper involved discrete data, correctly analysing using the chi-squared test. Thirteen papers (27 per cent) did not use statistics at all, 18 (37 per cent) used the t-test, 11 used the analysis of variance, and only a few used other methods. Covariance analysis was not used in this sample of experiments. Using the simple criteria listed above (i.e. the t-test is inappropriate with more than two treatments, and the one-way ANOVA with more than one factor, etc.), only 16/48 experiments were correctly analysed. However, no attempt was made to estimate whether the conclusions would have been different had a correct analysis been used.

Table 1.1. Results of a survey of experimental design and statistical analysis among 78 papers published in two toxicology journals

Item	Journal 1	Journal 2	Pooled	%	95% C.I.
Total papers studied	35	43	78	—	—
Number of papers using whole animals	14	19	33	42	29–52
Number of experiments, whole animals	21	27	48	—	—
Number of treatments					
2–5	8	18	26	54	41–64
6–10	13	4	17	35	23–46
> 10	0	5	5	10	3–17
Design					
Completely randomized	21	26	47	98	95–100
Randomized block	0	1	1	2	0–5
Treatment structure					
Single factor	13	18	31	65	54–75
Factorial	8	9	17	35	23–46
Statistical tests					
None	6	7	13	27	17–36
t-test	7	11	18	38	25–48
ANOVA	5	6	11	23	13–33
Non-parametric	2	1	3	6	2–11
Regression	1	0	1	2	0–5
Chi-squared	0	1	1	2	0–5
Not stated	0	1	1	2	0–5

The number of degrees of freedom for the error term among all 48 experiments is shown graphically in Fig. 1.2. About 31 per cent of papers had error degrees of freedom falling within the range of about 10–20 suggested by Mead (1988). Approximately 10 per cent had 10 or fewer, 30 per cent had more than 35 degrees of freedom for error.

1.4 Discussion

This survey was based on samples of papers from two toxicology journals which publish academic papers. It does not consider the number of animals used in screening experiments to fulfil government regulations, or unpublished studies in the pharmaceutical industry where there may be more consultation with professional statisticians than in academic institutes. As the results do not differ materially between the two journals, they have been pooled for this discussion.

Mead's (1988) suggestion that experiments with less than 10 degrees of freedom for error are too small and those with more than 20 are too large should not be taken too literally. Exactly where the cut-off points should be

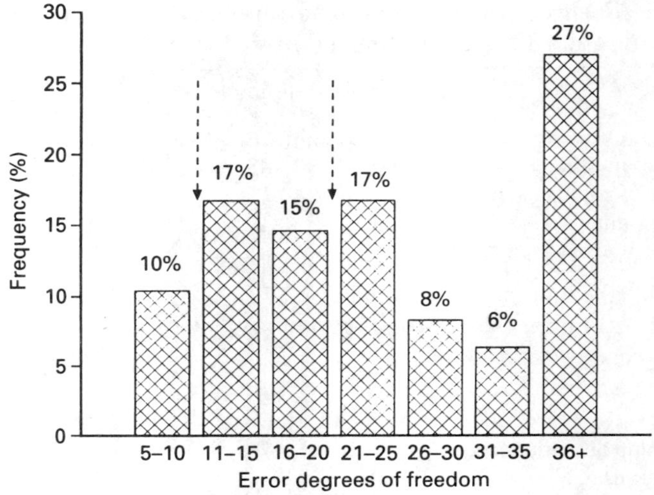

Fig. 1.2. A histogram showing the degrees of freedom for error among 48 experiments in 33 'animal' papers published in two toxicology journals. Mead (1988) suggested that experiments should be designed with 10–20 degrees of freedom for error (vertical arrows), although the cut-off points are somewhat arbitrary.

drawn is debatable, and depends largely on the cost of an experimental unit and possible type II errors. In all the experiments included in this survey the whole animal was the experimental unit, and so should be considered to have a relatively high cost financially and ethically. Only about 30 per cent of the papers studied in this survey would have been the 'right' size by these criteria. About 10 per cent of the experiments had less than ten degrees of freedom for error. Such experiments would involve a high probability of a type II error, and so would not be suitable as a basis for claiming that a given treatment has no effect. On the other hand, they would be quite acceptable as a basis for rejecting the null hypothesis at a stated probability level if in fact the treatment had a large effect. These criteria apply only to experiments involving quantitative data. However, only a single experiment involved discrete data (analysed by the chi-squared test).

About 30 per cent of the sample of experiments involved more than 35 degrees of freedom for error, and several of these may well have been unnecessarily large, particularly as many of the experiments were incorrectly analysed and there was a notable absence of block designs aimed at reducing experimental error. Thus, though only 4/48 experiments involved a comparison of two treatments, 18 of them were analysed using Student's *t*-test. Most scientists are intuitively aware of the importance of having 'enough' (say, between six and ten) degrees of freedom for error and may have chosen group sizes so that the experiment could be analysed using the *t*-test with this number of degrees of freedom for each comparison, rather than using the analysis of variance (with which they appear to be unfamiliar) with its pooled error term. Similarly, several factorial experiments were analysed by one-way rather than n-way ANOVA, and may have been designed so that each separate ANOVA was of a 'reasonable' size.

The almost universal practice of showing standard deviations or standard errors of means using an unpooled estimate of error for each individual mean may also, in the long run, inflate the numbers of animals used. In order to obtain 'reasonable' standard deviations, many scientists who use Student's t-test as their main statistical tool consider that minimum group sizes of about five or six are needed. They tend to design experiments by multiplying this minimum group size by the number of treatments. With a pooled estimate of error in experiments with more than two treatments which are analysed by the analysis of variance, smaller total numbers could be used without any loss of statistical power. However, with group sizes of, say, two or three animals, the unpooled standard deviations would be likely to fluctuate widely. Use of the pooled variance derived from the error mean square in the ANOVA would then be much more appropriate. The main advantage of presenting unpooled estimates of the standard deviations is that heterogeneity of variance may be detected. Although uncorrected heterogeneity of variance was not explicitly enumerated in this sample, several experiments might have been analysed more appropriately after a suitable numerical transformation.

In several cases, experiments were set up to investigate time or dose-level trends, and several animals were used at each dose level in order to give an estimate of variation at that level. However, most such experiments were analysed by comparing groups using a t-test or ANOVA; only one experiment was analysed using regression and none were designed and analysed using linear, quadratic, etc. orthogonal contrasts using the analysis of variance. Again, failure to extract all possible information from the data may have led to excessive use of animals.

A third (17/18) of the experiments involved a factorial design. This accounts for the surprisingly large number of treatments, averaging about six per experiment, though there was a wide spread between experiments. Most experiments still had less than the 10–50 degrees of freedom for treatments suggested by Mead (1988), although it would probably not be sensible to suggest using more treatments until existing ones are correctly analysed. In most cases the factors were a chemical treatment and a killing-time, though in a few cases sex or an additional chemical treatment were the factors. Unfortunately, few of the experiments were analysed as factorial designs. In seven cases a t-test was used and in six cases no statistical analysis was used, or the method used was not stated. A more detailed survey would be needed to find out whether the incorrect analyses led to incorrect conclusions.

Only one paper clearly had a randomized block experimental design, and in that case the data were not statistically analysed. Although randomized blocks are widely used in other branches or research, they appear to be rare in experiments with laboratory animals. The use of blocking should, in the long run, lead to more powerful experiments with fewer type II errors for a given size of experiments. Festing (1992) studied the relative efficiency of five randomized block experimentals using mice, involving 30 dependent variables, and found that they were often such more efficient than completely randomized designs and, in the samples he considered, were never significantly less efficient. However, such designs must be analysed correctly, with removal of the block effect, if these potential gains are to be realized. As only 16/48 experiments appear to have been correctly analysed, it seems unlikely that most research workers would handle the design and analysis of a randomized block experiment without statistical support.

The generally low level of statistical analysis revealed in this survey is in agreement with the findings of Sterling (1971), Benignus and Muller (1982), and Mitchell (1983), all of whom commented on the poor quality of statistical analysis in papers published in toxicological journals. Three specific examples were given by Festing (1994). In one case mongrel dogs of widely different body weights and both sexes had simply been assigned to the eight treatment groups of a 2×4 factorial design at random, with no attempt to control variability or maintain a balance of the sexes. The resulting data involving eight dependent variables were then inappropriately analysed using Student's *t*-test. Many other anomalies were also noted, and it was suggested that the experiment could have been done just as efficiently using half the number of carefully selected animals. In the second case, a single experiment involved two strains of mice, five time periods, and four dose levels in a $2 \times 5 \times 4$ factorial design, with between three and six mice per group. There was no indication of how the 120–240 mice had actually been used, and the reason for the unequal subclass numbers was unexplained. The experiment could probably have been done just as well with two blocks of 40 mice. The third example involved 80 mice in a 2×4 (sex $\times$ dose) factorial experiment, which had been analysed by the *t*-test, and had failed to detect a dose-level which was highly significant when analysed by the analysis of variance. The trend would still have been statistically significant ($p < 0.01$) using only 24 mice.

The present study has focused particularly particularly on whether animal experiments are the 'right' size. About a third appeared to be unnecessarily large. The survey supports previous studies in concluding that better experimental design and statistical analysis of animal experiments could lead to a reduction in animal use. There appears to be an urgent need for better training in the design and statistical analysis of animal experiments. Such training is ethically desirable and would probably be highly cost-effective in improving the overall quality of research, while making more efficient use of scarce resources.

References

Benigus, V. A. and Muller, K. E. (1982). Bad statistics are worse than none (letter). *Neurotoxicology*, **3**, 153–4.

Cohen, J. (1969). *Statistical power analysis for the behavioral sciences*. Academic Press, New York.

Festing, M. F. W. (1992). The scope for improving the design of laboratory animal experiments. *Laboratory Animals*, **26**, 256–67.

Festing, M. F. W. (1994). Reduction of animal use: experimental design and quality of experiments. *Laboratory Animals*, **28**, 212–21.

Mead, R. (1988). *The design of experiments*. Cambridge University Press, Cambridge.

Mitchell, C. L. (1983). 'Bad statistics' revisited (letter). *Neurotoxicology*, **4**, 157–9.

Russell, W. M. S. and Burch, R. L. (1959). *The principles of humane experimental technique*. Methuen, London (reprinted by the Universities Federation for Animal Welfare, 8 Hamilton Close, South Mimms, Potters Bar, Herts EN6 3QD, UK).

Sterling, T. D. (1971). Difficulty of evaluating the toxicity and teratogenicity of 2,4,5-T from existing animal experiments. *Science*, New York, **174**, 1358–9.

2 Estimating dose–response for toxic end-points

DAVID SALSBURG

'Only the dose makes a thing not a poison.'
Paracelsus

2.1 Introduction

The above quotation lies at the heart of almost all toxicological investigations. It tends to be ignored in the popular press and in political discussions of the consequences of these investigations, so we often read about 'toxic substances' that are 'the most toxic known to man' or that are 'very toxic'. The resulting political debates sometimes assume that some substances are 'toxic' and some are not. Then, the debate is over whether a particular substance belongs in that class. However, a little careful thought about the biological effects of chemicals will soon produce a Paracelsian conclusion. One molecule of anything is not going to produce damage to a living organism; and enough of anything, no matter how essential it may be to life, will kill. The ability of modern analytical chemistry to detect levels of contaminants down to the parts per billion level has made it essential that even the political debates come back to Paracelsus' insights.

Thus, although much of the toxicological literature deals with modes of toxicity or the development of methods to identify specific types of toxicity, the practical final use of toxicology rests on the ability of the science to develop believable dose–response estimates. The interface between toxicology and statistics has fallen short when it comes to this problem, although Williams (1972) provided a partial solution in his widely referenced article. Statistical techniques are often used to identify whether a compound produces a specific toxic lesion (through the use of significance tests—see Peto, 1974, for example) or to model fanciful 'dose–responses' beyond that range of observation (see Mantel and Bryan 1961), but there is very little in the literature that deals with methods for developing dose–responses that can be derived from experimental data and that are robust to unprovable assumptions in the model.

However, statistical theory is rich in methods of deriving dose–responses (Salsburg, 1990), and a great deal of recent work has been directed at problems that arise when the 'standard' assumptions of regression analysis are not met. This recent literature solves some of the problems that occur in toxicology and that have made application of statistical methods to dose–responses for toxic end-points difficult. This chapter attempts to address some of those problems and show how they can be solved.

Section 2.2 describes a traditional method of estimating dose–response, which developed early in toxicology and independently of formal statistical modelling. It is proposed here as a 'stalking horse' against which to compare statistically based dose–response estimates.

Statistical models of dose–response can be summarized as

$$Y = f(\text{dose}, x_1, x_2, \ldots, x_k) + E, \tag{2.1}$$

where Y is a measure of toxicity, $f(\ )$ is a function of dose and other variables, denoted by $x_1, x_2, \ldots, x_k$, and E, usually called 'error' or 'residual', represents a symmetric random variable that covers those things we cannot or did not observe.

Section 2.3 will describe various choices of Y, the measure of toxicity. Section 2.4 will describe various choices of $f(\ )$ and the effects of E on the usefulness of those choices.

2.2 A traditional 'dose–response'

During the 1940s and 1950s, a standard toxicology study was developed for pharmaceutical research, in conjunction with government regulators in the USA and the UK. I do not know who can claim priority, but the earliest printed reference I can find is in the 'Black Book' of the US Food and Drug Administration (1959). This study is now called a sub-chronic 90-day toxicity study, but it was originally developed as the longest-term animal toxicity study that would be used before taking a new drug into human trials.

The 90-day study was developed to determine:

(1) a 'safe dose' that could be used as an entering dose in human studies; and

(2) the nature of the toxic lesions that might be expected in human studies.

The usual design was to expose two sexes of a selected species to three or four doses of test compound, keeping an equal number for controls. The doses were selected so that the highest dose was sure to produce toxic lesions, and one or more of the lowest doses was expected to show no toxic effect.

Once the study was completed and all animals sacrificed, the toxicologist examined the pathology of the highest-dosed animals, along with records of blood chemistries and clinical observations taken while they were alive. This overall view of the high-dose animals was combined with a knowledge of what might be expected from the exaggerated pharmacology of the test compound and what had been seen with similar compounds. This careful examination led the toxicologist to devise a syndrome of toxicity that would be expected from the test compound. The controls were then examined to eliminate those aspects of the syndrome that appeared in any control animals and were, thus, the result of the experimental situation and not of the treatment. Finally, this syndrome of toxic lesions was projected back to establish putative precursors of those lesions.

The middle-dose groups were examined to find animals with this syndrome or its putative precursors. The highest dose that had no such animals was labelled a 'maximum safe dose'. The lowest dose which had any animals with such events was labelled a 'minimum toxic dose'. The 90-day toxicity study was usually run on three species. The lowest maximum safe dose was then divided by a safety factor, and the resulting dose was chosen as the entering dose in humans.

When first shown this procedure, the statisticians misunderstood what was happening. They assumed that there was some specific lesion that identified the toxic effect and that the toxicologists were declaring a dose 'safe' if no animals had that lesion. Put into a statistical model, this meant that the dose–response was taken as the probability of that lesion. The statisticians thought that the toxicologists were unaware of the fact that, with only N animals at a given dose, the probability of getting that lesion at that dose could be as high as $3/N$, even if no animals were seen with the lesion.

However, the toxicologists were dealing with more than a single well-defined lesion. They were looking at a syndrome of events (involving pathological lesions, clinical chemistries, and other measurements, along with putative precursors of the observed pathological lesions). A better statistical model would be one in which the toxicologists had developed a continuous measure of toxicity, and chose as the 'safe dose' one in which all of the treated animals had measures that were less than the minimum measure seen in the highest dose group. However, even that does not describe what was being done. To do so would involve Bayesian statistics and go outside the realm of formal significance tests.

The 90-day toxicity study has provided the pharmaceutical industry with a very useful tool. I know of no case in which serious damage has occurred to humans treated with an entering dose determined from the 'maximum safe dose' of a 90-day study. There has been unexpected toxicity to human subjects in drug studies, but this has occurred at doses higher than the projected entering dose. There have also been cases in which the 90-day toxicity study has not been run properly. Thalidomide is a prominent example. The drug was describe as being 'safe' because it was not possible to develop toxic lesions in animal trials. However, this runs contrary to the basic ideas behind the 90-day study. According to Paracelsus, all compounds are potential poisons. A proper 90-day study always includes a dose at which this happens. How else would the toxicologist be able to identify the syndrome of toxic events that is associated with that compound?

2.3 Measuring toxicity

Before we can produce a statistically based dose–response estimate, we need to have a measure of toxicity, Y in eqn (2.1). In any designed study, we have a 'unit of experimentation'. This is the basic material in which treatments can be randomly assigned. When animals are first treated post-weaning, the unit of experimentation is the animal. In teratology studies, the unit experimentation is the dam of F_0 generation (the original group of treated animals). In cell culture studies, the unit is the individual plate or well which has been seeded and then treated.

We can think of the unit of experimentation as contained information which will be converted into a one-dimensional number. The least informative number is a zero or one, depending upon whether or nor an event has occurred. Thus, we can take an animal and examine only if it has developed a liver tumour, ignoring other lesions on the same animal and the multiplicity or severity of the observed liver tumour(s). However, in most studies, more informative measures can be derived, because we often observe far more than event/no event in a unit of experimentation. In a teratology study, the measure might be the proportion of surviving pups with skeletal abnormalities. Alternatively, it might be an index of soft tissue effects that combines the number of corpora lutea, the number of pups that survive to X days, and the number of these with varying degrees of abnormalities.

If the unit of experimentation is used only to produce a zero or one, depending upon the occurrence of a given event, then the dose–response refers to the probability that the event will occur. This is an easily understood measure of toxicity. However, by using very little information in each unit of experimentation, it takes a large number of such units to provide reasonably narrow confidence bounds on the true probability of event at a given dose. For instance, if we wish to have a 95 per cent confidence bound on the probability of an event which does not include 1/1000, we need to observe 3000 units at that dose with none of them showing the event.

On the other hand, if the measure of toxicity is a continuous normally distributed random variable, with only 16 units at a given dose, the half-width of a 95 per cent confidence bound will be less than a half standard deviation from the observed response.

The problem with using more information to derive a measure of toxicity is that we need to agree about degrees of effect. For instance, is one benign tumour a less toxic event than three benign tumours, or than one malignant tumour? If the treatment induces nephropathy, can we order the pathology of the kidney to derive measures of effect? It is even more difficult to combine events across a syndrome of toxicity. Suppose that the compound induces elevated liver enzymes, associated with fatty deposits in the liver, with frank liver necrosis at higher doses, but also involving cardiac failure and ulcers of the forestomach.

One way to handle multiplicity of lesions across different organs and organ systems is to view each organ system separately. For instance, suppose that the compound causes gastric ulcers at high doses. We could order events starting with mild anaemia but no clear lesions, going on to inflammation of the stomach mucosa, then to minimal ulceration, to increasing size and number of ulcers.

The treated animals (all doses plus controls) can be ordered along this system of toxicity and given relative ranks. The animals could then be ordered in terms of lesions of another organ system and ranked again. This could be done for the several organ systems that are involved in the expected toxic effect of the compound.

Once we have ranked each animal along each of the several systems, we can apply a method due to O'Brien (1984). We let each animal's measure of toxicity be the average rank that animal has across all the systems. This average rank can then be used as a measure of overall toxicity. The disadvantage of using average rank is that it does not have any direct biological meaning. However, these numbers can be converted into something meaningful by examining the mean value of the average rank across all high-dosed animals and the mean value across all controls. Doses which produce values that are scattered about the mean value for controls could be called 'no effect' doses. The percentage distance from the mean for the controls to the mean for the high dose could characterize the level of toxicity for intermediate doses that cannot be called 'no effect' doses.

All of this would be an attempt to quantify the basic ideas of the 90-day toxicity study. It may be that no formal method of quantification will do as well as the judgment of a trained toxicologist. However, we should make the attempt.

In some cases, the unit of experimentation produces a more easily interpreted measure of toxicity. For instance, if we plate out 10 000 cultured embryonic cells and count how many remain after treatment, we can obtain a continuous measure for each plate. Several plates at a given dose provide us with a measure of random error. As in the use of simple event/no event values for the unit of experimentation, this measure can be interpreted as the mean probability of event at that dose. However, in this case, we can obtain a more precise measurement, based on the greater amount of information.

In teratology, we can derive an index of viability from counts of pups born, and surviving for different periods of time. Each dam will have such an index. A dose–response for that index will give us the expected average index of viability for a given dose. As with the average rank O'Brien statistic, we can examine the scatter of the indices in the control group to the scatter in any treated group and find a 'no effect' dose. However, this calls for a biological decision about what 'no effect' means; for we are now dealing with mean values, and there is no direct conversion of this to probability of event.

The main point of this section is that there are statistical techniques for examining a large contingency table of ordered events, which result in one-dimensional measures of 'effect'; and these can be used to derive dose–response curves. However, the statistical techniques are only methods for organizing data. The data result from toxicological experiments, so the measures that are developed have to be given biological interpretation.

One method for doing this was proposed in Salsburg (1992). We look at specific animals from a large number of studies and their derived measures of effect. The toxicologist uses her or his judgement to decide which of these animals shows a toxic effect and orders the level of toxicity. The measures of effect associated with those animals are then used to define mean values that represent 'not toxic effect', 'minimal toxic effect', and 'gross toxic effect'. These methods provide use with measures of toxicity that are more informative than modelling the probability of an effect. However, the price we have to pay for this greater level of information is a careful understanding of the biological events being examined.

2.4 The dose–response function

Most of the dose–response literature is based on the statistical concepts of regression where

$$Y = f(\text{dose}) + E \tag{2.2}$$

represents a well-defined mathematical function, e.g., with

$$f(\text{dose}) = \{1 + \exp[-(a + b\,\text{dose})]\}^{-1}. \tag{2.3}$$

These well-defined functions are usually constructed to match what is known of the dose response. For instance, the example given above matches the idea that Y is greater than zero, even when dose is zero, and that Y levels off no matter how high the dose. If the toxicity measure is known to result from enzyme kinetics, one could construct a dose–response curve that introduces parameters of those kinetics.

In some cases, we can model the dose–response in terms of a set of differential equations, as is done in a multicompartment model. There may not be a 'solution' for those differential equations that can be written down in a closed form, but computer algorithms have been developed that will estimate the parameters of those equations. For a probabilistic interpretation of such models, see McQuarrie (1967).

If the biological theory is inadequate to describe a dose response function, we can fit more general functions to the data. A great deal of the recent statistical literature deals with adaptive functions that may change their shape and form from one region of doses to another. These involve spline fits (Silverman 1985) and non-parametric kernel density based regression (Müller 1988), among others. Many widely used spreadsheet programs use spline fits and refer to the regression as 'smoothing'.

2.5 Confidence bounds and random noise

In the basic dose–response formula,

$$Y = f(\text{dose}, x_1, x_2, \ldots, x_k) + E,$$

we use the symbol E to denote those elements we do not understand and which cause the actual observed value of Y to be different from that predicted by the response function $f(\ )$. The degree to which Y differs from the predicted value provides us with a measure of the uncertainty associated with this type of prediction. This is true, whether the function $f(\ )$ is of a well-defined form or is a locally adaptive non-parametric regression. The greater the scatter of E, the greater the uncertainty associated with the prediction.

Thus, methods have been derived for fitting a band of uncertainty about the predicted dose–response. One way to derive a band of uncertainty is through the use of confidence bounds. Strictly speaking, 95 per cent confidence bounds provide us with a random band, into which we expect the true dose–response curve to fall for 95 per cent of the time. However, it is convenient to think of these bounds as providing a region of uncertainty, so we can say that we are reasonably sure that future dose–responses will fall within the 95 per cent confidence bounds and we have a 50:50 chance that future dose–responses will fall within the 50 per cent confidence bounds. Thus, the idea of a random additive error, E, provides us with a smear of uncertainty that can be used to derive conservative estimates of a 'no effect' dose.

How can these confidence bounds be derived? There are traditional algorithms that can be used if the dose–response function is a simple polynomial and if we assume that the error, E, is normally distributed. However, without those assumptions, we can use the Jackknife (Miller 1964), cross-validation (Salsburg 1992; Thall *et al.* 1992), or the Bootstrap (Efron and Tibshirani 1986; Hinkley 1988) to derive confidence bounds, without having to make these assumptions and allowing us to use adaptive local regression techniques. All of these are computer-intensive methods of analysis that have been developed in the past 15–20 years.

2.6 Conclusions

Toxicology as a science has failed to make use of recent computer–intensive statistical methods; yet those methods may well provide solutions to the real problem of toxicology—how to estimate safe doses. However, we need to derive continuous measures of toxicity and to make judgments about what degree of lesion or change is really 'toxic'.

If toxicologists are willing to make these types of decisions, statisticians stand ready to provide them with useful tools. In the end, we may be able to quantify the methods developed in the 90-day toxicity study and extend Paracelsus' insights to more complicated toxicity studies.

References

Efron, B. and Tibshirani, T. (1986). Bootstrap methods for standard errors, confidence intervals, and other methods of statistical accuracy. *Statistical Science*, **1**, 54–77.

Food and Drug Administration, US Department of Health and Human Services (1959). *Guidelines for toxicological testing*. US Government Printing Office, Washington, DC.

Hinkley, D. V. (1988). Bootstrap methods. *Journal of the Royal Statistical Society* (*B*), **50**, 321–37.

Mantel, N. and Bryan, W. R. (1961). "Safety" testing of carcinogenic agents. *Journal of the National Cancer Institute*, **27**, 455–470.

McQuarrie, D. A. (1967). Stochastic approach to chemical kinetics. *Journal of Applied Probability*, **4**, 413–78.

Miller, R. G. (1964). A trustworthy jackknife, *Annals of Mathematics and Statistics*, **35**, 1594–605.

Müller, H. C. (1988). *Nonparametric analysis of longitudinal data*. Springer-Verlag, Berlin.

O'Brien, P. C. (1984). Procedures for comparing samples with multiple endpoints. *Biometrics*, **40**, 1079–88.

Peto, R. (1974). Guidelines on the analysis of tumor rates and death rates in experimental animals. *British Journal of Cancer*, **29**, 101–5.

Salsburg, D. S. (1990). Estimating dose response in chronic toxicity studies; 24-month administration of acrylonitrile in drinking water of fischer 344 rats. *The Science of the Total Environment*. **99**, 289–305.

Salsburg, D. S. (1992). *The use of restricted significance tests in clinical trials*. p. 84. Springer-Verlag, New York.

Silverman, B. W. (1985). Some aspects of the spine smoothing approach to non-parametric regression curve fitting (with discussion). *Journal of the Royal Statistical Society (B)*, **47**, 1–52.

Thall, P. F., Simon, R., and Grier, D. A. (1992). Test-based variable selection with cross-validations. *Journal of Computational and Graphical Statistics*, **1**, 41–62.

Williams, D. A. (1972). The comparison of several dose levels with a zero-dose control. *Biometrics*, **28**, 519–31.

3 A literature review of statistical methods for the analysis of general toxicology data

ERYL SHIRLEY

3.1 Introduction

This review covers the analysis of standard general toxicology studies. The purpose of these studies is to test for possible toxic effects of drugs or other substances, such as agrochemicals. The studies are usually carried out on at least one rodent species and on either beagle dogs or monkeys. The decision as to whether to test a drug on humans or to introduce a substance into the environment will depend on the results of these studies. Previous acute toxicity studies on the same species will have been carried out in order to find non-lethal doses.

In each study there are a control group of animals, receiving a zero dose of the compound under test, sometimes a second control group which does not receive either the compound or the vehicle used for dosing the animals, and a number of groups dosed at increasing levels of the test compound. Most commonly there are three such groups, whose dose levels are on an approximate logarithmic scale. Occasionally, there is also a positive control group dosed with a standard compound already in use and thought to be similar in effect to the test compound. This group is dosed at a level which is considered to be equivalent to one of the doses of the test compound. Often, the low-dose equivalent is chosen. It is expected that the highest-dose group of the test compound will demonstrate some signs of toxicity, but it is hoped that none of the other groups will. The lowest dose level is chosen to be relatively close to the expected human dose level, but with a safety margin. In dog and monkey studies the group sizes are small—often only three or four of each sex. Group sizes in rodent studies are much larger—at least ten of each sex—often with increased replication in the zero-dose control group.

The studies last for from three to six months and, apart from noting visible signs of toxicity, blood samples are taken initially and at intervals for haematology and blood chemistry measurements to be made; urine samples are also analysed and regular body weight, food, and water consumption measurements are obtained. After death, the organs are examined and weighed. All these measurements and observations need to be analysed for evidence of toxicity.

Some of the statistical methods discussed in this review, such as transformation of data and analysis of covariance, have much broader applications than toxicity data analysis, while others, such as testing for a dose response, are more specialized. It is hoped that these discussions and the accompanying bibliography will assist statisticians and others in the analysis of this type of data.

3.2 Transformation of data

It has been shown (Lewi and Marsboom 1981; Sanderson and Phillips 1981; Sedlmayer and Hornacek 1984) that the biological variables measured on animals, particularly the haematology and blood chemistry observations, cannot be assumed to follow the normal distribution. The most common transformations found in the literature are the logarithmic, square root, and rank transformations. No single transformation has been found to be consistently suitable for any particular variable either in the literature or, in practice, by the author. Consequently, methods of examining data for its suitability for classical analysis of variance were investigated together with methods for choosing a suitable transformation.

The assumptions made by the classical least squares analysis of variance are that the errors are independently and normally distributed with zero mean and constant variance. In addition, any effects are assumed to be additive, i.e. the difference between two treatments will be a constant plus an error term. Fortunately, comparisons between means are not greatly affected by moderate departures from these assumptions, especially when the group sizes are equal. However, experiments with unequal group sizes are more sensitive to departures from the above assumptions, especially to heterogeneity of variance (see Kendall and Stuart 1977, Ch. 37). In addition, comparisons of means are more susceptible to lack of symmetry than they are to a difference in the value for kurtosis from that of the normal distribution (Kendall *et al.* 1991, Ch. 31). Very often a variance stabilizing transformation will not only normalize the errors but also cure lack of additivity of effects. The logarithmic transformation provides an excellent example. Data that are log-normally distributed are positively skewed, will demonstrate heterogeneity of variance (because the standard deviation is proportional to the mean), and the effects will usually be multiplicative, i.e. the difference between a treated group mean and the control group mean will be proportional to the control group mean. A logarithmic transformation can then solve all three problems.

Comparisons of variances are far more susceptible to departures from normality than are comparisons of means (Kendall *et al.* 1991, Ch. 31). These comparisons are very susceptible to the kurtosis of the underlying distribution. If the kurtosis is lower than that of the normal distribution, the comparisons between variances are conservative; and if the kurtosis is higher, then too many significant differences are found. This leads to problems when checking data for heterogeneity of variance prior to performing an analysis of variance and comparing mean values. The best known test for heterogeneity of variance is that proposed by Bartlett (1937), which is the likelihood ratio test based on the sample variance. Unfortunately, this test and others, such as that proposed by

Lehmann (1959), which are based on the sample variances, are very sensitive to kurtosis in the manner described above. Levene (1960) proposed a test based on the absolute values of the residuals. F-ratio tests are carried out on these values according to the study design. This test relies on the approximate normality of the group means of these absolute residuals since the individual values are not normally distributed. The test will also be sensitive to departures from normality and heterogeneity of variance in a similar way to the analysis of variance of the original observations. For example, if the standard deviation in one group is twice that in another, although the group means of the absolute residuals will differ by a factor of about two, so will their standard deviations.

A non-parametric method of comparing variances is described in Conover (1980) and is based on the ranked absolute deviations of the observations from their group mean values. Unfortunately, this test is not very powerful, with an asymptotic relative efficiency to the F-test (when two groups are being compared) of only 76 per cent when the actual underlying distribution is normal. Its asymptotic relative efficiency is 1.08 for a double exponential distribution and 1.0 for the uniform distribution.

If it is decided that the data needs to be transformed, then the most well known method of choosing a variance stabilizing transformation is that described by Box and Cox (1964). They consider the family of transformations

$$y = \{(x+b)^a - 1\}/a, \qquad a \neq 0,$$
$$y = \log(x+b), \qquad a = 0,$$

and apply maximum likelihood methods to obtain the values of a and b that will transform the observations to the desired normal model. Berry (1987) considered transformations of the form $\log(x+c)$, where c was chosen in order to minimize the sum of the absolute values of the skewness and kurtosis of the residuals (where the kurtosis was measured as a deviation from the value for the normal distribution, which is 3). These methods involve a considerable amount of computing and are not suitable for the hundreds of analyses involved in chronic toxicology studies. In practice, only the logarithmic, square root, and rank transformations are used routinely on toxicological data. Where values less that one are expected, the $\log(1+x)$ transformation is often chosen to prevent negative values or minus infinity, which occurs when x is zero (Snedecor and Cochran 1967, Ch. 11, pp. 329–30).

It should be noted that these preliminary tests on the data and the possible resulting transformations do not increase the type I errors, as do some other preliminary tests, which will be discussed in the next section. On the contrary, if gross violations of the assumptions involved in analysis of variance are left, type I errors may well increase considerably and the power may decrease.

3.3 The inclusion of covariates in the analysis

It has been shown by Shirley and Newnham (1984) and by Abeyasakera (1984) that is is not advisable to decide on whether or not to adjust for a covariate by a rule such as 'Adjust if the relationship between variate and covariate is significant at the 10 per cent level' or 'Adjust if the error mean square is reduced'. Firstly, such a rule increases the chance of finding a false positive result. Shirley and Newnham found that, in the case of organ weight analyses where the organ weight is adjusted for final body weight (see Section 3.10), this type I error could rise to about 12 per cent in some situations, where the nominal type I error was set at 5 per cent. Secondly, the inclusion of the covariate may be removing bias from the experimental results, and therefore not including it may give misleading results even when it does not appear to be significantly related to the variate in the current set of data, or does not improve the efficiency of the analysis.

It should be noted that the same principles apply to preliminary tests for the significance of blocking or other factors, and the consequent pooling of sums of squares, which reduces the residual mean square.

In both papers, it is recommended that the covariate always be included unless it is known (possibly from investigations of large sets of background data) that the covariate is not correlated with the variate. Also, Abeyasakera suggests the covariate should not be included if the covariate is very weakly correlated with the variate, and the degrees of freedom in the experiment are too few to estimate the regression coefficient with any accuracy.

3.4 Comparisons of treated groups with controls

When several increasing doses of a compound are to be compared with a control then, in the majority of cases, a monotonic response is expected. One exception to this monotonicity might be when the low dose has an effect—possibly beneficial—in one direction and the higher doses have effects in the opposite direction. More rarely, there might be an apparent lack of monotonicity at the highest dose levels, perhaps because the less resistant animals had died before the blood sampling procedures had taken place. Shirley (1985) and Hothorn (1989) showed that, if a monotonic trend with dose existed, tests for trend with dose performed very much better than comparisons between treated groups with controls which did not take the ordering of the means into account. A test for trend with dose is therefore recommended, preferably one which is fairly robust against violations of monotonicity.

Bartholomew (1959*a*, *b*, 1961) proposed the use of maximum likelihood estimates of group means, $m(1), \ldots, m(n)$, for n groups under the assumption that no $m(i) > m(i+1)$ for $i = 1$ to $n - 1$. These maximum likelihood estimates are easily calculated by a simple averaging procedure. Bartholomew's test is a likelihood ratio test for which he produced tables of critical values for equal group sizes. For details of the test statistic and its critical values, see the references above and also Barlow *et al.* (1972), Chacko (1963), and Robertson *et al.* (1988). Tables for increased replication in the control group can be found in Chase (1974).

Williams (1971, 1972) also calculated the maximum likelihood estimates of group means under order restrictions and produced statistics similar to the Student's t-statistic, based on the experimental residual mean square, for differences between the dosed groups and the controls. The numerators of his t-statistics were calculated as the differences between the $n-1$ dosed group estimated maximum likelihood means and the sample control mean. Starting at the highest dose level and moving sequentially down the dose levels, these t-type statistics are calculated until a non-significant difference is found. Tables of significance points for equal replication and for increased replication of the controls are given in the above references. Williams (1972) showed that his test was robust against other inequalities of replication, and calculated adjustments to be made to his significance points in cases of unequal replication amongst the dosed groups. He also showed that the most efficient allocation of a given number of animals to groups in a dose–response study was for there to be about $1.3\sqrt{(n-1)}$ as many animals in the control group as in each of the dosed groups.

Tukey *et al.* (1985) suggested testing for a response to increasing doses of a compound by using regression analysis with the pooled within-group estimates of variability as the error. They suggested regressing against different sets of values based on the doses, $X(i)$, for $i = 1$ to n, where $X(1)$ is the zero dose. The preferred sets were:

(1) the arithmetic doses, $X(i)$;

(2) the ordinal doses, $0, 1, 2, \ldots, n-1$;

(3) log doses except for group 1, the dose for which is calculated as

$$\log(X(2)) - (X(2) - X(1)) * [\log(X(3)) - \log(X(2))]/(X(3) - X(2)).$$

It is recommended that the smallest p-value resulting from these three regressions be taken as the significance level of the trend. This is considered to be 'conservative' in the sense that although there is an increased risk of finding false positives when the smallest of three p-values is chosen, there is also an increased chance of detecting any existing trend with dose.

Ragouzis and Ruberg (1987) describe two types of contrast which they consider useful for finding minimum and maximum effective doses. These are Helmert contrasts and Basin contrasts. Hermert contrasts compare the average of the first m treatment group means with the $(m+1)$st treatment mean, for $m = 1$ to $(n-1)$, when there are n groups altogether. Helmert contrasts for four groups are the vectors $(1, -1, 0, 0)$, $(-1, -1, 2, 0)$, and $(-1, -1, -1, 3)$. These contrasts do not seem suitable for toxicity studies in that, for each contrast, information from doses higher than the $(m+1)$st dose is ignored. Also, higher doses are compared with inflated 'control' values if there are even small effects at lower doses. Basin contrasts assume there is no effect until a certain dose level and that the trend with dose is linear from then on. This is too restrictive an alternative to the null hypothesis of no dose effect. Basin contrasts for four groups are the vectors $(-6, -2, 2, 6)$, $(-3, -3, 1, 5)$, and $(-1, -1, -1, 3)$. Williams' test and Bartholomew's test have been compared by Williams (1971), Shirley (1979, 1985), and Turnbul *et al.* (1987). Overall, it is agreed that Bartholomew's test is the more powerful, but Shirley found that Williams' test was more powerful at detecting low-dose effects. Turnbul found that Williams' test was more powerful when there was a gradual dose–response and Bartholomew's when there was a steep dose–response. He also found that Bartholomew's test improved in power compared with Williams' test the more groups there were in an experiment.

Turnbul *et al.* (1987) also compared Bartholomew's and Williams' tests with the Tukey *et al.* (1985) trend test. He found that when its type I error was adjusted to the correct nominal level, the last test was competitive with Bartholomew's and Williams' tests.

Ragouzis and Ruberg (1987) compared Williams' test with the Helmert contrasts and the Basin contrasts. They applied the Bonferroni correction to the significance levels of the Helmert and Basin contrasts, although the latter contrasts are not orthogonal, and so the correction produced a lower type I error than the nominal level. They found that the Basin contrasts performed well, but the configurations of means chosen for the computer simulations were tailor-made for these types of contrasts, and sets of means such as $(0, 0, 1, 1)$ and $(0, 1, 1, 2)$ were not used.

A robustness study was carried out by Hothorn (1989) on the behaviour of Williams' test under violation of the normality condition, lack of monotonicity, heterogeneity of variance, and unequal group sizes. The non-normal distributions considered were the Fleishman (1978) polynomial transformation of the normal distribution, $F(0, 1, \text{skewness} = 2, \text{kurtosis} = 7)$ and the exponential distribution, $\exp(1, 1)$. He considered group sizes of 5, 11, and 21 and the case of three dose levels being compared with a control group. He found that the type I experimentwise error was not influenced by non-normality, but that the comparisons between lower-dose groups and controls had very low type I errors which decreased with smaller sample sizes. He also found that the power of Williams' test was only slightly reduced where there was non-normality; e.g. when the highest dose level was compared with the control, the power was reduced from about 93 per cent for the normal distribution to 90 per cent for the Fleishman transformation with a group size of 5, to 91 per cent for this transformation and group sizes of 11 and 21; and to 89 per cent for the exponential distribution, group size of 5, and to 91 per cent and 92 per cent for group sizes of 11 and 21. It should be noted that Hothorn does not use one-sided tests at the lower dose levels, as recommended by Shirley (1979). Shirley proposes that if the highest dose level is found to be significant, whether by a one-sided or two-sided test of significance, the next dose level down should be tested by a one-sided test in the direction of highest dose level difference from the control. This increases the power of the test at lower dose levels while having a negligible effect on the type I error.

Hothorn showed that Williams' test was robust against moderate non-monotonicity of dose–response at the higher dose levels, comparing well with Dunnett's (1964) test, which does not assume monotonicity of dose response. He also carried out simulations in which all four groups were of size 5 or were of sizes 8, 4, 4, and 4, where the group variances were constant or were in the ratio 1 : 4 : 7 : 10 with increasing dose, and where the distribution was normal or Fleishman (0, 1, 2, 7), as described previously. When the underlying distribution was normal he found that the type I error was very close to 5 per cent except where both lack of balance and heterogeneity of variance existed, when it increased to about 10 per cent. Where the data follows the transformed distribution, the type I error went up to 6 per cent for unequal group sizes and to about 8 per cent when there were both unequal group sizes and heterogeneity of variance.

Generally, Williams' t-test is favoured in the literature because of its robustness to non-normality, lack of balance, and non-monotonicity of dose–response. Bartholomew's test comes a close second because of its superior power overall. However, Bartholomew's test does not allow for an effect at the low dose levels in the opposite direction to the general trend, which may happen quite frequently in toxicity studies.

3.5 Non-parametric methods

When the underlying distribution of a variable is grossly different from normal or there is considerable heterogeneity of variance, non-parametric methods of analysis, which do not assume any particular underlying distribution and have been shown to be more robust when there is heterogeneity of variance, are advisable (see Kruskal 1952).

Shorack (1967) produced a non-parametric version of Bartholomew's test and Shirley (1977a) produced a non-parametric version of Williams' test. Both tests were based on the ranks of the measurements. For the reasons given in the last section, Shirley's test is favoured for toxicity studies, although for strictly monotonic responses Shorack's test will be more powerful overall.

In Shirley's test the maximum likelihood estimators of the group mean ranks are calculated by the same simple averaging process described in Williams' test. Instead of calculating t-type values, Z-type values are obtained by dividing the difference between the maximum likelihood estimates of dosed groups and the control sample mean ranks by the standard error of this difference, based on the total mean square for the experiment. If the highest dose level is found to be significant then this group is excluded from the data set, the rest of the data re-ranked, and the highest dose level left tested for significance by a one-tailed test in the direction of the highest dose level. The process continues until a non-significant dose level is found.

Hothorn (1989) compared Williams' and Shirley's tests on normally distributed data, data transformed by Fleishman's polynomial (0, 1, 2, 7), constant variance or heterogeneity of group variances in the ratios 1 : 4 : 7 : 10, and on group sizes all equal to 5 or equal to 8, 4, 4, and 4. He found that Shirley's type I errors were around or below the nominal 5 per cent level, except in one configuration where there were unequal group sizes and heterogeneity of variance in normally distributed data. Williams' test had a 10 per cent type I error in this situation and Shirley's test a 7 per cent type I error. In the majority of cases with these small sample sizes, Shirley's had lower power than Williams' test, especially in the situation in which there were heterogeneity of variance, lack of balance, and normally distributed data. However, for non-normal distributions and equal group sizes, Shirley's test always had higher power for detecting the highest-dose effects; and, except for one configuration, where the group sizes were 5 and the underlying distribution was exponential, at detecting medium-dose effects. Shirley's test did not compare well with William's test at detecting low-dose effects, except when the sample size was greater than 11. However, it is not clear whether Hothorn used the modified version of Shirley's test, suggested by Williams (1986), in which the data is re-ranked at each sequential step. If he did not apply the modified Z-values this might explain the loss of power at the lower doses. (In fact, footnote 1 in Hothorn's paper implies that he did not use the modified procedure.)

House (1986) extended Shirley's non-parametric procedure, which was for a completely randomized design, to a randomized block design, using Friedman rank sums. Shirley (1987) showed how factorial designs could be analysed by taking one factor at a time, ranking the observations within levels of the other factors, and comparing rank sums. Shirley showed that when there were large effects in any of these other factors this method was more powerful than Bennett's method, which is described below.

Shirley (1981) presented a method for non-parametric analysis of covariance based on the methods of testing a general linear hypothesis described by Bennett (1968). The ranks of the variate are analysed and either the actual values of the covariate or its ranks may be used. The usual analysis of covariance procedures are carried out, but the residual mean square is replaced by the total mean square, the F-ratios are replaced with chi-square statistics and the t-tests are replaced with Z-tests. This method of analysis of covariance has an advantage over the methods proposed by Quade (1967) and Puri and Sen (1969), in that the covariate need not be identically distributed for each treatment group. There may be a treatment effect on the covariate. Also, this method of analysis may be extended to more complicated general linear models.

Conover and Iman (1976) suggest ranking all the data in the experiment and applying the usual analysis of variance procedures to these ranks. This method of analysis has not been theoretically justified but has been shown, empirically, to be efficient. However, the analysis does not guarantee that the type I error will remain at or below the chosen level of significance.

Papers pertaining to the analysis of frequency data in general toxicology studies were not found on this literature survey. However, it should be noted that the methods described in this section may be applied to frequency data after coding positives as 1 and negatives as 0.

3.6 Randomization tests

The non-parametric methods described above rely on large sample approximations to the normal distribution. For small sample sizes, randomization methods are available for developing equivalent tests which are either exact or very accurate at calculating levels of significance. See Edgington (1987) for a description of randomization methods and examples of computer routines.

3.7 Analysis of growth curves

The growth curves of animals generally show an initial fast growing period followed by a period of much slower growth, levelling out, and finally slowly declining. Lewis (1965) compared three methods of analysing the growth curves of rats in toxicological studies. He considered analysis of covariance, adjusting for baseline values at suitable times during the study and at the end of the study; Rao's method of analysis of rate of growth, which looks at the differences in body weight obtained over set intervals of time, e.g. daily differences, 14-day differences, etc.; and the analysis of the coefficients of orthogonal polynomials, usually of the fourth degree, leading to five analyses of variance, some of which are not very easy to interpret. Lewis concludes that the method of fitting orthogonal polynomials describes the curves most completely. In practice, in Lewis's example, analysis of covariance on the final body weight proved to be just as powerful at detecting differences in growth curves as the other methods.

3.8 Confidence limits and bounds

Schoenfeld (1986) considered confidence bounds for means of normal distributions under order restrictions. For random variables $y(1),\ldots,y(n)$ with ordered means $u(1),\ldots,u(n)$ such that no $u(i) > u(i+1)$ for $i = 1,\ldots,(n-1)$, he found a confidence bound for each $u(i)$ that took advantage of the ordering. The upper and lower limits are the maximum and minimum values of x such that the hypothesis that $x < u(i)$ and $u(i) < x$ are accepted by their respective likelihood ratio tests. These bounds are often more precise than the usual bounds and can be used to determine the safety of a toxin. The upper and lower bounds do not form a confidence interval. Tables of critical values are given for equal replication. Schoenfeld discusses simultaneous confidence bounds but only considers them useful for testing the fit of a parametric model. He also discusses an approach by Williams (1977), where the bound on $u(i)$ would be $u(i) + s'K(p)$, where $K(p)$ is the upper pth percentile of the distribution of $(u^*(i) - u(i))/s'$ computed under the hypothesis that $u(i) = u(j)$ for $j \geqslant i$ and $u(i) = -\infty$ otherwise. In this formula $u^*(i)$ is the maximum likelihood estimate of $u(i)$ under order restrictions and s' is the estimate of the residual standard deviation. Critical values of K are only given for equal group sizes and for the residual error degrees of freedom being greater than 8. It should be noted that the bounds and confidence limits described in this section do not allow for a lack of monotonicity at the low-dose level.

3.9 Analysis of organ weights

Stevens (1976) and Shirley (1977*b*) demonstrated theoretically, and also by computer simulation, that the analysis of organ weight relative to current body weight is only appropriate if the relationship between the two variables can be represented by a straight line which, where projected backwards, passes through the origin. If the relationship is linear and does not pass through the origin, analysis of covariance is the preferred method of analysis for detecting treatment effect on organ weights, since it takes into account any indirect effect via treatment effect on body weight. Within the body weight ranges encountered in toxicological studies, the relationship between body weight and organ weight has been found by the author to be linear, and rarely, when projected backward, passes through the origin. Before analysis of covariance is carried out, the lines representing the organ weight/body weight relationship for each treatment group should be tested for parallelism, in case the treatment has changed the relationship.

The precision of the analysis of covariance can be improved by using the average of the last few recorded body weights as the covariate rather than just the final body weight.

3.10 Multiple significance testing and multivariate methods

A problem that arises in toxicity studies is that of the multiple significance testing involved in the analysis of many biological variables. The number of false positives found increases with the number of separate significance tests performed.

One approach is to use multivariate methods, as suggested by Salsburg (1986) and Gad and Weil (1988). Here, a group of variates are considered simultaneously. However, these methods are either very conservative—lacking power at detecting treatment effects—or, in the case of methods such as principal component analysis, where the orthogonal linear combinations of the variates with maximum variance are sought, often difficult to interpret. Another method for reducing type I errors is to use the Bonferroni correction to the significance level (i.e. to divide it by the number of tests to be performed) for different sets of parameters such as haematology or organ weights. This will also produce results that are too conservative. Mantel (1980) suggested that for each set of parameters some of which are known to be correlated, the Bonferroni correction should be reduced by dividing the significance level by the square root of the number of parameters in the set. This was by way of being a 'hunch' rather than being based on any theory.

Acknowledgements

I should like to thank Glaxo Group Research for commissioning this review, and the Glaxo statisticians David Robinson and Richard Lyons and my colleague Helen Tate for their helpful comments and suggestions.

References

Abeyasakera, S. (1984). The desirability of covariance adjustments. *Applied Statistics*, **33**(1), 33–7.

Barlow, R. E., Bartholomew, D. J., Bremner, J. M., and Brunk, H. D. (1972). *Statistical inference under order restrictions*. John Wiley, New York.

Bartholomew, D. J. (1959*a*). A test of homogeneity for ordered alternatives. *Biometrika*, **46**, 36–48.

Bartholomew, D. J. (1959*b*). A test of homogeneity for ordered alternatives II. *Biometrika*, **46**, 328–35.

Bartholomew, D. J. (1961). A test of homogeneity of means under restricted alternatives. *Journal of the Royal Statistical Society B*, **23**, 239–81.

Bartlett, M. S. (1937). Properties of sufficiency and statistical tests. *Proceedings of the Royal Society A*, **160**, 268–82.

Bennett, B. M. (1968). Rank order tests of linear hypothesis. *Journal of the Royal Statistical Society B*, **30**, 483–9.

Berry, D. A. (1987). Logarithmic transformations in ANOVA. *Biometrics*, **43**, 439–56.

Box, G. E. and Cox, D. R. (1964). An analysis of transformations. *Journal of the Royal Statistical Society B*, **26**, 211.

Chacko, V. J. (1963). Testing homogeneity against ordered alternatives. *Annals of Mathematics and Statistics*, **34**, 945–56.

Chase, G. R. (1974). On testing for ordered alternatives with increased sample size for the control. *Biometrika*, **61**, 569–78.

Conover, W. J. (1980). *Practical nonparametric statistics*, Ch. 5, pp. 239–48. John Wiley, New York.

Conover, W. J. and Iman, R. L. (1976). On some alternative procedures using ranks for the analysis of experimental designs. *Communication in Statistics—Theory and Methods*, **A5**, 1349–68.

Dunnett, C. W. (1964). New table for multiple comparisons with a control. *Biometrics*, **20**, 482–91.

Edgington, E. S. (1987). *Randomization tests*. Statistics: textbooks and monographs, volume 77. Dekker, New York.

Fleishman, M. A. (1978). A method for simulating non-normal distributions. *Psychometrika*, **43**, 521–32.

Gad, S. and Weil, C. S. (1988). *Statistics and experimental design for toxicologists*. The Telford Press, Caldwell, New Jersey.

Hothorn, L. (1989). A robustness study on Williams and Shirley procedure with application in toxicology. *Biometrical Journal*, **31**(8), 891–903.

House, D. E. (1986). A non-parametric version of Williams' test for a randomized block design. *Biometrics*, **42**, 187–90.

Kendall, M. G. and Stuart, A. (1977). *The advanced theory of statistics*, vol. 3. Griffin, London.

Kendall, M. G., Stuart, A., and Ord, K. (1991). *The advanced theory of statistics*, vol. 2. Griffin, London.

Kruskal, W. H. (1952). A nonparametric case for the several sample problem. *Annals of Mathematics and Statistics*, **23**, 525–40.

Lehmann, E. L. (1959). *Testing statistical hypothesis*, p. 274. John Wiley, New York.

Levene, H. (1960). *Contributions to probability and statistics*, p. 278. Stanford University Press, Stanford, California.

Lewis, B. D. (1965). A survey of some of the available methods of analysis of the growth curves of rats in toxicological tests. *The Statistician*, **15**(1), 59–66.

Lewi, P. J. and Marsboom, R. P. (1981). *Toxicology reference data—Wistar rat*. Elsevier, Amsterdam.

Mantel, N. (1980). Assessing laboratory evidence for neoplastic activity. *Biometrics*, **36**, 381–99.

Puri, M. L. and Sen, P. K. (1969). Analysis of covariance based on general ranked scores. *Annals of Mathematics and Statistics*, **40**, 610–18.

Quade, D. (1967). Rank analysis of covariance. *Journal of the American Statistical Association*, **61**, 1187–200.

Ragouzis, L. P. and Ruberg, S. J. (1987). Estimating the minimum and maximum effective dose. *American Statistical Association, Proceedings of the Biopharmaceutical Section*, pp. 13–18.

Robertson, T., Wright, F. T., and Dykstra, R. L. (1988). *Order restricted statistical inference*. John Wiley, New York.

Salsburg, D. S. (1986). *Statistics for toxicologists*. Dekker, New York.

Sanderson, J. H. and Phillips, C. E. (1981). *An atlas of laboratory animal haematology*. Oxford Science Publications, Oxford.

Schoenfeld, D. A. (1986). Confidence bounds for normal means under order restrictions, with application to dose–response curves, toxicology experiments, and low-dose extrapolation. *Journal of the American Statistical Association*, **81**, no. 393. Theory and Methods, 186–95.

Sedlmayer, P. and Hornacek, J. (1984). Determination of reference biochemical values of the beagle breed of dogs. *Československa Farmacie*, **33**(7), 283–6.

Shirley, E. (1977*a*). A non-parametric equivalent of Williams' test for contrasting increasing dose levels of a treatment. *Biometrics*, **33**, 386–9.

Shirley, E. (1977*b*). The analysis of organ weight data. *Toxicology*, **8**, 13–22.

Shirley, E. A. C. (1979). The comparison of treatment and control group means in toxicological studies. *Journal of the Royal Statistical Society C*, **28**(2), 144–51.

Shirley, E. A. C. (1981). A distribution-free method for the analysis of covariance based on ranked data. *Journal of the Royal Statistical Society C*, **30**(2), 158–62.

Shirley, E. A. C. (1985). The value of specialised tests in studies where ordered group means are expected. *Statistics in Medicine*, **4**, 489–96.

Shirley, E. A. C. (1987). Application of ranking methods to multiple comparison procedures and factorial experiments. *Journal of the Royal Statistical Society C*, **36**(2), 205–13.

Shirley, E. A. C. and Newnham, P. (1984). The choice between analysis of variance and analysis of covariance with special reference to the analysis of organ weights in toxicology studies. *Statistics in Medicine*, **3**, 85–91.

Shorack, G. R. (1967). Testing against ordered alternatives in model I analysis of variance: normal theory and nonparametric. *Annals of Mathematics and Statistics*, **38**, 1740–52.

Snedecor, G. W. and Cochran, W. G. (1967). *Statistical methods*. Iowa State University Press, Ames, Iowa.

Stevens, M. T. (1976). The value of relative organ weights. *Toxicology*, **5**, 311.

Tukey, J. W., Ciminera, J. L., and Heyse, J. F. (1985). Testing the statistical certainty of a response to increasing doses of a drug. *Biometrics*, **41**, 295–301.

Turnbull, T. A., Malani, H., and Capizzi, T. P. (1987). The power of some tests for comparing several doses of a compound with a zero dose control. *American Statistical Association, Proceedings of the Biopharmaceutical Section*, pp. 76–80.

Williams, D. A. (1971). A test for differences between treatment means when several dose levels are compared with a zero dose control. *Biometrics*, **27**, 103–77.

Williams, D. A. (1972). The comparison of several dose levels with a zero dose control. *Biometrics*, **28**, 519–31.

Williams, D. A. (1977). Some inference procedures for monotonically ordered normal means. *Biometrika*, **64**, 9–14.

Williams, D. A. (1986). A note on Shirley's non-parametric test for comparing several dose levels with a zero dose control. *Biometrics*, **42**, 183–6.

Further reading

Baker, S. P. and Lew, R. A. (1987). Monte Carlo comparison of Turkey's and Bonferroni's methods with an optimised multiple comparison procedure in repeated measurements experiments. *American Statistical Association*, *Proceedings of the Biopharmaceutical Section*, pp. 23–9.

Chanter, D. O., Tuck, M. G., and Coombs, D. W. (1987). The chances of false negative results in conventional toxicology studies with rats. *Toxicology*, **43**, 65–74.

Hoel, D. G. (1979). Statistical approaches to toxicological data. *Environmental Health Perspectives*, **32**, 267–71.

Fligner, M. A. and Wolfe, D. A. (1982). Distribution-free tests for comparing several treatments with a control. *Statistica Neerlandica*, **36**(3), 119–27.

Hogg, R. V. (1981). On adaptive robust inference. In *Statistics and related topics* (ed. M. Csorgo), pp. 253–64. North Holland, Amsterdam.

Hothorn, L. (1989). On the behaviour of Fligner–Wolfe–Trend test: Control versus *k* treatments with application in toxicology. *Biom. J.*, **31**(7), 767–80.

Hothorn, L. (1990). *General statistical principles in toxicological studies*. Lecture Notes in Medical Informatics 43 (Statistical Methods in Toxicology), pp. 111–31. Springer-Verlag, Berlin.

Hothorn, L. and Lehmacher, W. (1991). A simple testing procedure control versus *K* treatments for one-sided ordered alternatives, with application in toxicology. *Biometrical Journal*, **33**, 179–89.

Ludin, E. (1985). A test procedure based on ranks for the statistical evaluation of toxicology studies. *Archives of Toxicology*, **58**, 57–8.

Padmanabhan, A. R., Puri, M. L., and Saleh, A. K. Md. E. (1981). A non-parametric test for equality against ordered alternatives in the case of skewed data with a biomedical application. In *Statistics and related topics* (ed. M. Csorgo), pp. 279–83. North Holland, Amsterdam.

Maul, A. (1990). *Determination of endpoints in acute and chronic toxicity tests by using generalized linear models*. Lecture Notes in Medical Informatics 43 (Statistical Methods in Toxicology), pp. 132–8. Springer-Verlag, Berlin.

Yamazaki, M., Noguchi, Y., Tanda, M., and Shintani, S. (1981). Statistical methods appropriate for general toxicological studies in rats. Algorthims for multiple comparisons of treated groups with controls. *Journal of the Takeda Research Laboratory*, **40**(3/4), 163–87.

4 Statistical analysis of genetic toxicology test data

D. P. LOVELL

4.1 Introduction

Genetic toxicology is the branch of toxicology which investigates the action of chemicals and physical agents on the genetical material of organisms. Ultimately, it is concerned with whether such agents may pose a risk to the human population. This chapter will briefly review the history of statistical involvement in genetic toxicology, outline David Williams' contributions to the field both through the UKEMS guidelines and his wider influences, discuss some of the more recent statistical developments, and outline some potential areas for statistical influence in the future.

4.2 The relevance of genetic toxicology

Genetic toxicology is the study of the interaction between chemical and physical agents and the processes of heredity. Damage to these processes can cause mutations, i.e. heritable changes in the genetic material, DNA. The discipline developed from the pioneering work of Müller (1927) and Auerbach *et al.* (1947), who induced mutations by irradiation and chemicals, respectively, in the fruit fly, *Drosophila*. Since then, the range of chemicals and organisms investigated has expanded enormously. Research was initially concerned with changes in genetic material in the germline which might lead to mutations, birth defects, and disabilities in the offspring of exposed individuals. The recognition that there is a genetic component to cancer has added to the relevance of results of genetic toxicology test data. Damage to the genetic material in the somatic, or non-germline, cells of the body has been shown to be associated with cancer, while there is an increasing understanding of the role that specific genes have in the development of cancers and differences in individual susceptibilities.

The terms 'genetic toxicology' and 'mutagenicity' sometimes appear to be used interchangeably, but there are some subtle differences in their precise meaning; imprecise use can lead to confusion. Mutations are changes in genetic material which are heritable in that they can be passed from generation to generation. Chemicals causing mutations are called 'mutagens'. Chemicals which cause damage to genetic material are termed 'genotoxins'. Genetic damage may be so severe that the changes resulting are not capable of being transmitted from generation to generation. Agents which cause genetic damage by breaking the chromosomes, the structures within the nucleus in which the DNA coding the specific genes is organized, rather than by altering the genetic material, are termed 'clastogens'. A further class of agents causes genetic damage by interfering with the mechanisms by which chromosomes move during cell division, by damaging the protein-based structures involved in these procedures; such damage often results in cells containing an incorrect number of chromosomes after cell division. Such chemicals are sometimes termed 'aneugens' or 'aneuploidogens'. Advances in molecular biology are increasing the understanding of the mechanisms within cells and identifying other forms of genetic damage. In some cases, this new knowledge is challenging the operational definitions given to terms such as mutagen and genotoxin.

4.3 Genetic toxicology tests

The realization that chemicals capable of damaging the genetic material may also cause cancer led to the development of short-term tests (STTs) for genotoxicity. One of the first of these, the *Salmonella*/microsome test, resulted in a publication by Ames *et al.* (1973) with the title 'Carcinogens are mutagens', suggesting there there was a very high association between chemicals which caused mutations in the bacterium *Salmonella* and chemicals which cause cancer in animals and man. This test offered the possibility of identifying potential carcinogens quickly and cheaply. It stimulated the development of many other STTs covering a wide range of end-points and organisms. They include tests for mutations in bacterial and mammalian cells in culture; tests for various types of chromosomal damage in both cultured cells (*in vitro* cytogenetics) and cells extracted from animals (*in vivo* cytogenetics); and tests for genetic damage in the offspring of treated males (the Dominant and the sex-linked recessive lethal tests in rodents and fruit flies, respectively). By 1987, the EPA Gene-Tox Database had data from over 70 STTs (Ray *et al.* 1987). Other authors have written of as many as 200 STTs (DeMarini *et al.* 1989).

In practice, the 'correlation' between carcinogens and mutagens is no longer considered so strong and it is recognized that there are ways in which chemicals can cause cancer other than by directly damaging the genetic material (Ames 1989). In general, the STTs fail to detect these 'non-genotoxic' carcinogens.

4.4 The purpose of genetic toxicology tests

The results from STTs are used in two ways; firstly, to predict the potential of a chemical to pose a carcinogenic hazard to the human population; and secondly, to predict whether the chemical poses a genetic hazard in terms of the potential to lead to inherited genetic changes

In the first case, the STT may either be predicting whether a chemical could cause cancer in a subsequent animal (usually rodent) cancer bioassay which in turn is used to predict a human carcinogenic hazard or the human hazard

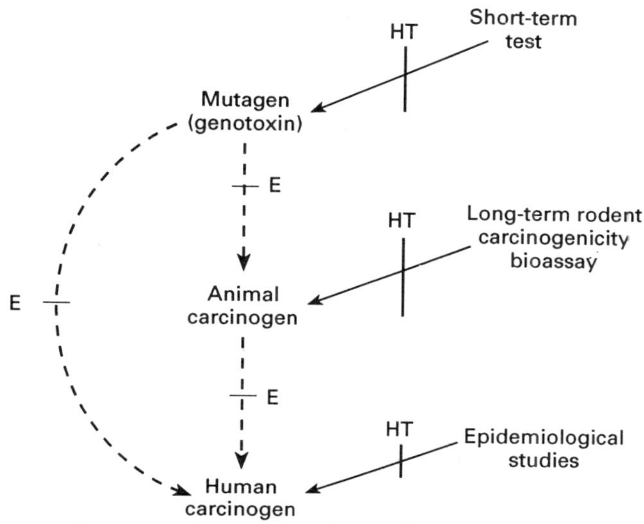

Fig. 4.1. The use of various methods to identify human carcinogens. HT indicates the use of hypothesis testing to identify the presence or absence of a hazard. E indicates the use of estimation approaches to estimate degree of risk.

directly (Fig. 4.1). These experiments may involve two types of statistical investigation: hypothesis testing, where the aim is to identify if a hazard exists or not; and the estimation of the size of the effect.

In practice, STTs have usually been used to identify hazards and considerations of hypothesis testing have predominated. Superficially, the type of errors occurring in 2×2 tables drawn up comparing the conclusions about whether a chemical is a mutagen or a carcinogen look similar to those produced by consideration of the Neyman–Pearson approach to hypothesis testing. False positives in one appear similar to type I errors in the other; and, similarly, false negatives and type II errors (Fig. 4.2). However, while type I and type II errors in a statistical test of a hypothesis have a stochastic interpretation, the false positives and false negatives of comparisons of animal cancer bioassays and STT results can arise from differences in metabolism between the species or differences in the routes of administration, or a failure of the STT to measure the appropriate type of genetic damage and, consequently, represent real biological differences. A failure to appreciate this difference in the interpretation of 2×2 type tables can lead to misunderstanding of the relevance of a statistical test by genetic toxicologists.

STTs are now being reassessed for their importance in determining whether a chemical has the potential to induce heritable mutations. In part, this reconsideration is a consequence of a growing requirement by regulatory authorities, particularly in the USA, for an assessment of the genetic risks associated with exposures to be carried out (Auletta *et al.* 1993). There is also the appreciation that the incidence of genetic diseases from identifiable genetic defects is about

(a)

Genotoxicity	Carcinogenicity: Carcinogen	Carcinogenicity: Non-carcinogen
Genotoxic	True positive	False positive
Non-genotoxic	False negative	True negative

(b)

Decision	Null hypothesis: False	Null hypothesis: True
Reject	Correct result	False rejection, type I error, significance level (α)
Accept	False acceptance, type II error (β), power ($1-\beta$)	True negative

Fig. 4.2. A comparison between (a) a 2×2 table of results using a short-term test (STT) to predict carcinogenicity and (b) a table representing the outcome of a Neyman–Pearson null hypothesis test.

1–3 per cent (Winston and Handyside 1993); that there are major chromosomal abnormalities in 1 in 200 live births, 1 in 20 perinatal and still births, and 1 in 2 early spontaneous abortions (Emery 1983); and that genetic and part-genetic diseases affect up to 1 in every 20 people at the age of 25 and up to two-thirds of people at some time in their life (British Medical Association 1992). There is also an increasing awareness of the potential importance of the involvement of mutations in other illnesses, such as cataracts and atherosclerosis (DeMarini *et al.* 1989).

4.5 Geneticists, mutations, and statistics

Mendel, of course, in his pioneering studies linking probability theory to inheritance, studied the inheritance of genetic differences arising from mutations in pure breeding lines of peas. Mutations provide the 'raw material' for the genetic variability. Galton developed correlation and regression while Pearson produced the chi-squared test to study this variability. Fisher linked the, then, rival schools of Biometricians and Mendelians and in the process laid the basis for the analysis of variance methodology (Piegorsch 1990). Concern over the potential increase in the 'genetic load' of detrimental mutations that might arise from exposure to mutagenic agents was a stimulus for developments in population genetics. Fisher, in fact, through his wide range of interests and experimental studies, was involved in many areas of work which subsequently became used in genetic toxicology. It comes as a surprise to many genetic toxicologists who have been isolated from a biometrical background to discover that someone who is known to them as the statistician who created the Fisher exact test and the F-test in the analysis of variance was also a geneticist who was involved in genetical studies on a wide range of organisms including mice; that he tried unsuccessfully to set up a pioneering bacterial genetics unit in the late 1940s; and that his colleagues called the virus-like particle which determines sex in *E. coli* the F-factor after him, in recognition of his postulation of its existence (Edwards 1990). Present-day statisticians and genetic toxicologists often no longer recognize the common interests and personalities who built the foundation of their modern disciplines.

4.6 The UKEMS guidelines

The importance of genetic events in carcinogenesis has led to the inclusion of a requirement for genetic toxicology testing to be included in the basic set of test data required to meet various regulatory requirements. Examples include the EC's Directive on the Labelling of Dangerous Substances (Commission of the European Communities 1992). Guidelines have been developed by organizations such as the OECD (1983). One particular response has developed from UKEMS, the United Kingdom Environmental Mutagen Society. UKEMS was founded in 1977 as the UK part of the European Environmental Mutagen Society (EEMS). The UK's Department of Health and Social Services guidelines for testing chemicals for mutagenicity (DHSS 1981) stimulated UKEMS to consider developing guidelines for the conduct of a series of STTs. It published two documents in the 1980s dealing with both the most commonly used tests and some lesser used supplementary methods (UKEMS 1983, 1984). (The UK Department of Health has since refined its guidelines (DoH 1989).)

In preparing the UKEMS guidelines it was considered that very few of the chapters adequately considered the statistical aspects either in experimental design or in terms of data analysis. Many of the existing guidelines, for example OECD (1983), were using phrases such as 'data should be analyzed using appropriate statistical methods' and 'biological and statistical significance should be taken into account'. The UKEMS Guidelines Sub-committee decided that part III of their reports should address the statistical evaluation of mutagenicity test data. The terms of reference were as follows.

The Sub-committee was asked to assess the various statistical approaches available for their suitability in evaluating data from the most widely used mutagenicity tests, such that practising genetic toxicologists would be better able to understand what was required of them by regulatory authorities in this respect, and be better advised as to which forms of analysis were preferred, and why. Specifically, for each of the test types, the following terms were to be considered:

1. How to determine the suitability of the data obtained from an assay for fitting a distribution; when the data are unsuitable; when and how should the data be transformed.

2. The types of statistical analyses that can be used with the assay data under consideration; which, if any, factors govern the choice of analysis; an order of preference if several types of analyses may be used

3. Some worked examples using real data to help the reader to understand points 1 and 2.

The Sub-committee set up eight working groups, consisting of between five and nine members. At least two statisticians were members of each group. In all, over 15 statisticians participated in the process. After the initial meetings of the groups, at which it became clear that there were a number of statistical issues which affected all the groups, the steering group of UKEMS members was augmented by three statisticians with experience of data in the field of genetic toxicology. The guidelines were published in 1989 (UKEMS 1989), and consisted of an introductory chapter and one chapter from each of the eight working groups (Table 4.1). Subsequently, UKEMS organized a Workshop, held at the University of Kent in September 1991, which was attended by about 40 people, including many of the participants in Working Groups, to discuss the guidelines. This Workshop maintained the close working relationships that had been built up between the statisticians and the genetic toxicologists.

Table 4.1. Mutagenicity tests covered by the eight Working Groups set up by the UKEMS Sub-committee on guidelines for mutagenicity testing (UKEMS 1989)

- Microbial colony assays (the Ames *Salmonella*/microsome test)
- Mammalian cell gene mutation assays based upon colony foundation
- Bacterial and mammalian fluctuation assays
- *in vitro* cytogenetic assays
- Sister chromatid exchange experiments
- *in vivo* cytogenetic assays (chromosomal aberrations and micronucleus tests)
- Dominant lethal assay
- Experiments with the fruit fly (*Drosophila melanogaster*)
  (the sex-linked recessive lethal)

4.7 David Williams' involvement

News of David's illness became known during the planning stage for the UKEMS Workshop. It was at that stage that it become clear how much influence David had brought to bear on the UKEMS guidelines. As well as being the co-author of the chapter on *in vitro* cytogenetics, he had been involved in discussions on various statistical aspects, as well as commenting on drafts of some of the chapters. His papers on procedures for making multiple comparisons in experiments in which there are planned dose comparisons (Williams 1971, 1972, 1986) influenced thinking in the Working Groups on the microbial colony assays and the dominant lethal assay. He provided advice to me on my introductory chapter. Those of us involved in the production of the guidelines will always remember the thoroughness that characterized his involvement and the consistency with which he argued for appropriate and informative statistical analyses. His early death has robbed us of a key figure in the development of statistical methods in this area of toxicology.

David wrote one paper arising from his involvement in the *in vitro* cytogenetics Working Group (Williams 1988*a*). The summary of the results of the UKEMS Working Group is given in Table 4.2. The paper involved the problem of testing the proportion of abnormal cells in a control sample compared with that in various treated samples. The number of cells examined in each culture at each dose level is low (100), reflecting both the cost of analysing individual cells

Table 4.2. Summary of the results of the UKEMS (1989) working group on *in vitro* cytogenetic assays

(a) A typical *in vitro* cytogenetic assay compares a solvent control, three dose levels of the test chemical, and a positive control, using at least two replicate cultures per treatment. From each culture a sample of at least 100 cells is scored and each structural aberration is categorized and recorded.

(b) The statistical analysis proposed here is appropriate after first reducing the information on each cell to a binary classification, each cell being classed as normal or aberrant. The experimenter has freedom to ignore certain categories of chromosome damage (e.g. achromatic gaps) when making this classification.

(c) In well-conducted assays there should be no extra-binomial variation between the proportions of aberrant cells in replicate cultures. This should be confirmed using a binomial dispersion test.

(d) Assuming that the variation between replicate cultures is binomial, the replicates can be combined to give a single proportion of aberrant cells for each treatment. Each treatment proportion is then compared with the negative control proportion using a Fisher exact test. Scientific judgement is needed when interpreting the results of these tests.

(e) Alternative statistical test procedures are available which take a more coherent view of the whole dose–response pattern, but these require greater statistical expertise.

Table 4.3. Data used by the UKEMS (1989) working group on *in vitro* cytogenetic assay

Dose (μg/ml)	Number of cultures	Number of aberrant cells in cultures	Total number of cells scored	Total aberrant
Assay A				
0	4	2, 1, 0, 0	400	3
20	2	4, 1	200	5
100	2	6, 8	200	14
200	2	3, 1	200	4
Assay B				
0	4	1, 0, 3, 1	400	5
62.5	2	0, 2	200	2
125	2	1, 1	200	2
250	2	0, 4	200	4
500	2	4, 3	200	7

for chromosomal abnormalities and the limited number of suitable cells for analysis. The background incidence of abnormalities is relatively low (usually below 2 per cent) and there is the added complexity that there is the potential for investigating different types of damage, such as breaks in or rearrangements of the chromosomes.

The paper used the data provided by the UKEMS Working Group (Table 4.3) to explore the small sample behavior of a range of statistical tests available for analysing this type of data. It showed that the inaccuracies associated with approximating these tests by continuous distributions can be avoided by using the exact conditional distribution of the test statistic. The paper described the calculation of the exact significance probabilities for eight tests and showed that the costs of computing the values are small relative to those of obtaining the data (Table 4.4). The paper concluded by making a strong case for the use of the mid-P value for discretely distributed test statistics. A program for IBM-compatible PCs, INVICTY, incorporated the tests developed in this paper plus some further modifications (Chanter, personal communication). The output of the package for one set of the UKEMS data set is illustrated in Fig. 4.3. INVICTY was just one of a number of software packages and papers which have been 'spin-offs' from the UKEMS guidelines process.

David Williams also produced an invited paper for the XIVth International Biometric Conference in Namur, Belgium, in which he discussed problems associated with the overdispersion of data and extra-binomial variation (Williams 1988*b*). It used data from a dominant lethal test to illustrate some approaches, and is very relevant to the problems associated with the analysis of the data from this test.

4.8 Developments in genetic toxicology

Many of the genetic toxicology tests have statistical problems which offer

Table 4.4. Exact P-values for eight test statistics applied to the in vitro cytogenetics data from Table 3 together with CPU time used in calculation as reported by Williams (1988*a*) (full details of the eight tests are given in the original paper)

Test statistic	P-value (%)	CPU time (s)
Assay A		
X^2	0.014	0.3
G^2	0.05	0.3
T_{CA}	1.28	0.2
$\bar{X}^2$	0.29	0.5
$\bar{G}^2$	0.10	0.5
$\bar{T}$	0.64	0.4
T_D	0.004	0.3
T'_D	0.04	0.3
Assay B		
X^2	23.9	1.4
G^2	30.2	1.3
T_{CA}	3.4	0.7
$\bar{X}^2$	3.6	2.1
$\bar{G}^2$	5.2	2.1
$\bar{T}$	3.7	1.6
T_D	12.0	1.2
T'_D	11.3	1.1

statisticians the possibility of becoming involved in design and analysis issues. A selection of these are discussed below for three different classes of tests. More detailed discussion is provided in the UKEMS guidelines (UKEMS 1989). Margolin (1985) reviews a series of statistical considerations in the context of the genetic toxicology programme carried out by the US National Toxicology Program, while Edler (1992) provides a recent review of the statistical methods used in genotoxicity testing.

4.8.1 *The Ames test*

The Ames test is the classical STT. It was initially devised as a qualitative test to determine if a chemical had mutagenic potential in bacteria. Refining and standardizing the design resulted in protocols amenable to statistical analysis. The data in the Ames test consists of the number of colonies of *Salmonella* bacteria on an agar plate. The strain of bacteria used cannot normally form colonies on the agar plate in the absence of the amino acid histidine; chemicals which cause mutations in bacteria result in mutant (or revertant) colonies being formed. The test usually includes an extract of mammalian liver as a source of

```
Version: 1.01 (August 1991)
Copyright 1991, D.O. Chanter, Brookwood Statistics

Run date: 1992/5/27   08:28


UKEMS Assay A data
==================


Data listing:
-------------

Group   Abnormal   Total    Proportion   Monotonic       Dose
number   cells     cells     affected   M.L. means      level

  1         3       400       0.007        0.007            0
  2         5       200       0.025        0.025           20
  3        14       200       0.070        0.045          100
  4         4       200       0.020        0.045          200

Totals     26      1000       0.026


Permutation test P-values (one-sided):
--------------------------------------

Test                           Minimum    Mid-P      Conventional

Heterogeneity (Pearson)        0.000122   0.000133   0.000144
Heterogeneity (lik. ratio)     0.000464   0.000468   0.000471
Cochran-Armitage (grp. no.)    0.00820    0.0105     0.0128
Cochran-Armitage (dose)        0.0525     0.0552     0.0580
Bartholomew's                  0.00280    0.00286    0.00292
Isotonic likelihood ratio      0.00100    0.00104    0.00107
Williams'                      0.00392    0.00514    0.00637
Modified Williams'             0.00501    0.00593    0.00686
All treated grps. >= control   0.0000967  0.000102   0.000108
Maximum excess                 0.0000263  0.0000401  0.0000540
Smoothed maximum excess        0.000145   0.000263   0.000381
Maximum paired product         0.00173    0.00175    0.00176
```

Fig. 4.3. Output of the INVICTY program, developed for analysing *in vitro* cytogenetic assay results.

mammalian drug-metabolising enzymes to mimic the action of the chemical in the whole animal.

A wide range of statistical methods have been developed, including various modelling approaches (Margolin *et al.* 1981, Myers *et al.* 1981), non-parametric procedures (Wahrendorf *et al.* 1985, Simpson and Margolin 1986) and non-linear regression methods (Krewski *et al.* 1993).

Statistical approaches that rely upon a test of the hypothesis that there is a treatment-related effect have resulted, in general, in the identification of effects which are not considered of biological importance by genetic toxicologists.

Various qualitative criteria, often based upon two- and three-fold increases over a background incidence, have been proposed by some genetic toxicologists. However, the protocols developed for the Ames test have the power to detect much lower-fold increases. For instance, assuming that the number of revertants on a plate follows a Poisson distribution and the control incidence is 20 colonies per plate, then a doubling to 40 per plate or a tripling to 60 per plate would, assuming a square root transformation, signify a 3.6 and 6.5 standard deviation unit increase over controls. Even experiments with sample sizes of three plates per dose would have a very high power for detecting such effects in a one-sided test using $P < 0.05$ as a criteria for significance.

In Table 4.5 are illustrated the differences in standard deviation units assuming a Poisson distribution between the negative control and the two- and three-fold increase levels based upon the negative control incidence supplied by UKEMS (1990). In all cases the differences are large and a sample size of three

Table 4.5. Power calculations for the Ames test based upon background colonies per plate and assuming a Poisson distribution

(i) The difference between the background and the two- and three-fold increases over the background (x_2 and x_3) are expressed in standard deviation units. The variance of a Poisson variable on a square root scale is 0.25; hence the standard deviation (S.D.) is 0.5:

		Mean number of revertants			S.D. units	
	UKEMS[a]	Control (C)	×2	×3	C v ×2	C v ×3
TA1535	3–37	20	40	60	3.7	6.5
TA1537	4–31	20	40	60	3.7	6.5
TA98	15–60	40	80	120	5.2	9.2
TA100	75–120	130	260	390	9.4	16.6
TA97	90–180	135	270	405	9.6	17.0
TA102	240–360	300	600	900	14.4	25.3

(ii) The sample sizes needed to detect a true difference between a control and treated group in a one-sided test at the 5 per cent significance level with 90 per cent power and $\beta = 0.10$ is calculated using the equation $n = (2\sigma^2/\delta^2)(Z_A + Z_B)^2$. For $\alpha = 0.05$ and $\beta = 0.10$, $(Z_A + Z_B)^2 = 8.6$; δ/σ is the ratio of the size of the difference to the standard deviation of the material. n is calculated below for different values of this ratio:

δ	σ	Ratio $\delta : \sigma$ (S.D. units)	$2\sigma^2/\delta^2$	n
1.5	0.5	3	0.22	1.9
2.0	0.5	4	0.12	1.1
2.5	0.5	5	0.08	0.7
3.0	0.5	6	0.06	0.5

[a] The range of background colonies/plate is taken from UKEMS (1990).

plates/dose would have a power of greater than 0.90 for detecting effects at a $P < 0.05$.

The ability to detect small effects which are not considered biologically important leads to the debate about whether a statistical analysis of the data is necessary. When a statistical analysis is carried out, various test approaches, including the use of multiple comparison approaches, such as those developed by David Williams, have been used. In practice, such approaches have mainly been aimed at 'damping' down the statistical significance level to reduce the number of findings flagged (or 'starred') as statistically significant. In the opinion of some genetic toxicologists, the use of such approaches still produces a test which is too sensitive.

Alternative approaches have been developed based upon estimation of the size of the mutagenic effect. This has involved estimating a linear component to the dose–response relationship usually at low doses (Margolin *et al.* 1981, Bernstein *et al.* 1982, Krewski *et al.* 1993). This has the advantage that it is concentrating attention on the size of any mutagenic effect. However, this type of result may be more difficult to fit into the requirement for a qualitative statement that the chemical is or is not a genotoxin. A further potential complication is that attempts have been made to use similar estimates as measures of mutagenic potency and, subsequently, to use these to predict carcinogenic potency. Early approaches were controversial (McCann *et al.* 1988, Piegorsch and Hoel 1988) and attempts to present the results from Ames tests in a quantitative form may be hampered because they re-awaken the criticism of the earlier studies.

4.8.2 *Cytogenetic assays*

Cytogenetic tests involve preparing cells from either animals or cell culture lines for microscopic examination of the chromosomes in the cell nucleus. This may involve looking for chromosomal damage such as breaks or rearrangements or counting the number of rearrangements, called sister chromosome exchanges (SCEs), seen in specially stained cells such as lymphocytes. Alternatively, the number of immature red blood cells (called polychromatic erythrocytes, PCEs) which contain a small amount of genetic material called a micronucleus may be counted. Micronuclei can be left behind after the nucleus is expelled during the normal differentiation of the red blood cell, as a consequence of damage to the genetic material.

The various cytogenetic assays illustrate the complications that can arise in the interpretation of standard protocols for test systems which have different statistical power. The data collected by the SCE test are, for instance, scores per cell, which can almost be considered as a continuous trait, the number of micronucleated PCEs in the micronucleus are, usually, in the control groups Poisson-distributed low scores, while the data for chromosomal abnormalities can be considered qualitative and 'scored' as either a normal or abnormal cell. All three approaches have a hierarchy of units (Fig. 4.4). In the case of *in vivo*

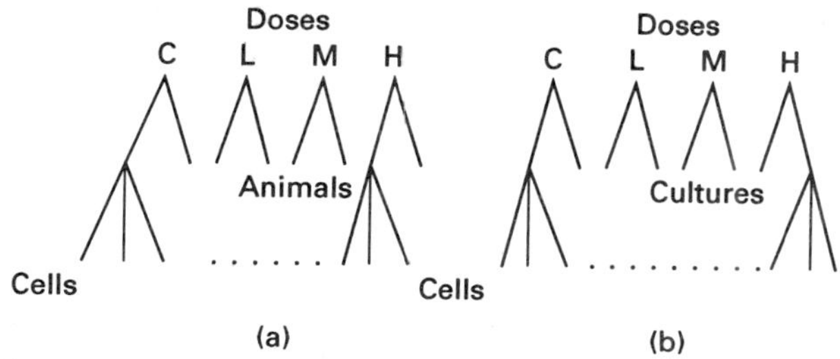

Fig. 4.4. The hierarchical designs in *in vivo* and *in vitro* cytogenetic assays. (a) Three levels of variability in the *in vivo* study; between doses, between animals within doses, and between cells within animals. (b) In the *in vitro* assay variability between animals is replaced by variability between cultures. C = control; L = low; M = medium; H = high.

studies, it is the doses, the animal, and the cell; correspondingly, in the *in vitro* studies, it is the doses, the cultures, and the cell. The experimental protocols usually specify the degree of replication and sample sizes needed.

The failure to appreciate the implication of the experimental structure, and the choice of units can lead to problems in the statistical analysis in the presence of appreciable inter-animal or inter-culture variability (Table 4.6). The combining of cells across animals or cultures can lead to spuriously significant effects in simple 2×2 tests or by the use of the Kastenbaum–Bowman tables familiar to many genetic toxicologists (Kastenbaum and Bowman 1970). These are tables of the conditional binomial test, and they assume homogeneity of the test material. The converse problem of carrying out analyses which assume homogeneity of variances in the presence of heterogeneity in the treated group is a loss of power. These are, of course, the same problems as encountered in the analysis of data from reproductive toxicology studies (Haseman and Hogan 1975). David Williams' paper at Namur considered the *in vivo* cytogenetic test as one example where permutation tests might be used for analysing data sets in toxicology with overdispersed or extra-bionomial variation (Williams 1988*b*).

The difference in the power of the designs of the different genotoxicity tests can result in the chromosomal aberration test apparently having lower sensitivity than other tests. Conversely, tests such as the SCE may be 'criticized' for being too sensitive. A simple illustration of the different power characteristics of the three tests is shown in Table 4.7. The calculations are simplistic and make, for instance, no attempt to incorporate between individual or culture variability. Nevertheless, it is clear that both the micronucleus and SCE tests have considerably greater power in terms of reduced animal use or technical effect than tests for chromosomal aberrations. This increased power may be considered by some to be a disadvantage, as it identifies statistical significances which are not considered biologically important. This is, therefore, another case in which an overemphasis on the use of statistical analysis for hypothesis testing can be counterproductive.

Table 4.6. An illustration, using artificial data, of the problems caused by overdispersion in a genetic toxicology test

Control	Treated
5/100	6/100
4/100	30/100
6/100	8/100
8/100	4/100
23/400	48/400

(i) Various different tests are made between a control and treated group, each of four animals, where, for instance, 100 cells are scored for chromosomal aberrations:

Fisher exact test (one-sided)	$P = 0.00132$	**
Chi-squared test = 8.903	$P = 0.0028$	**
$z = 2.984$	$P = 0.0014$	**
Two-sample pooled t-test	$P = 0.17$	NS
Mann–Whitney	$P = 0.28$	NS

(ii) Tests of the assumptions of homogeneity within the groups show that there is extra-binomial variability in the treated group:

F-test of ratio of variances	50.1 **
Heterogeneity chi-squared	
Control	1.61 NS
Treated	41.67 ***

An example of the characteristics of the different types of cytogenetic assays in practice comes from the work of Tice *et al.* (1987) on the genotoxic effects on mice exposed by inhalation to the industrial chemical 1,3-butadiene. Mice were investigated for the induction of chromosomal aberrations, SCEs and micronuclei. The sensitivity of the different end-points is shown in Table 4.8. Effects are detected using the SCEs and micronuclei at exposures down to 6.25 ppm, but were only found at 625 ppm in the case of chromosomal aberrations. In a case such as this, given the lack of power associated with the chromosomal aberration test, it is impossible to distinguish between no effect and an effect below the 'resolution' of the test. The point is further emphasized when the Dose for Unit Increase (DUI) in the cytogenetic damage is calculated. This is the dose which is estimated to increase the base level of SCE per cell by 1, the number of micronuclei per 1000 PCEs by 1, and the percentage of cells with chromosomal aberrations by 1 per cent.

The statistical power of the test is an important consideration in developing guidelines for the experimental designs used in genetic toxicology. The allocation of resources to an experiment are important both in terms of minimizing the number of animals needed to be used *in vivo* tests and also because 'scoring'

Table 4.7. An illustration of the power of different cytogenetic tests. The table shows the total number of cells needed to detect the difference between the control and treated mean in a one-sided test with a significance level (α) of 5 per cent and power ($1-\beta$) of 90 per cent. Calculations assume there there is no appreciable variability between animals in either of the groups. The units column is an indication of the number of animals that would need to be examined to obtain the total number of cells for the comparison; for example, 2000 polychromatic erythrocytes from each of six animals

	Control mean	Treated mean	Number of cells	Units
SCE (per cell)	10.0	12.0	42	2×25
Micronuclei (per 1000 PCEs)	2.0	4.0	12 500	6×2000
Chromosomal aberrations (%) abnormal cells	2.0	4.0	1 247	25×50

cells for assessment of cytogenetic damage is a skilled and time-consuming task. A trained technician will take about an hour to read 50 cells for chromosomal aberrations, half an hour to score 25 cells for SCEs and about 15–20 minutes to

Table 4.8. A comparison of results from three different end-points measured in the same experiment by Tice *et al.* (1987). The results show the order of sensitivity of the different indicators of chromosomal damage as SCE > MNT > CAB

	1,3-Butadiene (ppm) ($n = 12$)				Statistical test used by Tice *et al.*	Dose for Unit increase (DUI)
	0	6.25	62.5	625		
SCE per cell (25 cells per mouse)	5.51	6.49 ** †	10.88 ** †	35.09 *** †	One-sided t-test	12
MNT per 1000 PCEs (1000 PCEs per mouse)	3.75	5.50 *	8.36 *** †	30.0 *** †	One-sided Pearson's χ^2 test	15
CAB % abnormal cells (50 cells per mouse)	2.3	1.6	3.3	14.0 *** †	One-sided t-test	46

$^*P < 0.05$; $^{**}P < 0.01$; $^{***}P < 0.001$ using one-way analysis of variance methodology and least-significant difference tests for pairwise comparison with negative control group.
† Declared significant using Tice *et al.*'s criterion of $P = 0.017$ based upon the Bonferroni correction for three pairwise comparisons ($\alpha = 0.05/3$).

examine 1000 polychromatic erythrocytes for micronuclei. Increasing the number of cells that need to be analysed at each dose level—for example, from 1000 to 2000 in the micronucleus—will raise the cost of the test appreciably. Statisticians, therefore, can play an important role in helping genetic toxicologists to define the objectives of their assays and to optimize their designs. Murphy *et al.* (1992) provide an example of such an approach applied to SCE experiments.

4.8.3 *The dominant lethal test*

Dominant lethal tests entail the examination of the uterine contents of female rodents that have been mated to males exposed to or administered a potential mutagen. The data used in the analysis consists of the numbers of live and dead fetuses together with the number of small dark-coloured 'moles' (sometimes called resorptions) in the uterus. These are early deaths of embryos which have implanted in the uterus but failed to develop, as a result of chromosomal imbalances caused by genetic damage to the sperm of treated males.

The dominant lethal is important because it is the most widely used test for evidence of transmission of genetic damage from one generation to the next in mammals. Identification of such a hazard can then lead to further experiments aimed at estimating the risk associated with such damage. The US National Toxicology Program, for instance, has recently incorporated the dominant lethal study into part of its reproductive risk assessment program (Shelby *et al.* 1993)

The standard protocol consists of a negative control and up to three treated groups, each consisting of up to 25 males. Males are mated to two new females for up to eight weeks to ensure that sperm arising from cells exposed at different stages in the spermatogenic cycle are sampled. (Dominant lethal tests can also be conducted using exposed females, as there are female-specific germ-cell mutagens. However, this test is less often carried out.) The full protocol including a positive control group would involve over 2000 animals, not including the litters. Although this full protocol is now rare, any dominant lethal test obviously requires both ethical and economical justification. These constraints mean that an effective and informative approach to the analysis of the data is of crucial importance.

The statistical analyses suggested have varied from considerations of various Mutagenic Indices based upon the proportion of early deaths and which lacked a formal statistical test or consideration of inter-individual variability (Ehling *et al.* 1978) to the more sophisticated approaches of trying to model, in statistical terms, the various types of deaths observed, such as the methods reviewed by David Williams in his Namur paper (Williams 1988b). The UKEMS (1989) chapter, for instance, left the choice of the particular statistical analysis open. In part, this was because there may be a number of appropriate analyses that could be used, and the actual design used in the assay may vary from study to study.

The design is hierarchical in that there are fetuses, females, males, and dose groups. Some inappropriate approaches have in the past used the fetus as the unit and applied simple chi-squared tests. It is now usually accepted that the male is the unit in the analysis. However, Lockhart *et al.* (1991) have suggested that, in the majority of cases, carrying out an analysis using the female as the unit will not necessarily alter the results appreciably.

Multiple comparisons issues arise as the assay is designed to detect stage-specific effects, i.e. effects limited to just one or two weeks of testing. In the full protocol there are 48 possible comparisons between the control and the treated groups for each week. There are also multiple and correlated end-points for each litter: the total number of live fetuses, late deaths, and early deaths. The power of the test is, however, low and it is, consequently, difficult to distinguish between a genuine stage-specific effect and a type I error. Lockhart *et al.* (1992) have provided some indications of the power associated with the test.

Statistical analysis is further complicated because 'clusters' of deaths or abnormalities can occur within a litter. This is because an individual's development can be affected by its littermates. Consequently, the data can be over-dispersed or follow an extra-binomial distribution.

The statistical analysis of the dominant lethal assay, therefore, presents a challenge, because the analysis is not straightforward, different analyses can give conflicting indications of statistical significance, and there is a dichotomy between some genetic toxicologists who would prefer an extremely simple statistical test and statisticians who believe that the complex data set are suitable for more sophisticated analysis.

Modifications of the dominant lethal test are being used to try to identify agents which result in male-mediated congenital abnormalities, sometimes referred to as 'male teratogenicity' (Anderson *et al.* 1993). The dominant lethal test consequently straddles the fields of genetic, developmental, and reproductive toxicology. In practice, it is gradually being realized that the analysis of the dominant lethal shares many of the problems associated with the analysis of teratological and developmental toxicology studies. The statistical methods described (Ryan 1992) for developmental toxicology have obvious relevance. Statisticians have, for instance, previously pointed out the problem of correctly defining the unit for statistical analysis in teratology studies and the implications of incorrect approaches (Haseman and Hogan 1975).

4.9 Some future developments

Genetic toxicology continues to develop. New tests are being developed to fill gaps in the testing strategies, and advances in molecular biology are resulting in new approaches to testing chemicals. Statistical advice will be needed to ensure that appropriate designs are produced.

Unscheduled DNA synthesis (UDS) is a test which is increasing in use. Liver cells called hepatocytes are examined for evidence of DNA repair. Tritiated thymidine is used by the cell to repair DNA damage, and the subsequent radioactive decay is measured by counting the number of spots left on a photographic emulsion covering the cells. The test can be used for both *in vivo* and *in vitro* administration of a compound. These tests are often analysed by qualitative assessments and declared positive if the scores are above a certain number. However, the data are also suitable for analysis by statistical methods and the test proves to be very sensitive. The usual criteria for a positive result is in the order of five standard deviation units from the negative control. As a consequence, a large number of chemicals could be declared positive on the basis of a statistical test; falsely, in the view of the genetic toxicologist, because the effects of the chemicals would be considered of limited biological importance. This again is a problem of the over-reliance on hypothesis testing and statistical significance for the assessment of results.

Transgenic mice are another new development in mutation research: some genetic material from a bacterium is integrated into the mouse's genetic material by packaging it in a lambda shuttle vector using recombinant DNA technology. The bacterial DNA can be re-extracted using lambda phage particles and these used to infect a specific bacterial strain grown on plates. Mutations which have arisen in the bacterial DNA while it was integrated in the mouse's DNA can be detected by specific staining procedures. Although this assay uses new technologies, the problems relating to statistical analysis are familiar, such as: whether statistical analysis of the data is necessary; what the optimum number of animals and the 'phage' to sample are; what the appropriate methods for statistical analysis are, and what the criteria for positive responses are.

Another new assay is the COMET test. Individual cells from treated animals or cultures are placed on gels. An electric current is passed through the gel and the DNA is moved towards the anode. The degree of spread of the DNA is a measure of how much damage the treatment has caused to the DNA. Here again, the assay is being quantified and statistical issues will arise regarding design and analysis of the test.

4.10 Challenges for the future

Genetic toxicology has now become an accepted part of regulatory toxicology. Official guidelines have formalized the requirements for specific tests. Guidelines such as those of the OECD are being revised to take into account refinements to original tests and to include new tests such as the UDS assays. Even in those genetic toxicology tests which are now well developed, there are still many areas in which the statistician can play an important role in helping to interpret the results.

One is in clarifying the different roles of statistics for hypothesis testing or estimation by describing the properties of the tests in terms of statistical power. There is an increasing realization among genetic toxicologists that statistics can play an important role in estimating the size of effects rather than just relying on hypothesis testing. The statistician can help by characterizing the power of the designs and raising the question of whether the purpose of the test is to maximize the chance of identifying a hazard or to show that the chemical has cleared a 'reasonable hurdle'.

The statistician has an important role to play in helping to determine the optimum allocation of resources in the tests. This can represent a challenge, because there may be the conflicting pressures of tightly defined protocols and guidelines alongside the need to conduct innovative research experiments.

Statisticians should find many practical problems to interest them, such as determining appropriate analyses for the new assays such as the transgenic mouse, whether or not to incorporate historical control data into the analysis, or in developing approaches to the problem of overdispersion of data. The difficulty of a small number of 'responders' in a test causes considerable problems in identifying appropriate designs and analyses in genetic toxicology. David Williams' innovative work in this area, such as his Namur paper, needs to be developed further.

4.11 Conclusions

Genetic toxicology is still a developing science. It shares a common history with many aspects of modern statistics. There is a growing appreciation of the role of statisticians in the area, and the initiatives of organizations such as UKEMS have built up a considerable degree of interaction and communication between the two fields. The stimulus of attempts to harmonize guidelines, both to reduce unnecessary testing and to remove barriers to trade, is leading to a greater realization by genetic toxicologists that they need to define the purpose of their tests more clearly.

The new developments will raise statistical problems; most will probably be old problems in a different guise. A major problem facing statisticians will be how to balance the developments in statistics towards, for instance, methods which adopt modelling procedures, estimation, and data exploration against a background of prescriptive protocols heavily influenced by hypothesis testing, statistical significance, and probability levels.

Genetic toxicology offers a potentially fertile field for the teaching of the practical uses of statistics. There are many experimental design and statistical interpretation problems to test the student, together with the potential for abundant data. David Williams would have continued to be a major influence on the thinking of those involved in the development of the statistical analysis of genetic toxicology. His contributions to this area will remain as a foundation for some of the future exciting work in the area.

Acknowledgements

I would like to thank Peter Jenkinson, Diana Anderson, Stephen Blowers, and Ian Rowland for their comments and discussions on early drafts of this chapter.

References

Ames, B. N. (1989). Chemicals, cancers, casualties and cautions. *Chemtech*, **19**, 590–8.

Ames, B. N., Durston, W. E., Yamasaki, E., and Lee, F. D. (1973). Carcinogens are mutagens—a simple test system combining liver homogenates for activation and bacteria for detection. *Proceedings of the National Academy of Sciences*, **70**, 2281–5.

Anderson, D., Jenkinson, P. C., Edwards, A. J., Evans, J. G., and Lovell, D. P. (1993). Male-mediated F_1 abnormalities. In *Reproductive toxicology* (M. Richardson, ed.). VCH Verlagsgesellschaft mbh, Weinheim, pp. 101–16.

Auerbach, C., Robson, J. M., and Carr, J. G. (1947). The chemical production of mutations. *Science*, **105**, 243.

Auletta, A. E., Dearfield, K. L., and Cimino, M. C. (1993). Mutagenicity test schemes and guidelines: US EPA Office of Pollution Prevention and Toxics and the Office of Pesticide Programs. *Environmental and Molecular Mutagenesis*, **21**, 38–45.

Bernstein, L., Kaldor, J., McCann, J., and Pike, M. C. (1982). An empirical approach to the statistical analysis of mutagenesis data from the *Salmonella* test. *Mutation Research*, **97**, 267–81.

British Medical Association (1992). *Our genetic future: the science and ethics of genetic toxicology*. Oxford University Press, Oxford.

Commission of the European Communities (1992). Council Directive 92/32/EEC amending for the seventh time Council Directive 67/548/EEC on the approximation of laws, regulations and administrative provisions relating to the classification, packaging and labelling of dangerous substances: Annex III. *Official Journal of the European Communities* (L257), 13–33.

DeMarini, D. M., Lewtas, J., and Brockman, H. E. (1989). Utility of short-term tests for genetic toxicity. *Cell Biology and Toxicology*, **5**, 189–200.

DHSS (1981). *Guidelines for the testing of chemicals for mutagenicity*. Department of Health and Social Security, Report on Health and Social Subjects No. 24. HMSO, London.

DoH (1989). *Guidelines for the testing of chemicals for mutagenicity*. Department of Health, Report on Health and Social Subjects No. 35. HMSO, London.

Edler, L. (1992). Statistical methods for short-term tests in genetic toxicology: the first fifteen years. *Mutation Research*, **277**, 11–33.

Edwards, A. W. F. (1990). R. A. Fisher: Twice Professor of Genetics: London and Cambridge or "A fairly well-known geneticist". *Biometrics*, **46**, 897–904.

Ehling, U. H., Machemer, L., Buselmaier, W., Dycka, J., Frohberg, H., Kratochvilova, J., Lang, R., Lorke, D., Muller, D., Peh, J., Rohrborn, G., Roll, R., Schultze-Schencking, M., and Wiemann. H. (1978). Standard protocol for the dominant lethal test on male mice set up the Work Group "Dominant lethal mutations of the *ad hoc* committee chemicogenetics". *Archives of Toxicology*, **39**, 173–85.

Emery, A. E. H. (1983). *Elements of medical genetics* (6th edn). Churchill Livingstone, Edinburgh.

Haseman, J. K. and Hogan, M. D. (1975). Selection of the experimental unit in teratology studies. *Teratology*, **12**, 165–71.

Kastenbaum, M. A. and Bowman, K. O. (1970). Tables for determining the statistical significance of mutation frequencies. *Mutation Research*, **9**, 527–49.

Krewski, D., Leroux, B. G., Bleuer, S. R., and Broekhaven, L. H. (1993). Modelling the Ames *Salmonella*/microsome assay. *Biometrics*, **49**, 499–510.

Lockhart, A-M. C., Bishop, J. B., and Piegorsch, W. W. (1991). Issues regarding data acquisition and analysis in the dominant lethal assay. *Proceedings of the American Statistical Association, Biopharmaceutical Section*, pp. 234–7.

Lockhart, A-M. C., Piegorsch, W. W., and Bishop, J. B. (1992). Assessing over dispersion and dose response in the male dominant lethal assay. *Mutation Research*, **272**, 35–58.

Margolin, B. H., Kaplan, N., Zeiger, E. (1981). Statistical analysis of the Ames

Salmonella/microsome test. *Proceedings of the National Academy of Sciences*, **78**, 3779–83.

Margolin, B. H. (1985). Statistical studies in genetic toxicology: a perspective from the US National Toxicology Program. *Environmental Health Perspectives*, **63**, 187–94.

McCann, J., Gold, L. S., Horn, L., McGill, R., Graedel, T. E., and Kaldor, J. (1988). Statistical analysis of the *Salmonella* test data and comparison of results of animal cancer test. *Mutation Research*, **205**, 183–95.

Müller, H. J. (1927). Artificial transmutation of the gene. *Science*, **66**, 84–7.

Murphy, S. A., Tice, R. R., Smith, M. G., and Margolin, B. H. (1992). Contributions to the design and statistical analysis of *in vivo* SCE experiments. *Mutation Research*, **271**, 39–48.

Myers, L. E., Sexton, N. H., Southerland, L. I., and Wolff, T. J. (1981). Regression analysis of Ames test data. *Environmental Mutagenesis*, **3**, 575–86.

OECD (1983). *OECD guidelines for testing of chemicals. Genetic toxicology, No. 471–474.* Organisation for Economic Cooperation and Development, Paris, 26 May 1983.

Piegorsch, W. W. (1990). Fisher's contribution to genetics and heredity, with special emphasis on the Gregor Mendel controversy. *Biometrics*, **46**, 915–24.

Piegorsch, W. W. and Hoel, D. G. (1988). Exploring relationships between mutagenic and carcinogenic potencies. *Mutation Research*, **196**, 161–75.

Ray, V. A., Kier, L. D., Kannan, K. L., Haas, R. T., Auletta, A. E., Wassom, J. S., Nesnow, S., and Waters, M. D. (1987). An approach to identifying specialized batteries of bioassays for specific classes of chemicals: class analysis using mutagenicity and carcinogenicity relationships and phylogenetic concordance and discordance patterns. (I) Composition and analysis of the overall data base. A Report of Phase II of the US Environmental Protection Agency Gene-Tox Program. *Mutation Research*, **185**, 197–241.

Ryan, L. (1992). Quantitative risk assessment for developmental toxicity. *Biometrics*, **48**, 163–74.

Shelby, M. D., Bishop, J. M., Mason, J. M., and Tindall, K. R. (1993). Fertility, reproduction, and genetic disease: studies in the mutagenic effects of environmental agents in mammalian germ cells. *Environmental Health Perspectives*, **100**, 283–91.

Simpson, D. G. and Margolin, B. H. (1986). Recursive nonparametric testing for dose–response relationships subject to downturns at high doses. *Biometrika*, **73**, 589–96.

Tice, R. R., Boucher, R., Luke, C. A., and Shelby, M. D. (1987). Comparative cytogenetic analysis of bone marrow damage by multiple exposure to gaseous 1,3-butadiene. *Environmental Mutagenesis*, **9**, 235–50.

UKEMS (1983). *Sub-committee report on guidelines for mutagenicity testing. Report. Part I. Basic test battery* (ed. B. J. Dean). UKEMS, Swansea.

UKEMS (1984). *Sub-committee on guidelines for mutagenicity testing. Report. Part II. Supplementary tests, mutagens in food, mutagens in body fluids and excreta, nitrosation products* (ed. B. J. Dean). UKEMS, Swansea.

UKEMS (1989). *Sub-committee on guidelines for mutagenicity testing. Report. Part III. Statistical evaluation of mutagenicity test data* (ed. D. J. Kirkland). Cambridge University Press, Cambridge.

UKEMS (1990). *Sub-committee guidelines for mutagenicity testing. Report. Part I revised. Basic mutagenicity test. UKEMS recommended procedures* (ed. D. J. Kirkland). Cambridge University Press, Cambridge.

Wahrendorf, J., Mahon, G. A. T., and Schmuacher, M. (1985). A non-parametric approach to the statistical analysis of mutagenicity data. *Mutation Research*, **147**, 5–13.

Williams, D. A. (1971). A test for differences between treatment means when several dose levels are compared with a zero dose control. *Biometrics*, **27**, 103–17.

Williams, D. A. (1972). The comparison of several dose levels with a zero dose control. *Biometrics*, **28**, 519–31.

Williams, D. A. (1986). A note on Shirley's non-parametric test for comparing several dose levels with a zero-dose control. *Biometrics*, **42**, 183–6.

Williams, D. A. (1988*a*). Tests for differences between several small proportions. *Applied Statistics*, **37**, 421–34.

Williams, D. A. (1988*b*). Extra-binomial variation in toxicology. Invited paper, XIVth International Biometric Conference, Namur, July 1988, *Conference proceedings*, pp. 301–13.

Winston, R. L. and Handyside, A. H. (1993). New challenges in human *in vitro* fertilization. *Science*, **260**, 932–6.

PART II

OVERDISPERSION

5 Some observations on detecting extra-binomial variability within the beta-binomial model

KENNETH J. RISKO AND BARRY H. MARGOLIN

5.1 Introduction

The study of methods of analysis for over-dispersed binomial data has received much attention in the past decade. A substantial portion of that effort has centred on models in which the increased variability is attributable to the heterogeneity of the binomial parameter p across observations. The beta-binomial is one such model that affords both a degree of flexibility in the shape of the distribution of p and satisfactory analytical tractability. If p follows a beta distribution with parameters a and b, and n is the number of binary measurements summed in an observation, then the mean and variance of the beta-binomial distribution are $na/(a+b)$ and

$$nab(a+b+n)/[(a+b)^2(a+b+1)],$$

respectively. It will be convenient to make the transformation $\mu = a/(a+b)$ and $\theta = 1/(a+b)$, where $0 < \mu < 1$ and $0 \leqslant \theta$, so that $\mathrm{E}(Y) = n\mu$ and

$$\mathrm{Var}(Y) = [1 + \{(n-1)\theta/(1+\theta)\}]n\mu(1-\mu).$$

In this parametrization (Williams 1975) the binomial (n, μ) distribution is represented by $\theta = 0$ and extra-binomial variability is represented by $\theta > 0$, whereas in the original formulation, the binomial distribution is obtained in the limit as a and b tend to infinity with $a/(a+b)$ tending to μ and extra-binomial variability is achieved for $a+b$ finite. Interest here centres on ascertaining whether the over-dispersion is negligible, not whether there is under-dispersion. Consequently, the tests considered will all be one-tailed.

5.2 The cost of needless generalization

Although the beta-binomial sampling distribution is an attractive generalization of the binomial distribution, the cost of needlessly adopting the generalization can be significant. First, *vis-à-vis* the beta-binomial model, methods of analysis for binomially distributed data are more readily available and have been more extensively studied with regard to size and power. Examples of such well-studied procedures include Fisher's exact test and the binomial variance test for homogeneity of proportions. In many cases, tables of power are available to aid in the choice of sample size. Second, there is an attendant loss of power for detecting factor effects when excess variability is needlessly incorporated into the model. Finally, the ability to narrow one's focus to binomial sampling can also provide a valuable quality control tool. For example, if it can be established that a given laboratory is capable of routinely producing binomially distributed data, the appearance of data substantially more variable than binomial might be indicative of a new, controllable source of extraneous variability. An inexperienced laboratory technician, a change in protocol, or a new source or strain of laboratory animals are but a few examples of such sources. These same comments apply to inter-laboratory studies. The inability of one or more laboratories to achieve binomial sampling variability when the majority of laboratories in the study routinely obtain such variability is probably indicative of a need to improve laboratory procedures and practices, to investigate the source and quality of experimental materials, or to consider missing covariates. The excess variability, if not eliminated, can diminish power for detecting factor effects.

An actual quality control example involved the control data in Table 5.1, which arose as part of an international collaborative study (Margolin and Risko 1988). Presented in Table 5.1 are ten sets of daily control values for one laboratory, which tested five chemicals over ten days. The counts represent the number of cells with specific genetic defects (micronuclei) observed among 1000 red blood cells examined per animal. Aggregating the controls to estimate the daily spontaneous rate of the specific genetic defect can reduce the variability of this estimate and, consequently, increase the power of any procedure to detect a treatment effect.

The ten sets of control counts were subjected to a binomial variance test for homogeneity of proportions (Snedecor and Cochran 1967), and with each set (day) homogeneity is tenable. The right-most column of Table 5.1 displays the

Table 5.1. Example of a hidden[a] covariate

Day	Control animal counts (number of defective cells per 1000 scored)	Count total	Aggregate number of cells scored	Average proportion $\times 10^3$	p-value[b]
1	1, 5, 7, 4, 5	22	5000	4.4	0.36
2	6, 8, 3, 4, 8, 5	34	6000	5.7	0.58
3	9, 4, 6, 3, 5, 6	33	6000	5.5	0.56
4	5, 3, 2, 5, 6	21	5000	4.2	0.63
5	0, 2, 1, 1, 1	5	5000	1.0	0.74
6	1, 0, 3, 2, 3, 1	10	6000	1.7	0.49
7	3, 1, 1, 0, 2, 1	8	6000	1.3	0.55
8	1, 1, 1, 1, 1	5	5000	1.0	1.00
9	7, 4, 2, 8, 6, 4	31	6000	5.2	0.44
10	0, 1, 1, 1, 2, 1	6	6000	1.0	0.85

[a] A substantially different, but initially unrecorded, protocol was used on days 1–4 and 9.
[b] For the homogeneity of binomial proportions test.

resulting p-values. While the variance test may not be very powerful with such limited data, the fact that the same procedure, when applied individually to similar data of the 14 other laboratories comprising the study, never produced a p-value smaller than 0.31 provides compelling support for a binomial sampling model within laboratories and days. Next, the homogeneity of proportions across days within a laboratory was tested by aggregating controls within days and subjecting the resulting values to the binomial variance test. For the ten sets of data in Table 5.1 there is significant excess day-to-day variability and, moreover, the day-to-day component of variance is estimated to be more than eight times that of the within-day component. This finding was unexpected, since the same analysis applied to the 14 other laboratories demonstrated that day-to-day variability was insignificant. Investigation into the source of this anomaly led to a discovery that the laboratory in question had inadvertently neglected to note protocol differences among the experiments when the data were forwarded for analysis. (The other laboratories maintained a single protocol throughout the study, as per plan.) The control values on days 1–4 and day 9 were the result of one protocol, whereas the remaining control values were the result of a substantially different protocol. Applying the binomial variance test to each of these two subsets of control values produced p-values of 0.76 and 0.79, respectively, for the hypothesis of homogeneity of binomial proportions across days. As a result, the two subsets of aggregated control values were utilized separately for their respective protocols. Had the anomaly not been detected and the originally measured extra-binomial variability been assumed, a resulting loss of power in detecting treatment effects would almost certainly have occurred.

5.3 Detecting excess binomial variability

Although the beta-binomial distribution is most often utilized as the alternative of choice when an alternative model is specified, several other distributions are deserving of consideration for modelling variability in binomial probabilities. Most notable are the correlated binomial model of Kupper and Haseman (1978), which is identical to the additive generalization of the binomial model proposed by Altham (1978), and a multiplicative generalization by Altham (1978). Tarone (1979), using the $C(\alpha)$ procedure of Neyman (1959), derived tests for the goodness of fit of the binomial distribution that are asymptotically optimal against the correlated binomial alternatives of Kupper and Haseman (1978) and Altham (1978), as well as the beta-binomial alternative. The $C(\alpha)$ procedure has been demonstrated by Moran (1970) to be asymptotically equivalent to tests using maximum likelihood estimators, but it is usually easier to implement, since it involves parameter estimation only under the null hypothesis, in this case binomial sampling. The $C(\alpha)$ test statistic for the beta-binomial alternative is identical to that for the correlated binomial alternative (Tarone 1979). For an experiment in which the responses take the form of proportions

y_i/n_i, $i=0,\ldots,r$, the correlated binomial model log-likelihood function is

$$L_c(p,\phi)=K+\sum_{i=0}^{r}[y_i\log(p)+(n_i-y_i)\log(q)]$$
$$+\sum_{i=0}^{r}\log\left[1+\frac{\phi}{2p^2q^2}\{(y_i-n_ip)^2+y_i(2p-1)-n_ip^2\}\right],$$

where $q=1-p$, K is a constant involving only the observations, and ϕ is a parameter that corresponds to the correlation between observations. The $C(\alpha)$ test statistic for testing homogeneity of proportions [H_0: $\phi=0$] that is asymptotically optimal against correlated binomial alternatives [H_a: $\phi\neq 0$] is given by $X_c^2=Z_b^2$, where $\bar{p}=\Sigma y_i/\Sigma n_j$, $\bar{q}=1-\bar{p}$, and

$$Z_b=\frac{\left[\Sigma_{i=0}^{r}(y_i-n_i\bar{p})^2/(\bar{p}\bar{q})-\Sigma_{i=0}^{r}n_i\right]}{[2\,\Sigma_{i=0}^{r}n_i(n_i-1)]^{1/2}}. \tag{5.1}$$

Under H_0, X_c^2 will have an asymptotic chi-squared distribution with one degree of freedom.

For the beta-binomial model the log-likelihood function is given by

$$L_b(\mu,\theta)$$
$$=K+\sum_{i=0}^{r}\left[\sum_{m=0}^{y_i-1}\log(\mu+m\theta)+\sum_{m=0}^{n_i-y_i-1}\log(1-\mu+m\theta)-\sum_{m=0}^{n_i-1}\log(1+m\theta)\right]$$

and the $C(\alpha)$ test statistic for testing H_0: $\theta=0$ (binomial) against H_1: $\theta>0$ is given by Z_b in eqn. (5.1). This will have an asymptotic standard normal distribution, so that the test based on Z_b is the one-tailed version of the test based on X_c^2. Prentice (1986), in extending the beta-binomial distribution to allow for negative θ values, has shown that the $C(\alpha)$ test statistic for testing H_0: $\theta=0$ versus H_a: $\theta\neq 0$ is also given by eqn. (5.1). Tarone (1979) suggests that the $C(\alpha)$ test statistic in eqn. (5.1) may have the property of 'robustness of optimality' (Moran 1973) in the sense that it is optimal against several alternatives to the binomial distribution. The multiplicative generalization of the binomial distribution suggested by Altham (1978) is one distribution, however, for which the test statistic in eqn. (5.1) is not optimal (Tarone 1979).

In the equal sample size case, $n_i=n$ for all i, the standard variance test for homogeneity of binomial proportions (Cochran 1954) was shown by Gart (1970) to be optimal against beta-binomial alternatives. The binomial variance test is based on the statistic

$$X_v^2=\sum_{i=0}^{r}(y_i-n_i\bar{p})^2/(n_i\bar{p}\bar{q}), \tag{5.2}$$

which has an asymptotic chi-squared distribution with r degrees of freedom. Note in the equal sample size case that X_c^2 and X_v^2 are related by

$$X_c^2=\frac{n}{n-1}\left(\frac{X_v^2-(r+1)}{\sqrt{2(r+1)}}\right)^2,$$

and although it is clear that the test statistics X_c^2 and X_v^2 are simple functions of one another, the tests based on them are not equivalent because the referenced asymptotic distributions differ. Tarone (1979) undertook a small Monte Carlo study to investigate the small sample distribution of the test statistics X_c^2 and X_v^2 under the null hypothesis of binomial sampling, and reported that the observed significance levels for the test based on X_c^2 are significantly lower than nominal for the 5 per cent and 10 per cent levels, whereas the binomial variance test produced very good agreement between nominal and observed levels at all levels considered. For correlated binomial alternatives, Tarone (1979) has shown that the Pitman asymptotic efficiency of the binomial variance test relative to the score test is 95 per cent. Tarone (1979), however, did not present any results for the efficiencies of the tests against beta-binomial alternatives.

In an attempt to elucidate matters relating to detecting beta-binomial departures from a binomial model, a large-scale Monte Carlo study was undertaken to assess the size and power of several different possible tests. The tests considered are based on:

(1) the Fisher-standardized maximum likelihood estimate (F.s.m.l.e.) test statistic,

$$W_\theta = \hat{\theta}/I_{\theta\theta}^{-1/2}(\hat{\mu}, \hat{\theta}),$$

where $I_{\theta\theta}^{-1/2}(\hat{\mu}, \hat{\theta})$ is the appropriate square root of the diagonal element of the inverse of the Fisher information matrix evaluated at the maximum likelihood estimates $\hat{\mu}$ and $\hat{\theta}$, and reference is to a standard normal distribution;

(2) the sample-standardized maximum likelihood estimate (s.s.m.l.e) test statistic,

$$V_\theta = \hat{\theta}/H_{\theta\theta}^{-1/2}(\hat{\mu}, \hat{\theta}),$$

where $H_{\theta\theta}^{-1/2}(\hat{\mu}, \hat{\theta})$ is the appropriate square root of the diagonal element of the inverse of the observed information matrix evaluated at the maximum likelihood estimates $\hat{\mu}$ and $\hat{\theta}$, and reference is to a standard normal distribution;

(3) the likelihood ratio test statistic,

$$\Lambda_\theta = \left(2\{L_b(\hat{\mu}, \hat{\theta}) - L_b(\bar{p}, 0)\}\right)^{1/2},$$

referenced by a standard normal;

(4) the beta-binomial score test, Z_b, referenced by a standard normal; and

(5) the binomial variance test, X_v^2, referenced by a chi-square with r d.f.

All of these methods have previously been proposed to test the hypothesis of interest, but a comprehensive investigation into the relative merits of the procedures is presently wanting.

Since each of the test procedures (1)–(5) is asymptotically based, the first issue addressed is the quality of the asymptotic approximations to the Monte Carlo based levels. The test based on V_θ produced results virtually identical to those obtained with W_θ, and it was not considered further. Results for the equal sample size case $\text{Bin}(n, p)$, $i = 1, \ldots, N$, for the choices $n = 10, 20, 50, 100$, $N = 10, 20, 50, 100$, and $p = 0.1, 0.5$ are presented graphically in Fig. 5.1, wherein the deviations of the Monte Carlo based significance levels from the asymptotically based nominal levels are depicted by solid circles (observed significance level less than nominal significance level), and open circles (observed significance level greater than nominal significance level); the larger the circle, the greater the absolute deviation. All cases represented in Figure 5.1 are independent realizations and are based on 1000 replications each. Several immediate observations can be made from inspection of Fig. 5.1.

First, the comparison of the test statistic W_θ to a standard normal distribution produces an extremely conservative test for all sample sizes of practical interest. For example, the 0.05 nominal level test produced significance levels that never exceeded 0.01 for $N \leq 50$, and the observed levels for $N = 100$ were about half the nominal levels. In light of the results of Prentice (1986), the rather slow rate

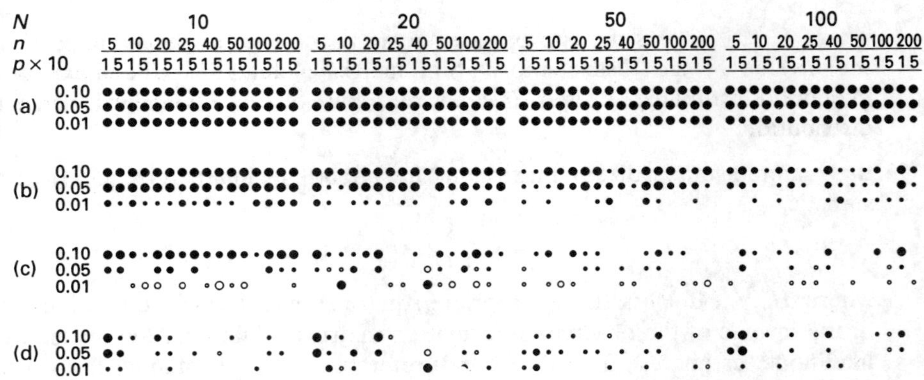

Fig. 5.1. A Monte Carlo study of the sizes of four procedures for detecting extra-binomial variability (equal sample size case). The four procedures are: (a) F.s.m.l.e., W_θ; (b) likelihood ratio, Λ_θ; (c) beta-binomial score, Z_b; and (d) the binomial variance test, X_v^2. Three levels of significance (0.10, 0.05, 0.01) are considered, and the size of each dot is indicative of the frequency of rejection of binomial variability in 1000 independent realizations. If α is the level of significance and if $s_\alpha = [1000\alpha(1-\alpha)]^{0.5}$, then the three sizes of dots, from smallest to largest, correspond to the absolute difference of the frequency of rejection and 1000α in the intervals $[s_\alpha, 2s_\alpha)$, $[2s_\alpha, 3s_\alpha)$, and $[3s_\alpha, \infty)$, respectively. Solid (hollow) dots represent cases in which the frequency of rejection is less (greater) than 1000α, and no dots are displayed if the frequency of rejection is in the interval $(-s_\alpha, s_\alpha)$. The data consist of N observations from the $\text{Bin}(n, p)$ distribution.

of convergence of the distribution of W to its asymptotic standard normal distribution cannot be attributed to the fact that $\theta = 0$ lies on the boundary of the parameter space. Indeed, when θ was chosen to produce beta-binomial data that was twice as variable as binomial data, the distribution of W_θ with $\hat{\theta} - \theta$ replacing $\hat{\theta}$ in the numerator of the test statistic showed the same degree of conservatism.

On the basis of Fig. 5.1, it is also clear that the likelihood ratio test statistic Λ_θ is very conservative for $N < 50$, where its size is approximately half the nominal asymptotically based level. It is less conservative for $N = 50$ and its size appears reasonable finally when $N = 100$. The score test statistic Z_b does produce reasonable sizes for $N \geq 20$, although there is a hint that the nominal 0.01 test is somewhat anti-conservative for $N \leq 20$ and that the nominal 0.10 level test is conservative for $N = 10$. It is the binomial variance test X_v^2 that produces sizes that are most nearly consistent with the asymptotically based approximations, even when there are as few as $N = 10$ observations. The relationship between X_c^2 $(= Z_b^2)$ and X_v^2 previously discussed suggests why Z_b^2 and X_v^2 may not share similar sizes when referenced to their respective asymptotic distributions, especially when N is small. Finally, the binomial parameter n appears to have little, if any, impact on the quality of the asymptotic approximation to the small sample distribution for all four test statistics while, not surprisingly, the number of observations N has a great impact. An explanation for this behavior is that since the parameter θ relates to the variance of the binomial probabilities from observation to observation, the number of binomial observations should greatly affect its estimation, whereas both n and N should affect the estimation of μ.

To investigate the power of the tests based on W_θ, Λ_θ, Z_b, and X_v^2, θ was chosen to produce beta-binomial data that are twice as variable as binomial data, i.e. $(n-1)\theta/(1+\theta) = 1$ for $\mu = 0.5$. The proportion of times that the tests rejected binomial sampling for nominal 0.05 level tests with $N = 10, 20$ is recorded in Table 5.2. The results for the 0.01 and 0.10 level tests (not presented) are qualitatively similar to the 0.05 level results, and the power of all 0.05 level procedures was virtually 1.0 for $N \geq 50$. It is clear that the test based on W_θ pays a heavy price in power for its extreme conservation in size. It is also indicated in Table 5.2 that the powers of the beta-binomial score test and the binomial variance tests are nearly equal, and that the power of the likelihood-ratio test (uncorrected for size) is slightly less than that of the other two tests. Had the three procedures been conducted at their empirical, rather than nominal levels, however, their powers would be virtually identical.

To assess the impact, if any, of unequal sample sizes on the quality of the asymptotic approximations, samples consisting of two different n-values were studied. For each choice of $k = 10, 20, 50, 100$, samples $(Y_1, \ldots, Y_N)$ were drawn with $Y_1, \ldots, Y_{tN} \sim \text{Bin}(k/2, p)$ and $Y_{tN+1}, \ldots, Y_N \sim \text{Bin}(2k, p)$, for $t = 0.2, 0.5, 0.7$ and $p = 0.1, 0.3, 0.5$. Presumably, any important differences in quality of the asymptotic approximations between equal and unequal sample sizes would begin to become evident in a Monte Carlo study of this design. The results of this

Table 5.2. A Monte Carlo study of the power[a] of four procedures for testing extra-binomial variability. Entries are the proportion of times in 1000 realizations that the hypothesis of binomial variability is rejected

N	n	F.s.m.l.e., W_θ	Likelihood ratio, Λ_θ	Score, Z_b	Binomial variance test, X_v^2
5	10	0	26	34	35
	50	0	21	28	32
	100	0	20	28	31
10	10	6	44	52	52
	50	4	38	46	47
	100	3	38	46	48
20	10	44	74	79	78
	50	39	67	73	73
	100	37	66	73	74

[a] The nominal level is 0.05 for all tests; $(n-1)\theta/(1+\theta)=1$; $\mu=0.5$.

additional study (not presented) closely resemble the equal sample size study, so the previous conclusions drawn regarding test size and relative power extend to unequal n_i.

5.4 Conclusions and recommendation

Various procedures for testing for the existence of extra-binomial variability, either against a specific alternative distribution or against a general alternative, have been studied with regard to their sizes and powers against beta-binomial alternatives. The results of the study suggest that: (i) the binomial variance test produces type I errors that are very close to nominal levels for even very small sample sizes; (ii) the s.m.l.e. test for extra-binomial variability is extraordinarily conservative, even for samples that are of considerably large size, whereas the likelihood ratio and score tests, although somewhat conservative for very small samples, produce reasonable agreement between observed and nominal levels; and (iii) the power of the binomial variance test against a beta-binomial alternative appears to be the best of all the tests considered and so is recommended when testing a beta-binomial alternative. In addition, its computation is simple, in contrast to the computer-intensive evaluation of the s.m.l.e. and likelihood ratio tests. The better performance of the binomial variance test is intriguing, since the other tests are tailored for the beta-binomial model, but the binomial variance test is not. This observation in a relatively simple setting suggests the need for further study of the comparable situation in more complex cases.

References

Altham, P. M. E. (1978). Two generalizations of the binomial distribution. *Applied Statistics*, **27**, 162–7.

Cochran, W. G. (1954). Some methods for strengthening the common X^2 tests. *Biometrics*, **10**, 417–51.

Gart, J. J. (1970). Some simple graphically oriented statistical methods for discrete data. In *Random counts in models and structures*, I (ed. G. P. Patil), pp. 171–91. Pennsylvania State University Press, University Park, Pennsylvania.

Kupper, L. L. and Haseman, J. K. (1978). The use of a correlated binomial model for the analysis of certain toxicological experiments. *Biometrics*, **34**, 69–76.

Margolin, B. H. and Risko, K. J. (1988). The statistical analysis of in vivo genotoxicity data: case studies of the rat hepatocyte UDS and mouse bone marrow micronucleus assays. In *Evaluation of short-term tests for carcinogenicity: report of the International Program on Chemical Safety Collaborative Study on In Vivo Assays*, Vol. I, Ch. 3. Cambridge University Press, Cambridge.

Moran, P. A. P. (1970). On asymptotically optimal tests of composite hypotheses. *Biometrika*, **57**, 47–55.

Moran, P. A. P. (1973). Asymptotic properties of homogeneity tests. *Biometrika*, **60**, 79–85.

Neyman, J. (1959). Optimal asymptotic tests of composite hypothesis. In *Probability and statistics: The Harald Cramér Volume* (ed. U. Grenander), pp. 213–34. Uppsala: Almgrist and Wiksell.

Prentice, R. L. (1986). Binary regression using an extended beta-binomial distribution, with discussion of correlation induced by covariate measurement errors. *Journal of the American Statistical Association*, **81**, 321–7.

Snedecor, G. W. and Cochran, W. G. (1967). *Statistical methods* (6th edn), p. 240. Iowa State University Press, Ames, Iowa.

Tarone, R. E. (1979). Testing the goodness of fit of the binomial distribution. *Biometrika*, **66**, 585–90.

Williams, D. A. (1975). The analysis of binary responses from toxicological experiments involving reproduction and teratogenicity. *Biometrics*, **31**, 949–52.

6 $C(\alpha)$ tests for homogeneity of proportions in toxicology in the presence of beta-binomial overdispersion

S. R. PAUL AND A. ISLAM

6.1 Introduction

Data in the form of proportions arise in toxicology and other similar fields. An important problem is to compare proportion of a certain characteristic in several groups. However, these proportions often exhibit variation greater than predicted by a simple binomial model (Williams 1975). Several parametric models are available for analysing binomial data with overdispersion (see, for example, Altham 1978, Haseman and Kupper 1979). The superiority of the beta-binomial (BB) model for the analysis of toxicological data in the form of proportions has been shown by many authors (Paul 1982, Pack 1986). For a fuller discussion of the methods of analysis of proportions in toxicology, see Haseman and Kupper (1979). A number of procedures are available for testing homogeneity of proportions in the presence of overdispersion. Of these, the likelihood ratio (LR) test has found prominence in the literature. For the homogeneity of proportions in two groups, Pack (1986) found, through simulation, that the likelihood ratio test was better than a range of others, including those based on simple transformation of proportions.

The purpose of this chapter is to derive $C(\alpha)$ (Neyman 1959) statistics for testing homogeneity of proportions in the presence of beta-binomial overdispersion. The $C(\alpha)$ test is based on the residual for a regression of the score function for the parameter(s) of interest on the score function for the nuisance parameters. The nuisance parameters are then replaced by $\sqrt{m}$ ($m =$ number of observations used in estimating the parameters) consistent estimators. For the definition of $\sqrt{m}$ consistency, see Neyman (1959). We derive two $C(\alpha)$ statistics; one based on the maximum likelihood estimators (mle's) and the other based on the method of moments estimators (mme's) of the nuisance parameters. The mle's and the mme's are $\sqrt{m}$ consistent. The $C(\alpha)$ statistic based on the mle's of the nuisance parameters is identical to the score statistic of Rao (1947). The score or $C(\alpha)$ statistic has been found to be useful for testing overdispersion in binomial and Poisson data (see, for example, Paul *et al.* 1989, Dean and Lawless 1990). Barnwal and Paul (1988) derived $C(\alpha)$ statistics for testing equality of Poisson means in presence of negative binomial variation.

In Section 6.2 we present the $C(\alpha)$ statistics; and a performance study, through simulations, for comparing the size and power of the $C(\alpha)$ statistics with the *LR* statistic is given in Section 6.3.

6.2 The $C(\alpha)$ statistics

Suppose that there are T treatment groups and that the ith group has m_i litters, $i = 1,\ldots,T$. The proportion responding in each litter is x_{ij}/n_{ij}, $j = 1,\ldots,m_i$; $i = 1,\ldots,T$. We assume that the binomial probability of response is distributed as a beta distribution over litters with mean π_i and variance $\pi_i(1-\pi_i)\theta_i/(1+\theta_i)$. The *BB* probability function is given by

$$P_r(X_{ij}=x_{ij}\mid n_{ij}) = \binom{n_{ij}}{x_{ij}} \frac{\Pi_{r=0}^{x_{ij}-1}(\pi_i + r\theta_i)\Pi_{r=0}^{n_{ij}-x_{ij}-1}(1-\pi_i+r\theta_i)}{\Pi_{r=0}^{n_{ij}-1}(1+r\theta_i)}, \quad (6.1)$$

$j = 1,\ldots,m_i$, $i = 1,\ldots,T$, $0 \leqslant \pi_i \leqslant 1$ and

$$\theta_i \geqslant \max\{-\pi_i/(n_{ij}-1), -(1-\pi_i)/(n_{ij}-1)\}$$

(Prentice 1985). Note that by allowing θ_i to be negative, we also allow the model to assume underdispersion. To make things simple, we assume homogeneous θ_i, i.e. we assume that $\theta_1 = \cdots = \theta_T = \theta$. Under this assumption we wish to test the hypothesis H_0: $\pi_1 = \cdots = \pi_T$ against H_A: not all π_i's are the same. This is the same as H_2 of Pack (1986). Under H_A the log-likelihood is

$$l = \sum_{i=1}^{T}\sum_{j=1}^{m_i}\left\{\sum_{r=0}^{x_{ij}-1}\log(\pi_i + r\theta) + \sum_{r=0}^{n_{ij}-x_{ij}-1}\log(1-\pi_i+r\theta) - \sum_{r=0}^{n_{ij}-1}\log(1+r\theta)\right\}. \quad (6.2)$$

Suppose that we let $\pi_i = \pi + \phi_i$ with $\phi_T = 0$. Then testing H_0 is equivalent to testing $\phi_i = 0$ for $i = 1,\ldots,T-1$ with π and θ treated as nuisance parameters. Tarone (1985) applied this technique to derive the $C(\alpha)$ statistic, to test the equality of several odds ratios. Barnwal and Paul (1988) and Paul (1989) applied this technique in similar situations.

Define $\phi = (\phi_1,\ldots,\phi_{T-1})$ and $\lambda = (\lambda_1, \lambda_2) = (\pi, \theta)$. Then we let

$$\psi_i = [\partial l/\partial\phi_i]_{\phi=0}, \qquad i = 1,\ldots,T-1$$

and

$$\gamma_k = [\partial l/\partial\lambda_k]_{\phi=0}, \qquad k = 1,2.$$

Now, let $\hat{\lambda}$ be some $\sqrt{n}$ consistent estimator of λ under the null hypothesis. Then the $C(\alpha)$ test is based on

$$S_i(\hat{\lambda}) = \psi_i(\hat{\lambda}) - \beta_{1i}\gamma_1(\hat{\lambda}) - \beta_{2i}\gamma_2(\hat{\lambda}), \qquad i = 1,\ldots,T-1,$$

where β_{1i} and β_{2i} are the partial regression coefficient of ψ_i on γ_1 and ψ_i on γ_2 respectively. The variance–covariance of $S(\lambda) = \{S_1(\lambda), \ldots, S_{T-1}(\lambda)\}'$ is $D - AB^{-1}A'$ and the regression coefficients $\beta = (\beta_1\ \beta_2) = AB^{-1}$, where $\beta_1 = (\beta_{11}, \ldots, \beta_{1T-1})'$, $\beta_2 = (\beta_{21}, \ldots, \beta_{2T-1})'$,

$$D_{it} = \mathrm{E}\left[\frac{-\partial^2 l}{\partial\phi_i \partial\phi_t}\bigg|_{\phi=0}\right], \qquad i, t = 1, \ldots, T-1,$$

$$A_{i_k} = \mathrm{E}\left[\frac{-\partial^2 l}{\partial\phi_i \partial\lambda_k}\bigg|_{\phi=0}\right], \qquad i = 1, \ldots, T-1, \quad k = 1, 2,$$

and

$$B_{ks} = \mathrm{E}\left[\frac{-\partial^2 l}{\partial\lambda_k \partial\lambda_s}\bigg|_{\phi=0}\right], \qquad k, s = 1, 2.$$

Using $\hat{\lambda}$ in S, A, B, and D, the $C(\alpha)$ statistic is given by $S'(D - AB^{-1}A')^{-1}S$, which is approximately distributed as chi-squared with $T-1$ degrees of freedom. Note that if we use the maximum likelihood estimate of λ, then $S_i(\hat{\lambda}) = \psi_i(\hat{\lambda})$, reducing the $C(\alpha)$ statistic to a score statistic (Rao 1947). Following Srivastava and Wu (1990) we derive the elements of S, D, A, and B in the context of the beta-binomial model. See the Appendix.

Note that under the null hypothesis the parameters π and θ are common across groups. Therefore, the estimation of π and θ from the T groups can be considered to be estimation from a single group consisting of the combined data in the T groups. The mle's and the mme's of π and θ have been shown to be consistent (Moore 1986). Denote the mle's of $\lambda = (\pi, \theta)$ by $\hat{\lambda}_m$ and the mme's by $\hat{\lambda}_{mm}$. If we use $\hat{\lambda}_{mm}$ in S, D, A, and B the $C(\alpha)$ statistic based on method of moments estimators is $C_{mm} = S'(D - AB^{-1}B')^{-1}S$. If $\hat{\lambda}_m$ is used in S, D, A, and B, then $S(\hat{\lambda}) = \psi(\hat{\lambda}_m) = (\psi_1(\hat{\lambda}_m), \ldots, \psi_{T-1}(\hat{\lambda}_m))^{\mathrm{T}}$ and the $C(\alpha)$ or the score statistic is $C_m = \psi'(D - AB^{-1}A')^{-1}\psi$.

6.3 Simulations

In this section we report on a small simulation study conducted to compare the performance, in terms of size and power, of the likelihood ratio statistic LR and the $C(\alpha)$ statistics C_m and C_{mm}. Maximum likelihood estimates of the parameters under the null and the alternative hypotheses were obtained by minimizing the negative of a relevant log-likelihood using the IMSL (IMSL 1987) subroutine BCONF. BCONF is a IMSL subroutine which minimizes a function of N variables subject to bounds on the variables using a quasi-Newton method and a finite difference gradient. Moment estimators of π and θ, under the null hypothesis, were obtained (following Kleinman 1973) as follows.

Define

$$\hat{p}_{00} = \sum_{i=1}^{T} \sum_{j=1}^{m_i} w_{ij}\hat{p}_{ij}/w_{00}$$

and

$$s = \sum_{i=1}^{T} \sum_{j=1}^{m_i} w_{ij}\left(\hat{p}_{ij} - \hat{p}_{00}\right)^2,$$

where $\hat{p}_{ij} = x_{ij}/n_{ij}$, $w_{ij} = n_{ij}/\{1 - \gamma(n_{ij} - 1)\}$, $w_{00} = \Sigma_i^T \Sigma_j^{m_i} w_{ij}$, and $\gamma = \theta/(1 + \theta)$. Then the estimates of π and γ are obtained iteratively from

$$\hat{\pi} = \hat{p}_{00},$$

$$\hat{\gamma} = \frac{s - \hat{\pi}(1-\hat{\pi})\Sigma_i^T \Sigma_j^{m_i} \dfrac{w_{ij}}{n_{ij}}\left(1 - \dfrac{w_{ij}}{w_{00}}\right)}{\hat{\pi}(1-\hat{\pi})\left[\Sigma_{i=1}^T \Sigma_{j=1}^{m_i} w_{ij}\left(1 - \dfrac{w_{ij}}{w_{00}}\right) - \Sigma_i^T \Sigma_j^{m_i} \dfrac{w_{ij}}{n_{ij}}\left(1 - \dfrac{w_{ij}}{w_{00}}\right)\right]}.$$

Once $\hat{\pi}$ and $\hat{\gamma}$ are obtained, $\hat{\theta}$ is obtained by $\hat{\theta} = \hat{\gamma}/(1 - \hat{\gamma})$. Note that all the estimates were obtained within the parameter space given in eqn. (6.1).

In this study we consider $T = 2$ groups. The litter sizes and numbers of litters were chosen as those of the control group ($m_1 = 27$) and low-dose treatment groups ($m_2 = 19$) of Paul (1982). Thus, for group 1 the litter sizes are $12, 7, 6, 6, 7, 8, 10, 7, 8, 6, 11, 7, 8, 9, 2, 7, 9, 7, 11, 10, 4, 8, 10, 12, 8, 7, 8$ and those for group 2 are $5, 11, 7, 9, 12, 8, 6, 7, 6, 4, 6, 9, 6, 7, 5, 9, 1, 6, 9$. Beta-binomial observations were generated by first generating a beta (π, θ) random variate p using the IMSL subroutine RNBET and then a binomial random variable with expectation $n_{ij}p$ ($i = 1, 2$, $j = 1, \ldots, m_i$) using IMSL subroutine RNBIN. Empirical levels were calculated based on 1000 replications for each combination of $\pi = 0.06, 0.08, 0.10, 0.12, 0.20, 0.30$ and $\theta = 0.02, 0.06, 0.10, 0.20$. The results are given in Table 6.1. For small θ ($\theta = 0.02$) the $C(\alpha)$ statistic C_{mm} shows some conservative behaviour; otherwise all the statistics produce empirical levels close to the nominal. For power comparison, we considered $\theta = 0.02, 0.06, 0.09, 0.12, 0.16$. For each value of θ empirical powers were calculated for (π_1, π_2): $(0.08, 0.10), (0.08, 0.15), (0.08, 0.20), (0.08, 0.30)$. The power results are given in Table 6.2. Again, except for very small θ the powers of the statistics do not show marked disagreement (see Table 6.2). For small θ ($\theta = 0.02$), the power of the statistic C_{mm} is to some extent smaller than that of the other two statistics LR and C_m. This is because the level of the C_{mm} for this value of θ is smaller than that of the other two. Either of the $C(\alpha)$ statistics are preferable, as they require estimates of the parameters only under the null hypothesis. The moment estimates are easier to obtain than the mle's, although for obtaining mle's under H_0 easily implementable subroutines are available, such as IMSL subroutine, BCONF or NEQNF or the subroutine by Smith (1983).

Table 6.1. $10^2 \times$ empirical levels: $\alpha = 0.05$, based on 1000 replications. $T = 2$ groups. $m_1 = 27$, $m_2 = 19$

θ	Test statistics	π 0.06	0.08	0.10	0.12	0.20	0.30
0.02	LR	4.3	5.4	5.7	5.2	4.4	4.9
	C_m	3.7	5.2	5.6	4.6	4.2	4.2
	C_{mm}	2.7	3.5	3.8	3.0	3.4	3.4
0.06	LR	6.0	7.0	6.2	4.9	6.0	6.7
	C_m	5.5	6.7	5.9	4.6	5.5	6.4
	C_{mm}	5.1	6.1	5.2	4.2	5.2	6.0
0.10	LR	5.4	5.6	5.8	5.8	5.2	6.2
	C_m	4.8	5.2	5.4	5.3	5.0	5.7
	C_{mm}	5.1	4.7	5.3	4.9	4.9	5.3
0.20	LR	4.8	6.3	8.0	5.8	6.4	6.3
	C_m	4.8	6.3	7.5	5.4	5.9	5.7
	C_{mm}	4.8	6.1	7.5	5.2	5.4	5.7

Pack (1986) indicated that it would be of interest to examine what effect allowing θ to be negative has on the properties of the hypothesis tests. We investigated this and found the effect to be negligible. The number of samples producing negative estimates of θ is small compared to the number of samples

Table 6.2. $10^2 \times$ empirical power: $\alpha = 0.05$, based on 1000 replications. $T = 2$ groups. $m_1 = 27$, $m_2 = 19$

θ	Test statistics	(π_1, π_2) (0.08, 0.10)	(0.08, 0.15)	(0.08, 0.20)	(0.08, 0.30)
0.02	LR	8.7	46.9	82.9	99.7
	C_m	8.8	47.0	83.6	99.7
	C_{mm}	7.0	40.7	78.3	99.4
0.06	LR	8.9	41.1	78.3	99.6
	C_m	9.0	40.1	78.3	99.5
	C_{mm}	7.0	38.8	76.2	99.4
0.09	LR	9.1	38.0	74.3	99.6
	C_m	10.1	37.9	74.1	99.0
	C_{mm}	9.9	37.3	73.0	98.9
0.12	LR	9.2	36.8	71.8	98.3
	C_m	8.4	36.5	70.7	98.2
	C_{mm}	8.4	36.7	71.2	98.1
0.16	LR	9.0	37.0	69.3	97.4
	C_m	8.4	36.1	68.9	97.1
	C_{mm}	9.0	36.7	69.5	97.1

used in the simulation study. This number becomes even smaller when we take a larger θ.

An alternative to the analysis of proportions based on the extended beta-binomial model is to consider semi-parametric models specified only by the first two moments, such as the quasi-likelihood (see Williams 1982). A detailed study of $C(\alpha)$ or score tests based on semi-parametric models such as that based on the quasi-likelihood and data simulated from other overdispersed binomial models will be reported in a further submission.

Acknowledgements

Dr Paul's research was partially supported by the Natural Sciences and Engineering Research Council of Canada (NSERC). Mr Islam's research was partially supported by Dr Paul's NSERC grant and a CIDA scholarship.

References

Altham, P. M. E. (1978). Two generalizations of the binomial distribution. *Applied Statistics*, **27**, 162–7.

Barnwal, R. K. and Paul, S. R. (1988). Analysis of one-way layout of count data with negative binomial variation. *Biometrika*, **75**, 215–22.

Dean, C. and Lawless, J. F. (1989). Tests for detecting overdispersion in Poisson regression models. *Journal of the American Statistical Association*, **84**, 467–72.

Haseman, J. K. and Kupper, L. L. (1979). Analysis of dichotomous response data from certain toxicological experiments. *Biometrics*, **35**, 281–93.

IMSL (International Mathematical and Statistical Libraries, Inc.) (1987). *IMSL manual.* IMSL, 2500 City West Boulevard, Houston, Texas 77042–3020, USA.

Kleinman, J. C. (1973). Proportions with extraneous variance: single and independent samples. *Journal of the American Statistical Association*, **8**, 46–54.

Moore, D. F. (1986). Asymptotic properties of moment estimators for over-dispersed counts and proportions. *Biometrika*, **73**, 583–8.

Neyman, J. (1959). Optimal asymptotic tests for composite hypotheses. In *Probability and statistics: The Harald Cramér Volume* (ed. U. Grenander), pp. 213–34. Uppsala: Almgrist and Wiksell.

Pack, S. E. (1986). Hypothesis testing for proportions with overdispersion. *Biometrics*, **42**, 967–72.

Paul, S. R. (1982). Analysis of proportions of affected foetuses in teratological experiments. *Biometrics*, **38**, 361–70.

Paul, S. R. (1989). Testing for the equality of several correlation coefficients. *Canadian Journal of Statistics*, **17**, 217–27.

Paul, S. R., Liang, K. Y., and Self, S. A. (1989). On testing departure from the binomial and multinomial assumptions. *Biometrics*, **45**, 231–236.

Prentice, R. L. (1986). Binary regression using an extended beta-binomial distribution, with discussion of correlation induced by covariate measurement errors. *Journal of the American Statistical Association*, **81**, 321–7.

Rao, C. R. (1947). Large sample tests of statistical hypothesis concerning several parameters with applications to problems of estimation. *Proceedings of the Cambridge Philosophical Society*, **44**, 50–7.

Smith, D. M. (1983). Maximum likelihood estimation of the parameters of the beta binomial distribution. Algorithm AMS/89. *Applied Statistics*, **32**, 196–204.

Srivastava, M. S. and Wu, Y. (1990). On beta-binomial model for extrabinomial variation. Technical report No. 16. Department of Statistics, University of Toronto.
Tarone, R. E. (1985). On heterogeneity tests based on efficient scores, *Biometrika*, **72**, 91–5.
Williams, D. A. (1975). The analysis of binary responses from toxicological experiments involving reproduction and teratogeneity. *Biometrics*, **31**, 949–52.
Williams, D. A. (1982). The extra-binomial variation in logistic linear models. *Applied Statistics*, **31**, 144–8.

Appendix: Derivations of the elements of S, D, A, and B for the $C(\alpha)$ test

Using the log-likelihood given in eqn. (6.2) we obtain for $i, t = 1, \ldots, T-1$,

$$\psi_i = \left[\frac{\partial l}{\partial \phi_i}\right]_{\phi=0} = \sum_{j=1}^{m_i}\left\{\sum_{r=0}^{x_{ij}-1}\frac{1}{(\pi+r\theta)} - \sum_{r=0}^{n_{ij}-x_{ij}-1}\frac{1}{(1-\pi+r\theta)}\right\},$$

$$\gamma_1 = \left[\frac{\partial l}{\partial \lambda_1}\right]_{\phi=0} = \sum_{i=1}^{T}\sum_{j=1}^{m_i}\left\{\sum_{r=0}^{x_{ij}-1}\frac{1}{(\pi+r\theta)} - \sum_{r=0}^{n_{ij}-x_{ij}-1}\frac{1}{(1-\pi+r\theta)}\right\},$$

$$\gamma_2 = \left[\frac{\partial l}{\partial \lambda_2}\right]_{\phi=0}$$

$$= \sum_{i=1}^{T}\sum_{j=1}^{m_i}\left\{\sum_{r=0}^{x_{ij}-1}\frac{r}{(\pi+r\theta)} + \sum_{r=0}^{n_{ij}-x_{ij}-1}\frac{r}{(1-\pi+r\theta)} - \sum_{r=0}^{n_{ij}-1}\frac{r}{(1+r\theta)}\right\},$$

$$\left(\frac{-\partial^2 l}{\partial \phi_i^2}\bigg|_{\phi=0}\right) = \sum_{j=1}^{m_i}\left\{\sum_{r=0}^{x_{ij}-1}\frac{1}{(\pi+r\theta)^2} + \sum_{r=0}^{n_{ij}-x_{ij}-1}\frac{1}{(1-\pi+r\theta)^2}\right\},$$

$$\left(\frac{-\partial^2 l}{\partial \phi_i \partial \phi_t}\bigg|_{\phi=0}\right) = 0, \qquad \text{for} \quad t \neq t,$$

$$\left(\frac{-\partial^2 l}{\partial \phi_i \partial \lambda_1}\bigg|_{\phi=0}\right) = \left(\frac{-\partial^2 l}{\partial \phi_i^2}\bigg|_{\phi=0}\right),$$

$$\left(\frac{-\partial^2 l}{\partial \phi_i \partial \lambda_2}\bigg|_{\phi=0}\right) = \sum_{j=1}^{m_i}\left\{\sum_{r=0}^{x_{ij}-1}\frac{r}{(\pi+r\theta)^2} - \sum_{r=0}^{n_{ij}-x_{ij}-1}\frac{r}{(1-\pi+r\theta)^2}\right\},$$

$$\left(\frac{-\partial^2 l}{\partial \lambda_1^2}\bigg|_{\phi=0}\right) = \sum_{i=1}^{T}\sum_{j=1}^{m_i}\left\{\sum_{x=0}^{x_{ij}-1}\frac{1}{(\pi+r\theta)^2} + \sum_{r=0}^{m_{ij}-n_{ij}-1}\frac{1}{(1-\pi+r\theta)^2}\right\},$$

$$\left(\frac{-\partial^2 l}{\partial \lambda_1 \partial \lambda_2}\bigg|_{\phi=0}\right) = \sum_{i=1}^{T}\sum_{j=1}^{m_i}\left\{\sum_{r=0}^{x_{ij}-1}\frac{r}{(\pi+r\theta)^2} - \sum_{r=0}^{n_{ij}-m_{ij}-1}\frac{1}{(1-\pi+r\theta)^2}\right\},$$

and

$$\left(\frac{-\partial^2 l}{\partial \lambda_2^2} \bigg|_{\phi=0} \right)$$

$$= \sum_{i=1}^{T} \sum_{j=1}^{m_i} \left\{ \sum_{r=0}^{x_{ij}-1} \frac{r^2}{(\pi + r\theta)^2} + \sum_{r=0}^{n_{ij}-x_{ij}-1} \frac{r^2}{(1-\pi+r\theta)^2} - \sum_{r=0}^{n_{ij}-1} \frac{r^2}{(1+r\theta)^2} \right\}.$$

Expectations of minus the second derivatives are given below, for $i, t = 1, \ldots, T-1$:

$$D_{ii} = \mathrm{E}\left(\frac{-\partial^2 l}{\partial \phi_i^2} \bigg|_{\phi=0} \right) = \sum_{j=1}^{m_i} \left\{ \sum_{r=0}^{n_{ij}-1} \frac{P(X_{ij} > r)}{(\pi + r\theta)^2} + \sum_{r=0}^{n_{ij}-1} \frac{P(X_{ij} < n_{ij} - r)}{(1-\pi+r\theta)^2} \right\},$$

$$D_{i1} = \mathrm{E}\left(\frac{-\partial^2 l}{\partial \phi_i \partial \phi_t} \bigg|_{\phi=0} \right) = 0, \qquad i \neq t,$$

$$A_{i1} = \mathrm{E}\left(\frac{-\partial^2 l}{\partial \phi_i \partial \lambda_1} \bigg|_{\phi=0} \right) = D_{ii},$$

$$A_{i2} = \mathrm{E}\left(\frac{-\partial^2 l}{\partial \phi_i \partial \lambda_2} \bigg|_{\phi=0} \right)$$

$$= \sum_{j=1}^{m_i} \frac{1}{\theta} \left\{ \pi \sum_{r=0}^{n_{ij}-1} \frac{P(X_{ij} > r)}{(\pi + r\theta)^2} - (1-\pi) \sum_{r=0}^{n_{ij}-1} \frac{P(X_{ij} < n_{ij} - r)}{(1-\pi+r\theta)^2} \right\},$$

$$B_{11} = \mathrm{E}\left(\frac{-\partial^2 l}{\partial \lambda_1^2} \bigg|_{\phi=0} \right)$$

$$= \sum_{i=1}^{T} \sum_{j=1}^{m_i} \left\{ \sum_{r=0}^{n_{ij}-1} \frac{P(X_{ij} > r)}{(\pi + r\theta)^2} + \sum_{r=0}^{n_{ij}-1} \frac{P(X_{ij} < n_{ij} - r)}{(1-\pi+r\theta)^2} \right\},$$

$$B_{12} = \mathrm{E}\left(\frac{-\partial^2 l}{\partial \lambda_1 \partial \lambda_2} \bigg|_{\phi=0} \right)$$

$$= \sum_{i=1}^{T} \sum_{j=1}^{m_i} \frac{1}{\theta} \left\{ -\pi \sum_{r=1}^{n_{ij}-1} \frac{P(X_{ij} > r)}{(\pi + r\theta)^2} + (1-\pi) \sum_{r=1}^{n_{ij}-1} \frac{P(X_{ij} < n_{ij} - r)}{(1-n+r\theta)^2} \right\},$$

and

$$B_{22} = \mathrm{E}\left(\frac{-\partial^2 l}{\partial \lambda_2^2} \bigg|_{\phi=0} \right) = \sum_{i=1}^{T} \sum_{j=1}^{m_i} \frac{1}{\theta^2}$$

$$\times \left\{ \sum_{r=0}^{n_{ij}-1} \pi^2 \frac{P(X_{ij} > r)}{(\pi + r\theta)^2} + \sum_{r=0}^{n_{ij}-1} (1-\pi)^2 \frac{P(X_{ij} < n_{ij} - r)}{(1-\pi+r\theta)^2} - \sum_{r=0}^{n_{ij}-1} \frac{1}{(1+r\theta)^2} \right\},$$

where, for example,

$$P(x > k) = \sum_{x=k}^{n} \binom{n}{x} \frac{\prod_{r=0}^{x-1}(\pi + r\theta)\prod_{r=0}^{n-x-1}(1 - \pi + \theta)}{\prod_{r=0}^{n-1}(1 + r\theta)}.$$

The expressions for the expectations of the quantities such as

$$\left(\frac{-\partial^2 l}{\partial \lambda_2^2}\bigg|_{\phi=0}\right)$$

are most easily obtained by rewriting l in terms of π and $c = \theta^{-1}$, calculating $\partial^2 l/\partial c^2$, and then noting that $\mathrm{E}(-\partial^2 l/\partial \theta^2) = \theta^{-4}\ \mathrm{E}(-\partial^2 l/\partial c^2)$.

7 Overdispersion in logistic-linear models

DAVID A. WILLIAMS

7.1 Introduction

The logistic-linear model is well established as the basis for analysing regression data, or data from a designed experiment, when the response variable is a proportion. Suppose that the data consist of a set of n cases. In the ith case r_i successes, $m_i - r_i$ failures, and a vector x_i of p explanatory variables are recorded. The logistic-linear model assumes that the r_i are realizations of random variables R_i distributed independently Binomial(m_i, θ_i), where θ_i is related to a linear predictor $\eta_i = \mathbf{x}_i^{\mathrm{T}}\beta$ through the logistic link logit$(\theta_i) = \log\{\theta_i/(1-\theta_i)\} = \eta_i$. An alternative link is the probit, given by probit$(\theta_i) = \Phi^{-1}(\theta_i) = \eta_i$, where Φ^{-1} denotes the inverse Normal distribution function.

Even when all available explanatory variables have been fitted, the residual variation may be too great to be attributable to pure binomial sampling variation. There are several possible explanations:

1. Some important explanatory variables may not have been recorded.
2. Some explanatory variables may have been measured subject to error.
3. There may be a source of extra-binomial random variation between cases.

This problem was first recognized at least 40 years ago (Cochran 1943; Finney 1947, Section 18). In Table 7.1 are given data from Table 9 of Finney (1947). The mortality of grain beetles is regressed on the log dose of ethylene oxide. After

Table 7.1. Response of grain beetles to ethylene oxide

log dose, x	Number of beetles m	Mortality, r	Expected mortality
0.033	24	0	1.2
0.167	31	10	8.1
0.199	30	17	10.8
0.225	31	12	14.0
0.260	27	7	15.6
0.314	26	23	19.5
0.322	30	22	23.1
0.362	31	29	26.6
0.391	30	30	27.0
0.394	30	23	27.1

Table 7.2. Numbers of deaths per litter from a mouse teratology experiment

Litter size, s	Dose in g/kg of body weight 0.0	0.75	1.5	3.0
3			3	
5			4	
7		0	4	
8			0	
9	12	2	22	225
10		0	0	16
11	0115	012		2
12	001	011	01123	00112225
13	0013	01125	0012	111
14	02	0124	123	24
15	012225	00015	022	33
16	022		2	29
17	3			
19		5		

fitting the logistic-linear regression on log dose the deviance is 36.2 with 8 df, the Pearson X^2 statistic is 33.2. There is significant heterogeneity, but comparison of observed and fitted mortalities reveals no systematic departure from the logistic-linear model.

Extra-binomial variation arises particularly often in studies using laboratory animals when the experimental units, i.e. the cases, are complete litters. A general review is provided by Haseman and Kupper (1979). Data from a teratology study comparing three dose levels of a test compound with a zero dose control are presented in Table 7.2. If the model DOSE × LITTER SIZE is fitted the deviance is 116.6 with 59 df, giving clear evidence of extra-binomial variation between replicate litters.

In such situations the standard GLIM analysis produces estimated standard errors which are too small. Any inferences based on the comparison of parameter estimates with their estimated standard errors, or on the comparison of deviance differences with χ^2 distributions, will be invalid. We need to base our analysis on a model which incorporates extra-binomial variation. In Section 7.2 I shall describe some models for extra-binomial variation. Some of these models make sufficient assumptions to permit the use of maximum likelihood estimation and likelihood ratio tests, but, as we shall see in Section 7.3, these likelihood methods can suffer a lack of robustness. Other models specify only the first two moments of the distribution, and can be analysed using quasi-likelihood methods. These are discussed in Section 7.4.

7.2 Models

For simplicity, I shall consider models incorporating only one component of extra-binomial variation, although some of the models considered readily extend to incorporate the several components needed to model hierarchically classified data. Moreover, the models considered here will all be binomial mixture models. Other approaches to modelling a set of m correlated binary responses include the use of models for 2^m symmetric contingency tables (Altham 1978), and dichotomizing the components of a symmetric m-dimensional multivariate Normal distribution (Ochi and Prentice 1984).

Binomial mixture models are derived by introducing latent variables P_i, with range $[0, 1]$, expectations $\mathrm{E}(P_i) = \theta_i$ and variances $\mathrm{Var}(P_i) = \phi_i \theta_i (1 - \theta_i)$. We then assume that the conditional distribution of R_i, given $P_i = p_i$, is Binomial(m_i, p_i). The consequent marginal distribution of R_i then satisfies

$$\mathrm{E}(R_i) = m_i \theta_i, \qquad \mathrm{Var}(R_i) = m_i \theta_i (1 - \theta_i)\{1 + \phi_i (m_i - 1)\}. \tag{7.1}$$

Here the new parameter ϕ_i measures the correlation between the binary responses of the ith case, so $0 \leqslant \phi_i \leqslant 1$ and $\phi_i = 0$ corresponds to pure Binomial variation. Equations (7.1) provide a general framework for discussing mixture models. Specific models are generated by considering the following questions:

1. How do we relate θ_i to $\mathbf{x}_i$?
2. How do we relate ϕ_i to θ_i or to $\mathbf{x}_i$?
3. What additional distributional assumptions, if any, do we make about the latent variables P_i?

The way we choose to answer questions 1 and 2 can depend on our answer to question 3. I shall consider four possible answers to question 3.

Answer 1: make no additional assumptions. Thus only the first two moments of R_i are specified. If is natural then to relate θ_i to the linear predictor $\eta_i = \mathbf{x}_i^{\mathrm{T}} \beta$ using the logistic link, although in certain situations other links such as the probit or the log–log might be preferred. The simplest assumption that we can make about ϕ_i is that it is a constant, but sometimes the data suggest that the value of ϕ_i should be linked to the value of θ_i. Williams (1982) considered three models, namely $\phi_i = 0$, $\phi_1 = \phi$, and $\phi_i = \phi\theta_i(1 - \theta_i)$, and all three are embraced by the two-parameter model

$$\phi_i = \phi\{\theta_i(1 - \theta_i)\}^{\delta}, \tag{7.2}$$

suggested by Moore (1987). In certain situations we might wish to relate ϕ_i to certain explanatory variables (Prentice 1986).

Answer 2: assume that P_i has a Beta distribution. The marginal distribution of R_i is then Beta-binomial with probabilities

$$\Pr(R = r)$$
$$= \binom{m}{r} \prod_{x=0}^{r-1} \{\theta(1 - \phi) + x\phi\} \prod_{x=0}^{m-r+1} \{(1 - \theta)(1 - \phi) + x\phi\} \Big/ \prod_{x=0}^{m-1} \{1 - \phi + x\phi\}.$$

Several references to the use of the Beta-binomial distribution in data analysis are given by Williams (1975). Crowder (1978) was the first to consider the application of the BB distribution to data more complex than a one-way classification. The parameters θ_i and ϕ_i can be related to $\mathbf{x}_i$ or to each other, as suggested in the previous paragraph.

Answer 3: assume that P_i has a Probit-normal distribution, i.e. the Probit transform of P_i is distributed Normal(μ_i, σ_i^2). Numerical integration is needed to determine the marginal Probit-normal-binomial (PNB) distribution of R_i. The PNB distribution is identical to the Correlated-probit distribution, obtained by Ochi and Prentice (1984) by assuming that the m_i binary responses are generated by dichotomizing, at the origin, the m_i components of a multivariate Normal($\mu_i\mathbf{1}, \mathbf{I} + \sigma_i^2\mathbf{1}\mathbf{1}^{\mathrm{T}}$) distribution. The natural assumptions about μ_i and σ_i^2 are those of the Normal linear regression model, namely

$$\mu_i = \mathbf{x}_i^{\mathrm{T}}\beta, \qquad \sigma_i^2 = \sigma^2.$$

It is of interest to know what these assumptions about the distribution of probit(P_i) imply for the moments of P_i itself. The value of θ_i is given exactly by

$$\text{probit}(\theta_i) = \mu_i/\sqrt{(1+\sigma^2)},$$

so θ_i is related to $\mathbf{x}_i$ by an exact probit-linear link. The parameter ϕ_i can be expressed as a function of μ_i and σ^2 using the tetrachoric series, and Gilmour *et al.* (1985) investigated the accuracy of the approximation which uses just the first term of this series. My own numerical investigations have shown that, provided that σ^2 is held constant, the relationship between ϕ_i and θ_i is well approximated by eqn. (7.2) with $0 \leqslant \delta \leqslant 1$.

Answer 4: Assume that P_i has a Logistic-normal distribution, i.e. the logistic transform of P_i is distributed Normal(μ_i, σ_i^2). Numerical integration is needed to determine the Logistic-normal-binomial (LNB) distribution of R_i. The LNB distribution was proposed by Pierce and Sands (1975) and was more recently used by Anderson and Aitken (1985) to model the interviewer variability in the analysis of survey questionaires. The Logistic-normal distribution has much earlier origins (Johnson 1965), and it is the univariate form of the distribution proposed by Aitchison (1986) for compositional data. Again it is natural to make the Normal linear model assumptions $\mu_i = \mathbf{x}_i^{\mathrm{T}}\beta$ and $\sigma_i^2 = \sigma^2$. A simple exact formula for θ_i is not obtainable, but a good approximation is provided by

$$\text{logit}(\theta_i) = \mu_i/\sqrt{(1+0.35\sigma^2)},$$

implying an approximate logistic-linear model. Again, the relationship between θ_i and ϕ_i is well approximated by eqn. (7.2).

If likelihood methods are to be used it is relevant to ask whether there are noticeable differences between the shapes of the BB, LNB, and PNB distributions when they share the same values of θ_i and ϕ_i. The BB and LNB distributions for the case $\theta_i = 0.1$, $\phi_i = 0.2$ are compared in Table 7.3. The PNB distribution is not included because it lies between the BB and LNB distributions. The shapes are broadly similar, and for $m_i = 5$ the differences are

Table 7.3. Comparison of the Beta-binomial and Logistic-normal-binomial distributions for $\theta_i = 0.1$, $\phi_i = 0.2$

	$m_i = 5$		$m_i = 10$		$m_i = 15$		$m_i = 20$	
	BB	LNB	BB	LNB	BB	LNB	BB	LNB
$r = 0$	0.692	0.686	0.573	[illegible]	[illegible]	[illegible]	0.458	0.406
$r = 1$	0.182	0.196	[illegible]	[illegible]	[illegible]	[illegible]	0.162	0.212
$r = 2$	0.077	0.071	[illegible]	[illegible]	[illegible]	[illegible]	[illegible]	0.120
$r = 3$	0.033	0.130	[illegible]	[illegible]	[illegible]	[illegible]	[illegible]	0.070
$r = 4$	0.012	0.013	[illegible]	[illegible]	[illegible]	[illegible]	[illegible]	0.045
$r = 5$	0.003	0.004	[illegible]	[illegible]	[illegible]	[illegible]	[illegible]	0.035
$6 \leqslant r \leqslant 10$			0.026	[illegible]	[illegible]	[illegible]	[illegible]	0.083
$11 \leqslant r \leqslant 15$					[illegible]	[illegible]	[illegible]	0.083
$16 \leqslant r \leqslant 20$							[illegible]	0.029

negligible. As m_i increases, however, so the finer differences between the Beta and Logistic-normal distribution are revealed, and for $m_i = 20$ the individual probabilities can differ by as much as 0.05. The LNB distribution here has the larger skewness and kurtosis.

7.3 Maximum likelihood estimation

If the BB distribution is assumed, the likelihood and its derivatives can be expressed in closed form, and inferences can be based on maximum likelihood (ML) estimates and asymptotic likelihood ratio (LR) tests. Several papers have investigated the performance of LR tests when used to compare two BB samples using m_i values typical of litter sizes in toxicology: see Pack (1986) for a survey and references. Two main conclusions can be drawn:

1. The LR tests have satisfactory type 1 error rates when the data are generated from a BB distribution and sample sizes are large (e.g. 40), but not when sample sizes are small (e.g. 12).

2. The type 1 error rates can deviate from the nominal error rates when the samples are drawn from real data sets, rather than from simulated BB distributions.

These conclusions are supported by results extracted from my own simulations and shown in Table 7.4. Here, 2000 samples of size 40 have been drawn from four distributions, each with $\theta = 0.1$ and $\phi = 0.2$; namely, the BB distribution, the LNB distribution, the two-point mixture with $\Pr(P_i = 0) = 0.643$, $\Pr(P_i = 0.28) = 0.357$, and the three-point mixture with $\Pr(P_i = 0) = 0.18$, $\Pr(P_i = 0.1) = 0.80$, $\Pr(P_i = 1) = 0.02$. Assuming a BB distribution, the ML estimates of θ and ϕ were calculated and the hypothesis $\theta = 0.1$ was tested using LR tests with nominal size 0.05.

Table 7.4. Performance of ML estimators assuming a BB distribution

Simulated distribution	Average $\hat{\theta}$	Average $\hat{\phi}$	Size of LR test
BB	0.099	0.193	0.055
LNB	0.099	0.175	0.068
Two point mix	0.092	0.281	0.019
Three point mix	0.108	0.125	0.190

We see that the estimates of both θ and ϕ can become noticeably biased when the incorrect likelihood is maximized. Even when the differences between the true and assumed distributions are as small as those between the BB and LNB distributions in Table 7.3, the estimate of ϕ can become sufficiently biased so as seriously to affect the type 1 error of the LR test.

A more subtle robustness problem is identified by Kupper *et al.* (1986) and Williams (1988). Even if the data are generated by a BB distribution, the ML estimators become biased if incorrect assumptions are made about ϕ. Thus, if we use ML to estimate β in the model $\text{logit}(\theta_i) = \mathbf{x}_i^{\mathrm{T}}\beta$, assuming that ϕ_i is constant, then the estimate of β becomes biased if in reality ϕ_i varies with θ_i. This contrasts with Normal linear models in which ML estimation of regression parameters remains unbiased when the variance is incorrectly modelled.

So far in this section we have considered ML estimation only for the BB distribution. ML estimation for the PNB and LNB distribution models is more difficult, because numerical integration is needed to evaluate the likelihood and its derivatives. Ochi and Prentice describe ML estimation for the PNB distribution using approximations for the symmetric multivariate Normal distribution function. Anderson and Aitken describe ML estimation for the LNB distribution using Gaussian quadrature. My own simulations, applying their method to samples generated by either a LNB or a BB distribution, suggest that the use of too few quadrature points leads to biased estimation. There is no reason to think that exact ML estimation of the PNB and LNB distributions will not suffer the same lack of robustness as exact ML estimation of the BB distribution. By increasing the number of quadrature points we expect to improve the estimates, but only if the distribution assumptions are correct. There is no point in increasing the number of quadrature points if this serves only to calculate an inappropriate likelihood more precisely.

7.4 Maximum quasi-likelihood estimation

Maximum quasi-likelihood (MQL) estimation has two advantages over ML estimation. Firstly, it is computationally simpler and can be more easily implemented using standard computing packages. Secondly, because it assumes only the structure of the first two moments of the response variable, i.e. only θ_i and ϕ_i, it avoids the robustness problems identified in Section 7.3.

Consider the model

$$\text{logit}(\theta_i) = \mathbf{x}_i^{\mathrm{T}}\beta, \qquad \phi_i = \phi. \tag{7.3}$$

The MQL estimate of β, for given values of ϕ_i, is obtained simply by using GLIM with Binomial error, logistic link, and prior weights

$$w_i = \{1 + \phi_i(m_i - 1)\}^{-1}.$$

Williams (1972) proposed an iterative procedure whereby β is estimated by MQL for given ϕ, and ϕ is then re-estimated by equating the Pearson generalized chi-squared statistic

$$X^2 = \Sigma w_i v_i^{-1}\left(r_i - m_i\hat{\theta}_i\right)^2, \qquad \text{where } v_i = m_i\hat{\theta}_i\left(1 - \hat{\theta}_i\right),$$

to its approximate expectation. The final value of X^2 is $n - p$, the residual degrees of freedom. The theoretical properties of this method were explored by Moore (1986). This method may be viewed as an extension of the weighted least squares method proposed by Cochran (1943) and developed by Kleinman (1973). There is some loss of efficiency relative to ML estimation when the distribution of the responses is known, but this loss is mainly confined to the estimation of ϕ, unless ϕ is large.

The method of estimation outlined above provides point estimates $\hat{\beta}$ and $\hat{\phi}$ and an estimate $(\mathbf{X}^{\mathrm{T}}\mathbf{WVX})^{-1}$ of the variance matrix of $\hat{\beta}$. Here $\mathbf{W}$ and $\mathbf{V}$ are diagonal matrices with elements w_i and v_i, respectively, and $\mathbf{X}$ is the matrix of explanatory variables. Using the asymptotic Normality of $\hat{\beta}$, confidence intervals for single components of β, or single linear combinations of β, are formed in the usual way using the point estimate, its estimated standard error, and the appropriate Normal deviate. More general linear hypotheses about β can be tested by comparing Wald statistics with χ^2 distributions. The results of McCullagh (1983) suggest that hypotheses can alternatively be tested by comparing with a χ^2 distribution the increase in deviance when β is re-estimated by MQL, subject to the constraints imposed by the hypothesis and using the original estimate of ϕ. When there is no extra-binomial variation and we use GLIM to fit a logistic-linear model there are reasons for basing inferences on deviance differences rather than Wald statistics. The same may not be true when we allow for extra-binomial variation. I have compared the performance of the Wald test and the deviance test in simulations involving (a) testing the value of logit(θ) in a single sample and (b) comparing the values of logit(θ) between four samples. My results suggest that the deviance test is more liberal than the Wald test, the type 1 error of the Wald test being closer to the nominal significance level.

Nelder and Pregibon (1987) proposed an extended quasi-likelihood function which permits a more integrated analysis, allowing us to make inferences about both β and ϕ in model (7.3) and allowing us to entertain more complex models in which ϕ_i is a function of $\mathbf{x}_i$ and/or θ_i involving unknown parameters. The ith component of the extended log quasi-likelihood is

$$-\tfrac{1}{2}\log[2\pi\{1 + \phi_i(m_i - 1)\}r_i(1 - r_i/m_i)] - \tfrac{1}{2}d_i/\{1 + \phi_i(m_i - 1)\},$$

where d_i is the binomial deviance. For the simplest case, in which model (7.3) is assumed and the m_i are all equal, ϕ is estimated by equating $1 + \phi(m - 1)$ to $D/(n - p)$, where D denotes the deviance from fitting the Binomial model. This contrasts with the estimate obtained by equating $1 + \phi(m - 1)$ to $X^2/(n - p)$ suggested by Williams (1982). Clearly, the mean deviance estimate is inconsistent (as n increases for fixed m), and this inconsistency must extend to estimating the variance parameters of more general models. Analysis based on the extended quasi-likelihood cannot therefore be recommended unless the m_i are large, for the estimates of the variance parameters can be seriously biased, leading to invalid inferences about β.

Suppose, then, that we wish to fit the model

$$\text{logit}(\theta_i) = \mathbf{x}_i^{\mathrm{T}}\beta, \qquad \phi_i = \phi g(\theta_i, \mathbf{x}_i, \delta), \tag{7.4}$$

where g is a known function and δ is a set of unknown parameters. Suppose that we wish to make no additional assumptions, and the m_i values are too small to rely on the extended quasi-likelihood method of Nelder and Pregibon (1987). It seems that the only approach open to us is to iterate between estimation of β for given ϕ and δ by MQL, and estimation of ϕ and δ for given β by regressing squared residuals on their expectations. The following iterative scheme could be used, where $\tilde{\beta}$, $\tilde{\phi}$, and $\tilde{\delta}$ denote the current estimates and $\tilde{\theta}_i$ and $\tilde{\phi}_i$ are given by $\text{logit}(\tilde{\theta}_i) = \mathbf{x}_i^{\mathrm{T}}\tilde{\beta}$, $\tilde{\phi}_i = \tilde{\phi} g(\tilde{\theta}_i, \mathbf{x}_i, \tilde{\delta})$.

1. Using weights $w_i = \{1 + \tilde{\phi}_i(m_i - 1)\}^{-1}$, determine the new estimates $\hat{\beta}$ of β using MQL.
2. Calculate $v_i = m_i\hat{\theta}_i(1 - \hat{\theta}_i)$, the diagonal elements $\mathbf{q}_i$ of $\mathbf{X}(\mathbf{X}^{\mathrm{T}}\mathbf{WVX})^{-1}\mathbf{X}^{\mathrm{T}}$, and the squared standardized residuals
$$z_i = w_i\big(r_i - m_i\hat{\theta}_i\big)^2 v_i^{-1}(1 - w_i v_i q_i)^{-1}.$$
The z_i have expectations $w_i\{1 + \phi_i(m_i - 1)\}$.
3. Estimate ϕ and δ by minimizing
$$\Sigma\big[w_i^{-1}z_i - 1 - \phi g\big(\hat{\theta}_i, \mathbf{x}_i, \delta\big)(m_i - 1)\big]^2.$$

Step 3 can possibly be made more efficient by use of weighted least squares, or more robust by use of absolute residuals. See Davidian and Carroll (1987) for a general discussion of this kind of estimation problem.

We must recognise that reliable estimation of δ will only be possible in large data sets, and it will rarely be sensible to entertain a model in which δ comprises more than one parameter. Moreover, if $g = \{\theta_i(1 - \theta_i)\}^{\delta}$, as in eqn. (7.2), it will not be possible to estimate δ reliably unless the θ_i values cover a wide range which extends into at least one of the extremes, i.e. close to 0 or close to 1. Estimation of δ may be unnecessary when the aim of the analysis is to make inferences about β, e.g. testing treatment differences, when it is sufficient to confirm that these inferences are unchanged when different values of δ are assumed.

Acknowledgements

I thank Dr Bern Schwetz of the National Toxicology Program, NIEHS, Research Triangle Park, NC, and Drs Carole Kimmel and Dorothy Wellington of the Environmental Protection Agency, Washington, DC, for help in obtaining the teratology data, which was collected by Research Triangle Institute on contract with the NTP.

References

Aitchison, J. (1986). *The statistical analysis of compositional data*. Chapman and Hall, London.

Altham, P. M. E. (1978). Two generalizations of the binomial distribution. *Applied Statistics*, **27**, 162–7.

Anderson, D. A. and Aitken, M. A. (1985). Variance component models with binary response: interviewer variability. *Journal of the Royal Statistical Society, B*, **47**, 203–10.

Cochran, W. G. (1943). Analysis of variance for percentages based on unequal numbers. *Journal of the American Statistical Association*, **38**, 287–301.

Crowder, M. J. (1978). Beta-binomial ANOVA for proportions. *Applied Statistics*, **27**, 34–7.

Davidian, M. and Carroll, R. J. (1987). Variance component estimation. *Journal of the American Statistical Association*, **82**, 1079–91.

Finney, D. J. (1947). *Probit analysis*. Cambridge University Press, Cambridge.

Gilmour, A. R., Anderson, R. D., and Rae, A. L. (1985). The analysis of binomial data by a generalized linear mixed model. *Biometrika*, **72**, 593–9.

Haseman, J. K. and Kupper, L. L. (1979). Analysis of dichotomous response data from certain toxicological experiments. *Biometrics*, **35**, 281–93.

Johnson, N. L. (1965). Systems of frequency curves generated by methods of translation. *Biometrika*, **36**, 149–76.

Kleinman, J. C. (1973). Proportions with extraneous variance: single and independent samples. *Journal of the American Statistical Association*, **68**, 46–54.

Kupper, L. L., Portier, C., Hogan, M. D., and Yamamoto, E. (1986). The impact of litter effects on dose-response modelling in teratology. *Biometrics*, **42**, 85–98.

McCullagh, P. (1983). Quasi-likelihood functions. *Annals of Statistics*, **11**, 59–67.

Moore, D. F. (1986). Asymptotic properties of moment estimators for overdispersed counts and proportions. *Biometrika*, **73**, 583–8.

Moore, D. F. (1987). Modelling the extraneous variance in the presence of extra-binomial variation. *Applied Statistics*, **36**, 8–14.

Nelder, J. A. and Pregibon, D. (1987). An extended quasi-likelihood function. *Biometrika*, **74**, 221–32.

Ochi, Y. and Prentice, R. L. (1984). Likelihood inference in a correlated probit regression model. *Biometrika*, **71**, 531–43.

Pack, S. E. (1986). Hypothesis testing for proportions with overdispersion. *Biometrics*, **42**, 967–72.

Pierce, D. A. and Sands, B. R. (1975). Extra-binomial variation in binary data. Technical report 46. Department of Statistics, Oregon State University.

Prentice, R. L. (1986). Binary regression using an extended Beta-binomial distribution, with discussion of correlation induced by covariate measurement errors. *Journal of the American Statistical Association*, **81**, 321–7.

Williams, D. A. (1972). The comparison of several dose levels with a zero dose control. *Biometrics*, **28**, 519–31.

Williams, D. A. (1975). The analysis of binary responses from toxicological experiments involving reproduction and teratogenicity. *Biometrics*, **31**, 949–52.

Williams, D. A. (1982). Extra-binomial variation in logistic linear models. *Applied Statistics*, **31**, 144–8.

Williams, D. A. (1988). Estimation bias using the Beta-binomial distribution in teratology. *Biometrics*, **44**, 305–8.

PART III

LD_{50} ESTIMATION

8 On likelihood and Bayesian methods for interval estimation of the LD_{50}

ANDREW P. GRIEVE

8.1 Introduction

The controversy surrounding the validity, and usefulness, of acute toxicity experiments in which interest centres on determining an estimate of the median lethal dose (LD_{50}) reached a climax in the 1980s. On the one hand, animal rights groups questioned the biological relevance of such tests, quoting examples in which only insignificant information was able to be extracted. The scientific objections were generally supported by toxicologists (e.g. Zbinden and Fluri-Roversi 1981), while at the same time they emphasized the need to quantify the toxic potential of a chemical and simultaneously encouraged the development of procedures designed to limit the number of animals required to give an assessment of lethality.

The fixed-dose procedure put forward by the British Toxicology Society (1984), a modified version of which was the subject of an international validation study (van den Heuvel 1990) and which is discussed by Whitehead and Curnow (1996) in this volume, has largely supplanted the classical acute toxicity test with its associated LD_{50} estimate. Indeed, the process of international harmonization is likely to ensure the complete demise of LD_{50} estimation within one or two years.

In the light of the likely demise of what might be termed the LD_{50} test, it could be argued that continuing interest in LD_{50} estimation is only of academic interest. There are, however, a number of reasons for continued interest. First, there are drugs, for example cytotoxic drugs, for which clinicians involved in the earliest human studies require an animal LD_{50} estimate as an aid to determining 'safe' dose levels, although this is not a regulatory requirement. Second, until LD_{50} is completely abandoned then, as Finney (1985) has argued, it is incumbent upon statisticians to ensure that the most efficient statistical methods should be used for their analysis. This argument is closely akin to Fisher's reason for developing the maximum likelihood estimate in the first place (Box 1978, p. 272). Third, while LD_{50} studies are rapidly disappearing in toxicity testing, they are still conducted in the original setting considered by Trevan (1927); namely, in the testing of vaccines. An example of this is given by Thraenhart (1986), who considers the testing of batches of rabies vaccine (see also Berres 1991); a second, more recent, example is described by Bolwell *et al.*

Table 8.1. Results from an inhalation acute toxicity experiment carried out to assess the toxic potential of an agrochemical product in powder form

Dose (mg/kg)	Number of animals	Number of deaths
422	5	0
744	5	1
948	5	3
2069	5	5

(1992) who consider problems concerning the testing of foot-and-mouth vaccines. Finally, there are many *in vivo* and *in vitro* models in drug screening which, while not concerned with lethality, have essentially similar problems when considering interval estimation of ED_{50} for small numbers of experimental units.

In Section 8.2 the model under consideration is introduced, as are the experimental data which are used for illustration. In Section 8.3 properties of the fiducial interval for the LD_{50} based on Fieller's Theorem are reviewed. In Section 8.4 the idea of the likelihood ratio (LR) interval is introduced and applied to the LD_{50}, and in Section 8.5 one property of it is derived. In Section 8.6 Cox and Reid's (1987) conditional profile likelihood (CPL) is investigated as a means of avoiding the pitfalls associated with the LR interval, and in Section 8.7 this approach is compared and contrasted with the Bayesian approach proposed by Grieve (1988).

8.2 Data and model

For the purposes of illustrating the ideas considered in this paper the experimental results shown in Tables 8.1 and 8.2 are used. Both sets of data arose from studies involved in the testing of agrochemical products. The data in Table 8.1 have been considered previously by both Aitkin (1986) and by Racine *et al.* (1986), while the data in Table 8.2 have also been considered by Smith *et al.* (1985), Aitkin (1986), and Grieve (1988).

Table 8.2. Results from a standard acute toxicity experiment carried out to classify an agrochemical substance according to the 1983 Swiss poison regulation

Dose (mg/ml)	Number of animals	Number of deaths
500	5	1
1000	5	2
2500	5	3
5000	5	2

In traditional acute toxicity tests the design consists of k dose levels on an appropriate scale. The experiment is characterized by the triplets $\{d_i, n_i, r_i\}$, where d_i is the dose administered to n_i animals of which r_i respond in the ith group. A mathematical dose–response model relating the probability of response, θ_i, to the dose d_i, is specified; for the purposes of the investigation in this chapter the logit model $\log[\theta_i/(1-\theta_i)] = \alpha + \beta x_i$ is used, where $x_i = \log(d_i)$, although similar results could be derived for the probit model $\theta_i = \Phi[\alpha + \beta x_i]$, where $\Phi(\cdot)$ is the standard normal distribution function. For either model, the $\log(LD_{50})$ is given by $\mu = -\alpha/\beta$.

8.3 Fiducial interval estimate of the LD_{50} and its properties

The standard approach to providing an interval estimate for μ is based upon the asymptotic normality of the maximum likelihood (ML) estimates of α and β and Fieller's Theorem (Fieller 1954). Let $\hat{\alpha}$ and $\hat{\beta}$ be the ML estimates of α and β obtained by maximizing the log-likelihood

$$l(\alpha, \beta) = \sum_{i=1}^{k} (r_i \log(\theta_i) + (n_i - r_i)\log(1-\theta_i))$$

(for convenience, this will in general be denoted by l); then at convergence the asymptotic covariance matrix of these estimates is given by

$$\begin{pmatrix} \hat{\sigma}_\alpha^2 & \hat{\sigma}_{\alpha\beta} \\ \hat{\sigma}_{\alpha\beta} & \hat{\sigma}_\beta^2 \end{pmatrix} = -\begin{pmatrix} \partial^2 l/\partial\alpha^2 & \partial^2 l/\partial\alpha\partial\beta \\ \partial^2 l/\partial\alpha\partial\beta & \partial^2 l/\partial\beta^2 \end{pmatrix}^{-1}.$$

Clearly, $\hat{\mu} = -\hat{\alpha}/\hat{\beta}$ is the ML of μ. A 'confidence interval' for μ is available from Fieller's Theorem as follows. From the asymptotic normality of $\hat{\alpha}$ and $\hat{\beta}$, and from standard properties of normal distributions, we have

$$\frac{\hat{\alpha} + \hat{\beta}\mu}{\sqrt{\hat{\sigma}_\alpha^2 + 2\mu\hat{\sigma}_{\alpha\beta} + \mu^2\hat{\sigma}_\beta^2}} \sim N(0,1). \qquad (8.1)$$

From this asymptotic property a $(1-\gamma)$ per cent interval for μ may be obtained by setting the left-hand side of eqn. (8.1) equal to the $(1-\gamma/2)$ percentile of the normal distribution and solving for μ. This procedure gives rise to a quadratic equation in μ which does not necessarily have real roots. To understand how this may occur, take the square of eqn. (8.1) and denote it by χ^2. As a function of μ, the curve thus formed is in general similar to that shown in Fig. 8.1, which is based on the data in Table 8.1. The curve has the following characteristics:

(1) it has its minimum at the ML estimate $\hat{\mu} = -\hat{\alpha}/\hat{\beta}$;

(2) it has an asymptote with value $\chi_{asy}^2 = \hat{\beta}^2/\hat{\sigma}_\beta^2$; and

(3) it has a maximum at $\mu^* = (\hat{\alpha}\hat{\sigma}_{\alpha\beta} - \hat{\beta}\hat{\sigma}_\alpha^2)/(\hat{\beta}\hat{\sigma}_{\alpha\beta} - \hat{\alpha}\hat{\sigma}_\beta^2)$ for which the value of χ^2 is $\chi_{\max}^2 = \chi_{asy}^2 + (\hat{\beta}\hat{\sigma}_{\alpha\beta} - \hat{\alpha}\hat{\sigma}_\beta^2)^2/(\hat{\sigma}_\beta^2(\hat{\sigma}_\alpha^2\hat{\sigma}_\beta^2 - \hat{\sigma}_{\alpha\beta}^2))$.

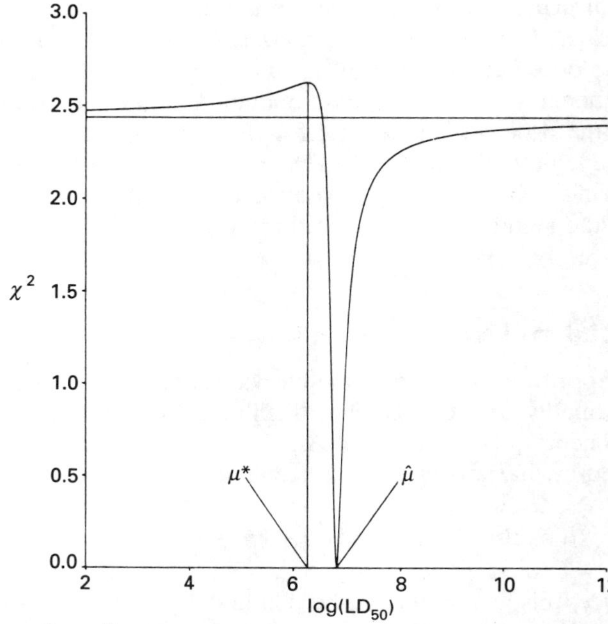

Fig. 8.1. The χ^2 statistic as a function of μ for the data in Table 8.1.

These characteristics imply the following: (i) if the $(1-\gamma)$ percentile of the χ^2 distribution with one degree of freedom, $\chi_1^2(1-\gamma)$, is less than χ_{asy}^2, then $(1-\gamma)$ per cent fiducial limits for μ exist; (ii) if $\chi_1^2(1-\gamma)$ is greater than χ_{asy}^2 but less than $\chi_{\max}^2$, then the $(1-\gamma)$ per cent fiducial limits are exclusive in the sense that they are of the form $\mu \leqslant \mu_L$ and $\mu \geqslant \mu_U$, where $\mu_L < \mu_U$; and (iii) if $\chi_1^2(1-\gamma)$ exceeds $\chi_{\max}^2$, then the fiducial interval for μ is the whole real line. In practice, therefore, useful fiducial limits based on Fieller's Theorem only exist if $\chi_1^2(1-\gamma)$ is less than χ_{asy}^2; that is, when there is significant evidence for the regression of $\log[\theta_i/(1-\theta_i)]$ on x_i. For the concrete case of the data in Table 8.1, $\chi_1^2(0.95)$ is greater than $\chi_{\max}^2$ and therefore the fiducial interval encompasses the whole real line.

8.4 Likelihood ratio interval estimate of the LD_{50}

In discussion of Racine *et al.* (1986), Ross, Bailey and Gower, and Cox all suggest that the failure of the traditional method of setting confidence intervals based on Fieller's Theorem to give an adequate result for the data in Table 8.1 is a direct result of the invalidity of the normal approximation to the binomial for small numbers of animals. They conclude that the use of likelihood ratio intervals, also known as profile likelihood or relative likelihood intervals, solves the problem. This approach was explicitly suggested independently by Williams (1986) and Aitkin (1986). In this section we summarize the basic ideas of the general approach as it applies to the problem of LD_{50} estimation.

DEFINITION. Suppose $L(\phi, \psi | X)$ is a two-parameter likelihood. Then the profile likelihood of ϕ, $P(\phi)$, is defined as

$$P(\phi) = L\big(\phi, \hat{\psi}(\phi) \,|\, X\big),$$

where $\hat{\psi}(\phi)$ is the solution to $\partial L(\phi, \psi | X)/\partial\psi = 0$. The $(1-\gamma)$ per cent LR, or profile likelihood, interval for ϕ is given by the solutions to

$$2\log\big[P(\hat{\phi})/P(\phi)\big] = \chi_1^2(1-\gamma), \tag{8.2}$$

where $\chi_1^2(1-\gamma)$ is the appropriate percentile of the chi-square distribution with one degree of freedom.

In order to apply this approach to the LD_{50} we need to reparametrize the logit model in terms of μ and β. Since by definition $\mu = -\alpha/\beta$ then, clearly, in terms of μ and β the model becomes $\log[\theta_i/(1-\theta_i)] = \beta(x_i - \mu)$. The procedure for determining the profile likelihood function, $P(\mu)$, in the case of the LD_{50} is simple. For a large number of values of μ, say μ_j, the likelihood is maximized with respect to β to give $\hat{\beta}_j$. The likelihood value at $\{\hat{\beta}_j, \mu_j\}$ is the profile likelihood value at $\mu = \mu_j$. Both Williams (1986) and Aitkin (1986) describe how this procedure may be simply carried out in GLIM. In practice, the resulting tabulation of $P(\mu)$ may be used to determine the solution of eqn. (8.2) to sufficient accuracy. For example, in Fig. 8.2 we display $\log(P(\mu))$ as a function of μ for the data in Table 8.1. It is then easy to determine the 95 per cent LR interval for μ as 6.59–7.11. While this procedure is extremely simple to

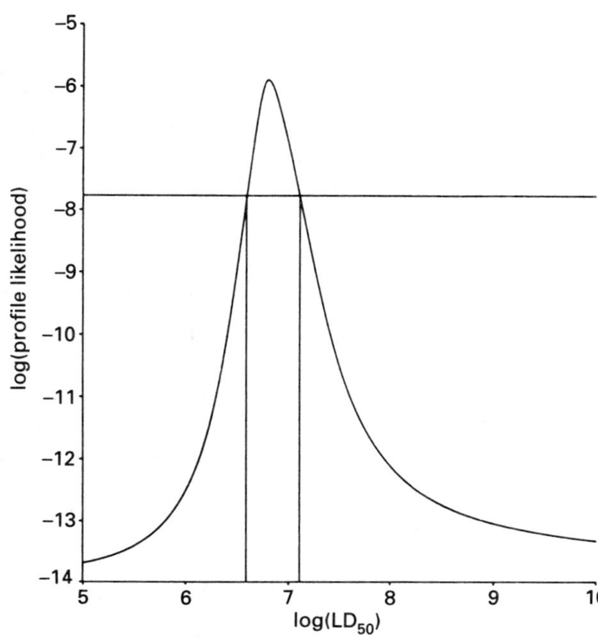

Fig. 8.2. The log (profile likelihood) function for the data in Table 8.1.

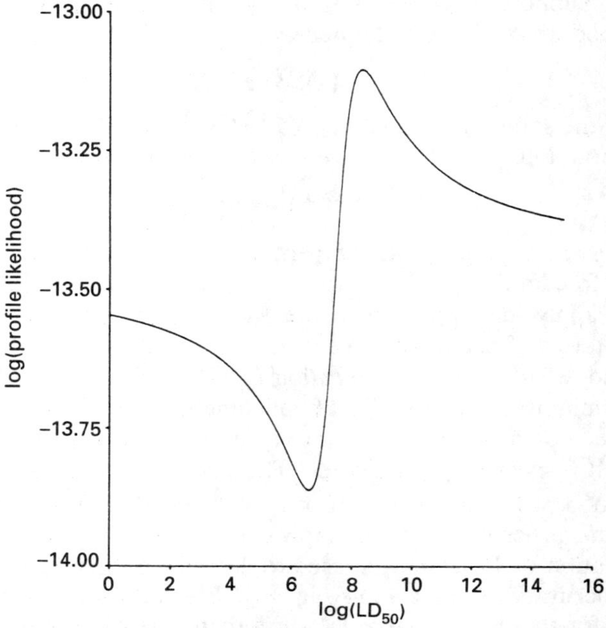

Fig. 8.3. The log (profile likelihood) function for the data in Table 8.2.

implement, a direct solution of eqn. (8.2) may be obtained from the algorithm proposed by Venzon and Moolgavkar (1988).

It would appear from Fig. 8.2 that the discussants of Racine *et al.* (1986) were correct in asserting that the use of the LR interval in place of an interval based on the asymptotic approximation represented by Fieller's Theorem circumvents the problems associated with the latter. A similar view was expressed by Williams (1986) who, when comparing the confidence properties of the LR interval with those of Fieller's fiducial interval, wrote:

> the modest shortfall in the true confidence probability of (the) LR interval may be judged as a small price to pay for an interval that can always be determined.

Unfortunately, as noted by Aitkin (1986), it is not true that the LR interval is always determinable. To illustrate, in Fig. 8.3 we display $\log(P(\mu))$ for the experimental results of Table 8.2. Two features of this display are of particular interest. First, $\log(P(\mu))$ varies by no more than approximately 1.5 over the whole range and therefore no 95 per cent LR interval exists. Second, $\log(P(\mu))$ has both a maximum and a minimum. We consider the implications of this latter observation in the next section.

8.5 A property of the LR interval estimate of the LD_{50}

In the previous section we saw that there exist experimental configurations of data for which $\log(P(\mu))$ has both a maximum and a minimum. In this section we show that an implication of this observation is that, in exactly the same way as with the fiducial intervals based on Fieller's Theorem, there always exists a 'confidence level' for which this likelihood method fails to produce an interval. We establish this result for the logit model which we have used throughout, although the same result may be empirically demonstrated for the probit model.

THEOREM. *The profile likelihood for μ for a logit response model has a minimum given by*

$$\mu^* = \frac{\sum_{i=1}^{k} x_i(r_i - n_i/2)}{\sum_{i=1}^{k} (r_i - n_i/2)}, \qquad \beta(\mu^*) = 0.$$

Proof. See the Appendix

This result implies that the profile likelihood function for μ always has both a maximum and a minimum. Thus the profile likelihood can be characterized, for convenience, using the log of the profile likelihood, as in Fig. 8.4. The behaviour of the profile likelihood function evidenced in this figure is mirrored in the plots of $L(\mu_0)$, the likelihood ratio statistic, given by Williams (1986), and has also

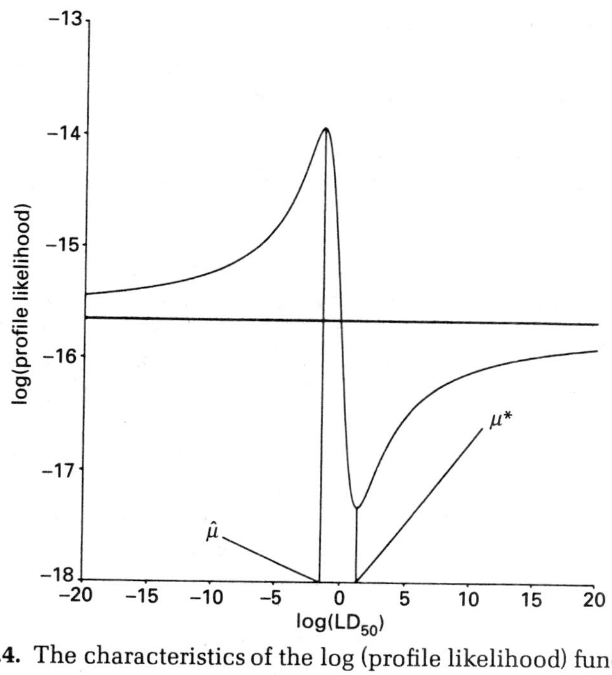

Fig. 8.4. The characteristics of the log (profile likelihood) function.

been described explicitly by Aitkin (1986). The horizontal asymptote represents the log of the profile likelihood for zero slope and corresponds to

$$l(\infty, \hat{\beta}(\infty)) = r\log(r/n) + (n-r)\log(1-r/n),$$

where

$$r = \sum_{i=1}^{k} r_i, \qquad n = \sum_{i=1}^{k} n_i.$$

Thus $\log(P(\mu))$ has precisely the same characteristic form as does Fieller's χ^2 function noted in Section 8.3. The implication of the form of $\log(P(\mu))$, which was apparently not appreciated by either Williams (1986) or Aitkin (1986), is that there will always be a level γ for which the likelihood interval will comprise the whole real line. The level at which this occurs will be less than that at which Fieller's Theorem applied to the asymptotic normal approximation breaks down, but it will always occur. This may clearly be seen in Fig. 1 of Williams (1986), in which the likelihood ratio statistic always lies above the asymptotic approximation. Aitkin (1986) concluded that the behaviour of $\log(P(\mu))$ in the specific case of the data in Table 8.1 was because evidence for regression of $\log[\theta_i/(1-\theta_i)]$ on x_i was weak. However, as we have seen, this behaviour is an inherent characteristic of the LR interval and only depends upon the 'weakness' of the evidence for regression for a given $(1-\gamma)$.

8.6 A modified profile likelihood approach

The profile likelihood, or relative likelihood approach, has a second major defect. As Kalbfleisch and Sprott (1969) point out:

> ...the maximum relative likelihood does not take account of the uncertainty due to lack of knowledge of β and so can be misleading in terms of both precision and location.

This comment relates to an implicit assumption within the framework of profile likelihoods that, for fixed μ, β is known to be equal to the value of $\hat{\beta}$ obtained by maximizing the likelihood for that particular value of μ. In this section we consider a modified profile likelihood approach which addresses this issue.

Cox and Reid (1987) consider problems associated with making inferences about a scalar parameter ϕ in the presence of one or more nuisance parameters ψ using likelihood inference. In particular, they consider whether a likelihood ratio statistic constructed from the conditional distribution of the data given the ML estimate of ψ is preferable to the profile likelihood. Under the assumption that ϕ is orthogonal to ψ, they show that the effect of conditioning is to modify the profile likelihood from $L(\phi, \hat{\psi}(\phi) \mid X)$ to

$$L(\phi, \hat{\psi}(\phi) \mid X)\left|nj_{\psi\psi}(\phi, \hat{\psi}(\phi))\right|^{-1/2}, \qquad (8.3)$$

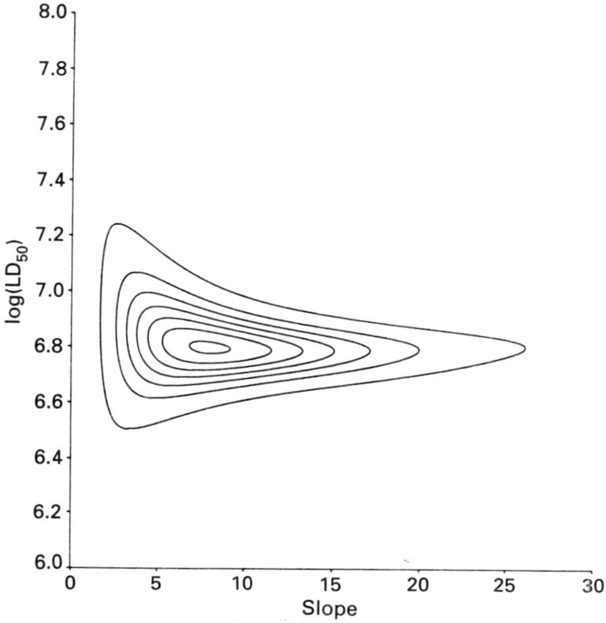

Fig. 8.5. Likelihood contours for the data in Table 8.1.

where $j_{\psi\psi}(\phi, \hat{\psi}(\phi))$ is the observed information for ψ given fixed ϕ. This is the conditional profile likelihood (CPL). The effect of the modifying factor $|nj_{\psi\psi}(\phi, \hat{\psi}(\phi))|^{-1/2}$ is 'to penalize values of ϕ for which the information about ψ is relatively large' (Cox and Reid 1987), thereby addressing exactly the problem identified by Kalbfleisch and Sprott.

We noted above that Cox and Reid assume that ϕ and ψ are orthogonal, which separates their approach from the modified profile likelihood of Barndorff-Nielsen (1983). Empirically, one often finds that in a logit model μ and β are approximately orthogonal. For example, in Fig. 8.5 we display contours of the likelihood function in this parametrization for the data of Table 8.1 which show evidence of approximate orthogonality. Cox and Reid define parameter orthogonality by $(1/n)\mathrm{E}(-\partial^2 l/\partial\phi\partial\psi) = 0$, so that support for approximate orthogonality will be given by small values of $\mathrm{E}(-\partial^2 l/\partial\phi\partial\psi)$. In the μ and β parametrization the mixed partial derivative has the form

$$-\frac{\partial^2 l}{\partial\mu\partial\beta} = \sum_{i=1}^{k} [(r_i - n_i\theta_i) - \beta n_i\theta_i(1-\theta_i)(x_i - \mu)],$$

so that

$$\mathrm{E}\left(-\frac{\partial^2 l}{\partial\mu\partial\beta}\right) = -\beta\sum_{i=1}^{k} n_i\theta_i(1-\theta_i)(x_i - \mu),$$

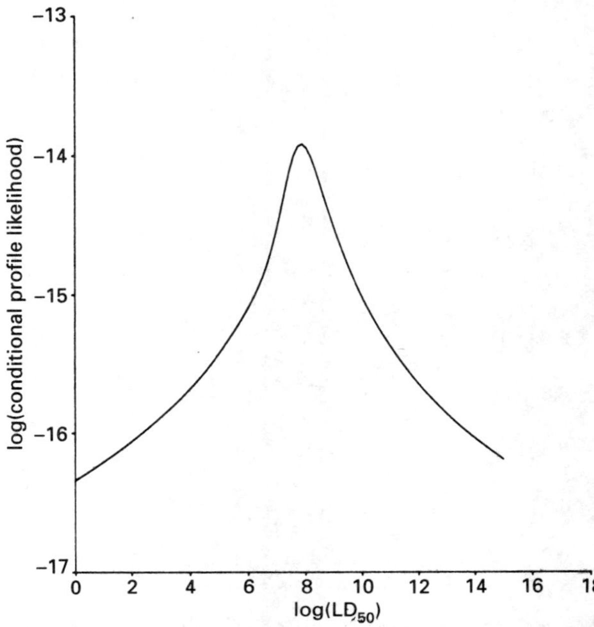

Fig. 8.6. The log (conditional profile likelihood) function for the data in Table 8.2.

which will tend to be small, as the doses will be chosen to span μ and thus $\Sigma_{i=1}^{k}(x_i - \mu)$ will generally be small.

Were it not the case that μ and β were approximately orthogonal, it would still have been possible to use Cox and Reid's results, since they show that if ϕ is a scalar then it is always possible to find a transformation $(\phi, \psi) \rightarrow (\phi, \eta)$ such that ϕ and η are orthogonal. The fortunate circumstance that μ and β are approximately orthogonal obviates the need to determine η.

In Figure 8.6 we display the logarithm of the CPL for the data in Table 8.2. As before, this graphical display is sufficient to allow the determination of a 95 per cent interval for μ, which in this case is 3.4–13.0.

8.7 The relationship of modified profile likelihood results to Bayesian methods

Thus far, we have concentrated on likelihood alternatives to the 'classical' approach based on Fieller's fiducial limits. We have seen that the profile likelihood method has similar problems to the fiducial approach, in that there is always a confidence level for which no interval can be determined. The modified profile likelihood approach takes into account the uncertainty regarding the nuisance parameters which is ignored in the basic profile likelihood method. The Bayesian analysis developed by Grieve (1988) also takes account of this uncertainty in the following way (see also Racine *et al.* 1986).

Suppose again that we have two parameters ϕ and ψ, and we wish to make inferences about ϕ. For a uniform prior on both parameters, an asymptotic approximation to the posterior distribution of ϕ has been developed by Tierney and Kadane (1986) in the form

$$p(\phi|X) \approx \left(\frac{\left|j_{\phi,\psi}(\hat{\phi},\hat{\psi})\right|}{2\pi n \left|j_{\psi\psi}(\phi,\hat{\psi}(\phi))\right|} \right)^{1/2} \frac{e^{l(\phi,\hat{\psi}(\phi))}}{e^{l(\hat{\phi},\hat{\psi})}},$$

where $\hat{\phi}$ and $\hat{\psi}$ are the global maximum likelihood estimates, $j_{\phi,\psi}(\hat{\phi}, \hat{\psi})$ is the observed information for ϕ and ψ and, as before, $\hat{\psi}(\phi)$ is the maximum likelihood estimate of ψ for fixed ϕ and $j_{\psi\psi}(\phi, \hat{\psi}(\phi))$ is the associated observed information. The profile likelihood function, $\exp[l(\phi, \hat{\psi}(\phi))]$, is weighted in the above expression by $j_{\psi\psi}(\phi, \hat{\psi}(\phi))$, which represents the uncertainty in $\hat{\psi}(\phi)$ measured by the curvature of the log-likelihood at that point.

The similarity between this Bayesian analysis and the modified profile likelihood method is manifest. However, the development above was based on a uniform, so-called uninformative prior. The Bayesian development in Grieve (1988) for an analysis of the LD_{50} was based upon an assumption of a uniform prior for α and β which, in the more useful parametrization μ and β, is no longer uniform but has the form

$$p(\mu,\beta) \propto \beta, \qquad -\infty<\mu<\infty, \quad 0<\beta.$$

Returning, then, to the general case with parameters ϕ and ψ, suppose that their joint prior $p(\phi, \psi)$ is written in the form $p(\phi, \psi)=p(\psi|\phi)p(\phi)$. Then the posterior for ϕ may be expressed as

$$p(\phi|X) \propto \int L(\phi,\psi|X)p(\psi|\phi)p(\phi)\,d\psi.$$

Sweeting (1987) shows that, given this structure, then if ϕ and ψ are orthogonal the Tierney and Kadane expansion for $p(\phi|X)$ has the form

$$p(\phi|X) \propto p(\hat{\psi}(\phi)|\phi)L(\phi,\hat{\psi}(\phi)|X)\left|j_{\psi\psi}(\phi,\hat{\psi}(\phi))\right|^{-1/2}. \qquad (8.4)$$

Sweeting further shows that, to the same order of approximation in $p(\hat{\psi}(\phi)|\phi)$, $\hat{\psi}(\phi)$ may be replaced by $\hat{\psi}$ so that (3) and (4) are equal whenever ϕ and ψ are taken to be *a priori* independent.

We saw above (i) that μ and β in the logit model are approximately orthogonal and (ii) that in Grieve's (1988) Bayesian development they are *a priori* independent. Therefore, Grieve's Bayesian development when applied to the logit model is approximately the same as the CPL approach.

8.8 Discussion

In this chapter we have, in a sequential manner, investigated a number of methods for interval estimation of the LD_{50}. The main conclusions of these investigations are as follows:

1. For experiments with small numbers of animals per dose group, it is inappropriate to use Fieller's Theorem to set a 'confidence' interval for μ.
2. As numerous discussants of Racine *et al.* (1986) have suggested, a profile likelihood approach to interval estimation is preferable to Fieller's method.
3. The profile likelihood method suffers the same defect as does Fieller's method, but at a higher level of 'confidence'.
4. The CPL method, which takes account of uncertainty in estimating β, overcomes the problem noted in 3 above.
5. The CPL is approximately the same as the posterior distribution derivable from the Bayesian approach developed by Grieve (1988).

There are cases involving small numbers of animals per group in which degeneracy of maximum likelihood estimation occurs, in the sense that $\hat{\beta} = \infty$. In an effort to overcome this defect, Williams (1986) proposed that the slope be constrained to be no greater than some arbitrary upper limit β_{max}. Williams commented that this informal use of prior information might be thought of as 'a small step in a Bayesian direction'.

Another perspective on this problem may be gained by considering the meaning of $\hat{\beta} = \infty$. We could clearly not expect an infinite slope, and therefore we may conclude that the estimate is biased away from zero. Recent work by Firth (1993) has shown that the first-order term of the asymptotic bias of the maximum likelihood estimates may be removed by a suitable modification to the score function. In exponential families, under a canonical parametrization, the effect is to penalize the likelihood by Jeffreys' invariant prior.

We have seen that—from two different perspectives—attempts to overcome difficulties associated with likelihood estimation of the LD_{50} lead to Bayesian solutions.

References

Aitkin, M. (1986). Statistical modelling: the likelihood approach. *The Statistician*, **35**, 102–13.

Barndorff-Nielsen, O. (1983). On a formula for the distribution of the maximum likelihood estimator. *Biometrika*, **70**, 343–65.

Berres, M. (1991). Eine effektive Methode zur Schätzung und zum Vergleich der ED_{50} bei kleinen Fallzahlen. *Journal of Experimental Animal Science*, **34**, 21–9.

Bolwell, C., Parry, N. R., and Rowlands, D. J. (1992). Comparison between *in vitro* neutralization titres and *in vivo* protection against homologous and heterologous challenge induced by vaccines prepared from two serologically distinct variants of foot-and-mouth disease virus, serotype A22. *Journal of General Virology*, **73**, 727–31.

Box, J. F. (1978). *R. A. Fisher, the life of a scientist*. John Wiley, New York.

British Toxicological Society (1984). A new approach to the classification of substances and preparations on the basis of their acute toxicity. *Human Toxicology*, **3**, 85–92.

Cox, D. R. and Reid, N. (1987). Parameter orthogonality and approximate conditional inference (with discussion). *Journal of the Royal Statistical Society, Series B*. **49**, 1–39.

Fieller, E. C. (1954). Some problems in interval estimation. *Journal of the Royal Statistical Society, Series B*, **16**, 175–85.

Finney, D. J. (1985). The median lethal dose and its estimation. *Archives of Toxicology*, **56**, 215–8.

Firth, D. (1993). Bias reduction of maximum likelihood estimates. *Biometrika*, **80**, 27–8.

Grieve, A. P. (1988). A Bayesian approach to the analysis of LD_{50} experiments. In *Bayesian Statistics* 3 (eds. J. M. Bernardo, M. H. deGroot, D. V. Lindley, and A. F. M. Smith). Oxford University Press, Oxford.

Kalbfleisch, J. D. and Sprott, D. A. (1969). Application of likelihood methods to models involving large numbers of parameters (with discussion). *Journal of the Royal Statistical Society, Series B*, **32**, 175–208.

Racine, A., Grieve, A. P., Flühler, H., and Smith, A. F. M. (1986). Bayesian methods in practice: experiences in the pharmaceutical industry. *Applied Statistics*, **35**, 93–150.

Smith, A. F. M., Skene, A. M., Shaw, J. E. H., Naylor, J. C., and Dransfield, M. (1985). The implementation of the Bayesian paradigm. *Communications in Statistics—Theory and Methods*, **14** (5), 1079–102.

Sweeting, T. J. (1987). In discussion of Cox and Reid (1987), op. cit.

Thraenhart, O. (1986). Wertbemessung von Gewebekultur-Impstoffen gegen Tollwut für Mensch und Hund. Habilitationsschrift, University of Essen.

Tierney, L. and Kadane, J. B. (1986). Accurate approximations for posterior moments and marginal densities. *Journal of the American Statistical Association*, **81**, 82–6.

Trevan, J. W. (1927). The error of determination in toxicity. *Proceedings of the Royal Society, Series B*, **101**, 483–514.

van den Heuvel, M. J., Clark, D. G., Fielder, R. J., Koundakjian, P. P., Oliver, G. J., Pelling, D., Tomlinson, N. J., and Walker, A. P. (1990). The international validation of a fixed-dose procedure as an alternative to the classical LD50 test. *Food and Chemical Toxicology*, **28**, 469–82.

Venzon, D. J. and Moolgavkar, S. H. (1988). A method for computing profile-likelihood-based confidence intervals. *Applied Statistics*, **37**, 87–94.

Whitehead, A. and Curnow, R. N. (1996). Statistical evaluation of the fixed-dose procedure. In this volume.

Williams, D. A. (1986). Interval estimation of the median lethal dose. *Biometrics*, **42**, 641–5.

Zbinden, G. and Flury-Roversi, M. (1981). Significance of the LD_{50}-test for the toxicological evaluation of chemical substances. *Archives of Toxicology*, **47**, 77–99.

Appendix

From the log-likelihood $l(\mu, \beta(\mu))$ which, for convenience, we denote by l and regard as a function of μ alone, we have

$$\frac{\partial l}{\partial \mu} = \sum_{i=1}^{k} (r_i - n_i\theta_i)\left[(x_i - \mu)\frac{\mathrm{d}\beta(\mu)}{\mathrm{d}\mu} - \beta(\mu)\right].$$

When $\beta(\mu)=0$ it follows that $\theta_i=1/2$ and, therefore, substitution of $\mu=\mu^*$ gives $\partial l/\partial\mu=0$. Differentiation of $\partial l/\partial\mu$ gives

$$\frac{\partial^2 l}{\partial\mu^2}=\sum_{i=1}^{k}(r_i-n_i\theta_i)\left[(x_i-\mu)\frac{\mathrm{d}^2\beta(\mu)}{\mathrm{d}\mu^2}-2\frac{\mathrm{d}\beta(\mu)}{\mathrm{d}\mu}\right]$$
$$-\sum_{i=1}^{k}n_i\theta_i(1-\theta_i)\left[(x_i-\mu)\frac{\mathrm{d}\beta(\mu)}{\mathrm{d}\mu}-\beta(\mu)\right]^2.$$

At the turning point μ^*, $\beta(\mu^*)=0$ and $\theta_i=1/2$, so that

$$\frac{\partial^2 l}{\partial\mu^2}=-2\frac{\mathrm{d}\beta(\mu^*)}{\mathrm{d}\mu}\sum_{i=1}^{k}(r_i-n_i/2)-\tfrac{1}{4}\sum_{i=1}^{k}n_i(x_i-\mu^*)^2\left[\frac{\mathrm{d}\beta(\mu^*)}{\mathrm{d}\mu}\right]^2. \quad \text{(A1)}$$

By definition, $\beta(\mu)$ is defined as an implicit function of μ by the equation

$$\frac{\partial l}{\partial\mu}=\sum_{i=1}^{k}(x_i-\mu)(r_i-n_i\theta_i)=0.$$

A second differentiation with respect to μ gives

$$-\sum_{i=1}^{k}(r_i-n_i\theta_i)-\sum_{i=1}^{k}n_i\theta_i(1-\theta_i)(x_i-\mu)\left[(x_i-\mu)\frac{\mathrm{d}\beta(\mu)}{\mathrm{d}\mu}-\beta(\mu)\right]=0,$$

implying

$$\frac{\mathrm{d}\beta(\mu)}{\mathrm{d}\mu}=\frac{\beta(\mu)\sum_{i=1}^{k}n_i\theta_i(1-\theta_i)(x_i-\mu)-\sum_{i=1}^{k}(r_i-n_i\theta_i)}{\sum_{i=1}^{k}n_i\theta_i(1-\theta_i)(x_i-\mu)^2}.$$

At the turning point μ^*, $\beta(\mu^*)=0$ and $\theta_i=1/2$, so that

$$\frac{\mathrm{d}\beta(\mu)}{\mathrm{d}\mu}=\frac{\sum_{i=1}^{k}(r_i-n_i/2)}{\tfrac{1}{4}\sum_{i=1}^{k}n_i(x_i-\mu^*)^2}.$$

Substituting this into eqn. (A1) gives

$$\frac{\partial^2 l}{\partial\mu^2}=\frac{8\left[\sum_{i=1}^{k}(r_i-n_i/2)\right]^2}{\sum_{i=1}^{k}n_i(x_i-\mu^*)^2}-\frac{4\left[\sum_{i=1}^{k}(r_i-n_i/2)\right]^2}{\sum_{i=1}^{k}n_i(x_i-\mu^*)^2}=\frac{4\left[\sum_{i=1}^{k}(r_i-n_i/2)\right]^2}{\sum_{i=1}^{k}n_i(x_i-\mu^*)^2},$$

which is clearly positive, so that the turning point is a minimum.

9 The analysis of grouped longitudinal mortality data allowing for variable natural mortality

R. J. O'HARA HINES AND W. G. S. HINES

9.1 Introduction

One of David Williams' many interests was the analysis of data from toxicological studies in which groups of animals were exposed to different treatment conditions and the resulting proportions responding or exhibiting some symptom or behaviour were recorded. For example, in Williams (1987), he discussed deletion diagnostics and residuals for the detection of influential observations and outliers when generalized linear models are fitted to such data. In Williams (1982, 1988), variance models which account for the presence of extra-bionomial variation in the proportions were presented. He was also interested in interval estimation of the median lethal concentration (LC_{50}) in toxicological studies in which the recorded response recorded was death (Williams 1986). Additionally, in a study of exposure time on the susceptibility of a certain species of snail (Boyce and Williams 1967), Williams estimated the median mortality time for a given toxicant concentration (LT_{50}) using independent groups of animals at the different observation times. In contrast, the present chapter considers studies in which mortalities in the same groups of animals are recorded at a number of observation times.

Williams' work, along with the work of other authors cited in Section 9.3, has provided guidance for the analysis of data gathered from a somewhat more complex type of toxicological experiment. In these experiments, mortality counts are recorded at a number of observation times for each group of animals exposed to one of the treatment conditions. Such experiments are often labelled as grouped (or interval-censored) longitudinal mortality studies, and may be analysed by using survival analysis models (Prentice and Gloeckler 1978; Pierce *et al.* 1979; Lawless 1982, Section 7.3; Aranda-Ordaz 1983; Tibshirani and Ciampi 1983; Finkelstein 1986; Petkau and Sitter 1989; Preisler 1989) or multinomial generalized linear models (McCullagh 1980; Green 1984; McCullagh and Nelder 1989, Ch. 5; O'Hara Hines and Hines 1992; O'Hara Hines *et al.* 1992; O'Hara Hines and Lawless 1993). Pack and Morgan (1990) and Farewell (1982) used mixture models which combined a survival model for animals affected by the toxicant with another model which accounted for long-term survivors to analyse interval-censored survival data.

Further comparison of the survival analysis approach for grouped survival data and the generalized linear model approach that we will be using shows that the essential difference has less to do with any considerable difference in modelling than with the contrasting objectives of the two approaches: We are interested in this paper in determining 50 per cent mortality conditions (LC_{50} for a specific observation time and LT_{50} for a given toxicant concentration), while survival analysis studies focus more on survival and hazard functions. For example, Aranda-Oradaz (1983) estimated the survivor function using a proportional-hazards model for grouped survival data (see equation (6) in his paper). His model and the one we use, however, are quite similar except that he used a complementary log–log link on the conditional probability of failure in a particular interval given survival up to that interval, while we will be using a logit link on cumulative proportions over time.

In this chapter we will discuss the analysis of a grouped longitudinal mortality study using a cumulative multinomial generalized linear model. The diagnostic tools described in O'Hara Hines *et al.* (1992) will be used to check its fit, and the methods detailed in O'Hara Hines and Lawless (1993) to account for any extra-multinomial variation which might be present. Our analysis has additional features. We show how suitable new plots of the Cook statistics can reveal patterns of influence among the treatment conditions. Additionally, in toxicological studies such as these, natural mortality, with animals dying from natural causes—independently of the effects of the toxicant—may also be present, and this mortality can vary because of treatment conditions other than the toxicant level. Toxicologists are interested in studying the effects of the toxicant only, unobscured by natural mortality. We will therefore also discuss a method of adjusting for natural mortality.

9.2 The longitudinal mortality study data set

An experiment on the toxicity of copper on white sucker larvae was carried out in the Department of Biology at the University of Waterloo (Munkittrick and Dixon 1989). Tanks containing roughly ten white sucker larvae were set up under varying conditions. The eggs from which the larvae hatched were obtained from two lakes in Northern Ontario, Lake Manitouwadge and Loken Lake. Lake Manitouwadge was contaminated by runoff from mine tailings and, as a result, had elevated levels of copper and zinc. Loken Lake was used as a reference lake since it was considered to be relatively unpolluted. The toxicologist was interested in whether these elevated levels of zinc and copper in Lake Manitouwadge had detrimental effects on the white sucker larvae. Roughly half of the test tanks contained larvae from Lake Manitouwadge, while the other tanks contained larvae from Loken Lake.

The ages of the exposed larvae also varied from tank to tank. These ages were 9, 13, 17, 21, 25, 29, and 37 days posthatch. Additionally, larvae in roughly half the tanks were fed until the onset of the exposure to the treatment, while the others were left unfed. However, since the larvae were nourished by the contents of their egg yolk sacs up to roughly 20 days of age, at about which time they were also observed to start feeding, only those unfed tanks containing larvae aged 21 days or older could be considered starved (i.e., roughly one quarter of the tanks). All the other tanks were regarded as fed in terms of the treatment applied. (It is standard practice in these tolerance studies not to feed the larvae during the actual exposure (144 hours) to the toxicant. This complication was not addressed in the model fitted below.)

Eight concentrations (0, 150, 300, 450, 600, 900, 1200 and 2200 μg Cu l^{-1}) of copper were used for each combination of lake type, age of larvae and feeding practice. The tanks with a concentration of 0 μg Cu l^{-1} were called control tanks, and were used to measure natural mortality. The other tanks were referred to as treated tanks. The resulting design was fairly well balanced except for the fed-starved condition, with only one quarter of the tanks being starved. In addition, the starvation condition resulted in high mortality in the untreated larvae by the end of the experiment. Most of the starved larvae from Lake Manitouwadge were dead by 29 days posthatch, while some from Loken Lake survived without food until age 42. This caused even more imbalance in the study of the feeding practice condition, since no treatments were run with starved tanks at age 37; and age 29 for Lake Manitouwadge had only one starved tank, a tank with the highest concentration of copper. (While the possible bias resulting from this censoring is ignored in the following analysis, the toxicologist should keep it in mind in his overall interpretation.) Altogether, 195 tanks were set up over a period of several months—170 treated tanks and 25 control tanks. Observed median mortality times for all the treatment combinations used in the study are given in Table 9.1.

Mortality counts were taken at 2, 4, 6, 8, 11, 12, 16, 20, 21, 24, 28, 32, 44, 45, 48, 52, 55, 68, 70, 72, 80, 84, 96, 108, 120, 128, and 144 hours after the start of each run. A fairly detailed, but highly redundant, record of cumulative mortality counts at most of these times was taken for each tank. A referee has noted that the use of just a few of the time points—say, using times 24, 48, 72, 96, 120, and 144 hours—would reduce that redundancy. Our approach, however, was to allow for it explicitly, by removing all observations which simply confirmed that no new mortality had occurred, and by recording the new cumulative mortalities after all times at which additional mortalities had occurred. This approach had the advantage of extracting the informative part of the data record while avoiding the loss of information that would result if the set of time points used had simply been reduced as suggested by the referee. For the analysis described in the next section, our method resulted in records of mortality counts with the number of observation times varying between one and nine.

A referee also asked about problems that the retention of redundant observations might cause in diagnostic plots, in estimates of overdispersion, in standard errors of model terms, and in the numerical methods used. Our experience has been that while the presence of redundant observations became quite apparent

Table 9.1.
(a) Observed median mortality times (hours) for Loken Lake

	Concentration (μg Cu l^{-1})							
Age	0	150	300	450	600	900	1200	2200
Fed tanks								
9	>	>	>	>	>	>	>	34
	>	>	>	>	>	>	>	20
13	>	>	>	>	>	132	>	29
	>	>	>	>	>	>	129	47
17	>	>	>	>	144	124	87	34
	>	>	>	>	138	90	96	26
21	>	>	>	>	108	107	83	24
25	96	>	>	144	72	77	67	16
29	>	>	96	112	76	47	55	28
37	131	107	—	41	20	22	21	13
Starved tanks								
21	>	>	>	144	125	83	86	21
25	>	>	>	>	100	90	83	13
29	>	>	>	61	107	42	35	11
37	—	—	—	—	—	—	—	—
(b) Observed median mortality times (hours) for Lake Manitouwadge								
Fed tanks								
9	>	>	>	>	>	>	—	44
	>	>	>	>	>	>	—	40
13	>	>	>	>	>	>	>	82
	>	>	>	>	>	>	>	82
17	>	>	>	>	>	117	136	44
	>	>	>	>	120	92	107	56
21	>	>	120	127	83	77	87	24
25	120	>	>	108	114	72	72	30
29	104	>	96	99	96	87	55	24
37	120	132	53	144	103	63	20	11
Starved tanks								
21	87	127	86	107	69	77	72	19
25	59	24	33	48	24	27	33	17
29	—	—	—	—	—	—	—	6
37	—	—	—	—	—	—	—	—

>, Observed LT_{50} greater than 144 hours.
—, Treatment combination not run.

in some diagnostic plots, there was little or no effect on the numerical methods used. Retention of redundant observations can, however, increase the degrees of freedom associated with a Pearson chi-square based measure of overdispersion, and reduce the apparent size of that measure, and hence the corresponding estimates of standard errors. Note, however, that these replies should be regarded as tentative rather than definitive since, in our research to date, we have not explicitly addressed those issues as yet.

9.3 Analysis of the data

9.3.1 *Fitting procedure*

It was decided to fit separate, more parsimonious, models to the treated and the control tanks. The reasons for this decision were several: the sole purpose of measuring control mortalities was to use them to adjust for background mortality, so that a combined model with its many interaction terms reflecting the differences between treatment and control would be of little interest and would unnecessarily complicate the analysis; in practice, background mortality data might well be measured from separate studies; and the use of separate models for the treated and control data sets simplified the process for obtaining confidence intervals for estimated LC_{50}s and LT_{50}s, adjusted for natural mortality.

In a standard longitudinal mortality study, a single multivariate observation is obtained when a total of n animals are exposed to one experimental condition and their mortalities are observed only at the discrete time points $-\infty < t_1 < t_2 < \cdots < t_m < \infty$. Under the assumption that their deaths are statistically independent for the given experimental condition, the numbers of animals responding in the time intervals $(-\infty, t_1]$, $(t_1, t_2], \ldots, (t_{m-1}, t_m]$ jointly follow a multinominal distribution. Since one of the assumed objectives of the study is to estimate the LT_{50}, it proves to be more convenient to deal with the cumulative numbers or cumulative proportions of animals responding up to each time point. Let R_j be the proportion of animals responding by time t_j, and define

$$\mathbf{R}^{\mathrm{T}} = (R_1, R_2, \ldots, R_m), \qquad 0 \leqslant R_1 \leqslant R_2 \leqslant \cdots \leqslant R_m \leqslant 1,$$

where the superscript T denotes a matrix transpose. Correspondingly, let $p_j = \mathrm{E}(R_j)$ denote the probability that an individual animal responds by t_j, and let $\mathbf{p} = \mathrm{E}(\mathbf{R})$. It is readily shown from multinominal distribution results (e.g. McCullagh and Nelder 1989, p. 167) that the covariance matrix of $\mathbf{R}$ is $\mathrm{Var}(\mathbf{R}) = V(\mathbf{p})$, where $V(\mathbf{p}) = (v_{hj})$, with

$$v_{hj} = v_{jh} = p_h(1 - p_j)/n, \qquad 1 \leqslant h \leqslant j \leqslant m.$$

Now suppose that there are a total of K cumulative responses, with the kth response $(k = 1, \ldots, K)$ having m_k observation times. The model fitted separately to the treated and control data sets was a cumulative multinomial generalized linear model which, for the kth observation, can be written as

$$\boldsymbol{\eta}_k = g(\mathbf{p}_k) = \mathbf{X}_k \boldsymbol{\beta},$$

where $\eta_{kj} = g(p_{kj})$, $j = 1, \ldots, m_k$, with $g()$ representing the logit link function and $\boldsymbol{\beta}$ the $q \times 1$ vector of regression coefficients. With the logit link, we were assuming that the underlying response–time distribution and, for the treated data, the tolerance distribution at specified values of the other covariates, are logistic. In the $m_k \times q$ covariate matrix $\mathbf{X}_k$, for the rows corresponding to proportions within one tank, only those columns of the matrix corresponding to time-dependent covariates (observation time, possibly transformed, and any needed interaction terms with observation time) differed from row to row; the time-independent covariates (lake type, feeding practice, age of larvae, concentration, and any needed interaction terms among these covariates) were constant within tanks, and only differed for proportions corresponding to different tanks.

The maximum-likelihood equations for $\hat{\boldsymbol{\beta}}$, based on the observed cumulative proportions $\mathbf{r}_k$, follow from eqn. (5.16) of McCullagh and Nelder (1989, p. 172) and can be written as

$$\sum_{k=1}^{K}\left[\frac{\mathrm{d}\mathbf{p}_k}{\mathrm{d}\boldsymbol{\beta}^{\mathrm{T}}}\right]\mathbf{V}_k^{-1}\mathbf{S}_k = \sum_{k=1}^{K}\mathbf{X}_k^{\mathrm{T}}\left[\frac{\mathrm{d}\boldsymbol{\eta}_k}{\mathrm{d}\mathbf{p}_k^{\mathrm{T}}}\right]^{-1}\mathbf{V}_k^{-1}\mathbf{S}_k = \mathbf{0},$$

where $[\mathrm{d}\boldsymbol{\eta}_k/\mathrm{d}\mathbf{p}_k^{\mathrm{T}}]$ is an $m_k \times m_k$ diagonal matrix with diagonal elements $\mathrm{d}\eta_{kj}/\mathrm{d}p_{kj}$, $\mathbf{V}_k = \mathbf{V}(\mathbf{p}_k)$, and $\mathbf{S}_k = \mathbf{r}_k - \mathbf{p}_k$. Iterated re-weighted least squares (Green 1984; McCullagh and Nelder 1989, Section 2.5) can be used to solve for $\hat{\boldsymbol{\beta}}$. If we define

$$\mathbf{Z}_k = \mathbf{X}_k\hat{\boldsymbol{\beta}}^{(i)} + \left[\frac{\mathrm{d}\boldsymbol{\eta}_k}{\mathrm{d}\mathbf{p}_k^{\mathrm{T}}}\right]\mathbf{S}_k \quad \text{and} \quad \mathbf{W}_k = \left[\frac{\mathrm{d}\boldsymbol{\eta}_k}{\mathrm{d}\mathbf{p}_k^{\mathrm{T}}}\right]^{-1}\mathbf{V}_k^{-1}\left[\frac{\mathrm{d}\boldsymbol{\eta}_k}{\mathrm{d}\mathbf{p}_k^{\mathrm{T}}}\right]^{-1},$$

where the superscript (i) denotes the ith iteration and where $[\mathrm{d}\boldsymbol{\eta}_k/\mathrm{d}\mathbf{p}_k^{\mathrm{T}}]$, $\mathbf{S}_k$, and $\mathbf{V}_k$ are all evaluated at $\mathbf{p}_k^{(i)}$, then the iterative equations for estimating $\boldsymbol{\beta}$ are

$$\hat{\boldsymbol{\beta}}^{(i+1)} = \left(\sum_{k=1}^{K}\mathbf{X}_k^{\mathrm{T}}\mathbf{W}_k\mathbf{X}_k\right)^{-1}\sum_{k=1}^{K}\mathbf{X}_k^{\mathrm{T}}\mathbf{W}_k\mathbf{Z}_k.$$

If we assume that $[\mathrm{d}\boldsymbol{\eta}_k/\mathrm{d}\mathbf{p}_k^{\mathrm{T}}]$, $\mathbf{S}_k$, $\mathbf{W}_k$, and $\mathbf{V}_k$ are all evaluated at $\hat{\mathbf{p}}_k$, the estimated asymptotic covariance matrix of $\hat{\boldsymbol{\beta}}$ is then

$$\mathrm{Var}(\hat{\boldsymbol{\beta}}) = \left(\sum_{k=1}^{K}\mathbf{X}_k^{\mathrm{T}}\mathbf{W}_k\mathbf{X}_k\right)^{-1}.$$

Further details of the fitting procedure can be found in O'Hara Hines *et al.* (1992) or O'Hara Hines and Lawless (1993).

9.3.2 *Diagnostic checks*

Diagnostic tools for univariate generalized linear models have been developed by Pregibon (1981), Landwehr, Pregibon and Shoemaker (1984), Cook (1986), Williams (1987), and O'Hara Hines and Carter (1993). Diagnostics tools for the cumulative multinomial generalized linear model applied to grouped longitudinal mortality data are described in O'Hara Hines *et al.* (1992). In contrast

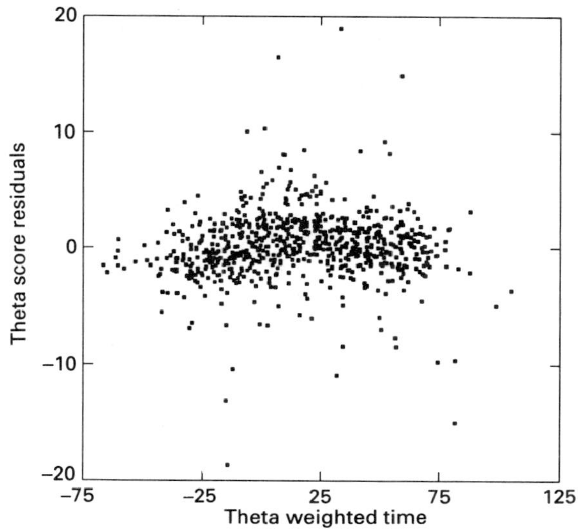

Fig. 9.1. Time-dependent covariate plot for observation time with the initial model for the treated data, a model with the covariates lake type, age of larvae, feeding practice, concentration, and observation time.

to that paper, in which the multinomial categories were inherently ordered, Lesaffre and Albert (1989) have extended the influence diagnostics of Williams and Pregibon to multiple-group logistic regression, using a multinomial generalized linear model in which the categories are not necessarily ordered.

The same fitting procedure was followed for both the treated and control data. The first model fitted to the data contained the covariates lake type (0 for Loken Lake, 1 for Lake Manitouwadge), feeding practice (0 for fed, 1 for starved), and linear terms in age of larvae, concentration (for the treated data only), and observation time. Diagnostics were then used to check the fit of the model. As usual, with diagnostic scatter plots, we were looking for very unusual points or signs of structure in what should be featureless plots. Often, when changes are made to a proposed model—for example, transforming a covariate—it helps to examine these diagnostics plots before and after the model change to see if the change has improved the scatter. Some of the plots included with this chapter are such pairs.

Residual plots to detect misspecification of time-dependent covariates indicated a slight amount of curvature for the covariate observation time in both the treated and control data (Figs. 9.1 and 9.2). (These plots involve a process termed 'theta weighting', which consists of transforming the score residuals and weighting and transforming the observation times in a manner which both compensates for the potentially high correlations among observations taken over time and does so with comparatively little of the unavoidable consequent distortion of the time axis; see O'Hara Hines *et al.* (1992). Logging time

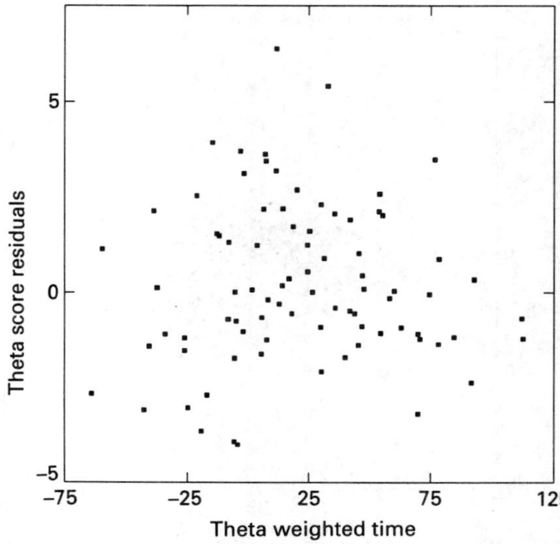

Fig. 9.2. A time-dependent covariate plot for observation time with the initial model for the control data, a model with the covariates lake type, age of larvae, feeding practice, and observation time.

provided a slightly better fit, as shown by the resulting time-dependent covariate plots (Figs. 9.3 and 9.4), and by the fact that the deviances and Pearson

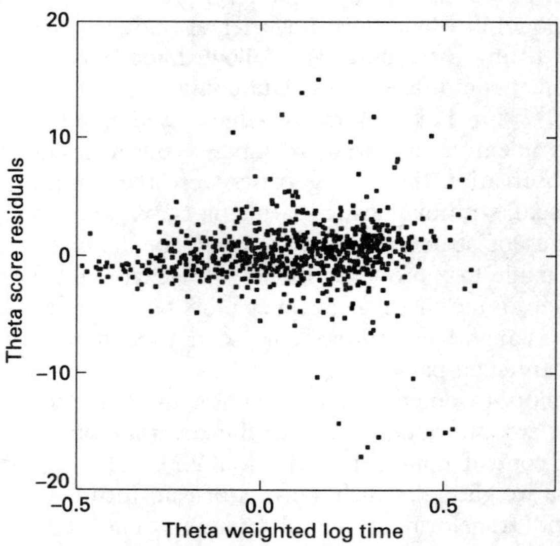

Fig. 9.3. A time-dependent covariate plot for log observation time with the initial model for the treated data, but with log observation time replacing observation time.

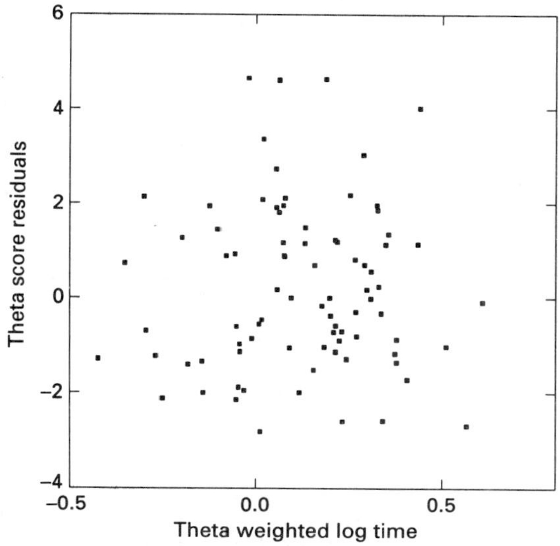

Fig. 9.4. A time-dependent covariate plot for log observation time with the final model for the control data, a model with the covariates lake type, age of larvae, feeding practice, and log observation time.

chi-squared values of the associated models were smaller with the logged time scale than with the raw time scale. (We do note that transformed treated data shown in Fig. 9.3 has more kurtosis than that for the untransformed treated data in Fig. 9.1.) In addition, our assessment that the use of log-time produces a somewhat better model is consistent with the common practice in toxicology of using that time scale.

Time-independent covariate plots, residual plots which check for the misspecification of time-independent covariates, indicated that neither the age of the larvae nor the concentration level needed to be transformed. (These time-independent covariate plots have one point per multinomial observation, called a constant-over-time component, which is the result of a linear combination of the cell residuals over time; see O'Hara Hines *et al.* (1992).) Often in this type of study, it is expected that the response is linearly related to the log of the concentration level rather than to concentration level itself; however, that is not true for this study. When log concentration is included in the model for the treated data, the time-independent plot showed a systematically poorer fit, indicating that concentration was better left unlogged. The time-independent plots indicated that two interaction terms between the time-independent covariates—lake-by-concentration and lake-by-feeding practice, both for the treated model—were needed. As can be seen from the plots for assessing the lake-by-concentration interaction, the pattern—a slightly negative trend—is weak (Fig. 9.5) but does appear to be less structured (i.e. more scattered) after the lake-by-concentration interaction term is added (Fig. 9.6). However, in contrast

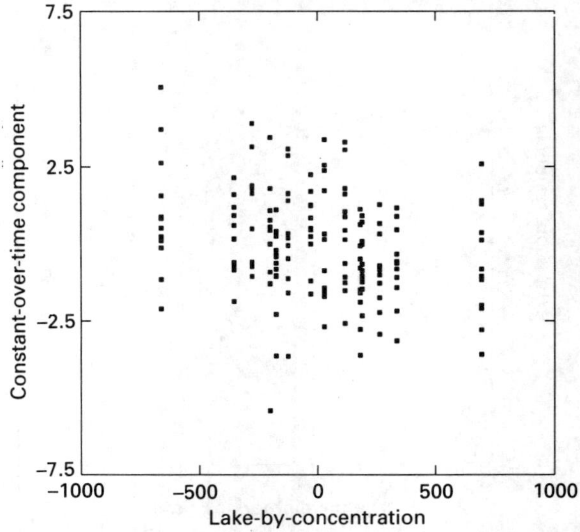

Fig. 9.5. A time-independent covariate plot for lake-by-concentration with the initial model for the treated data, but with log observation time replacing observation time.

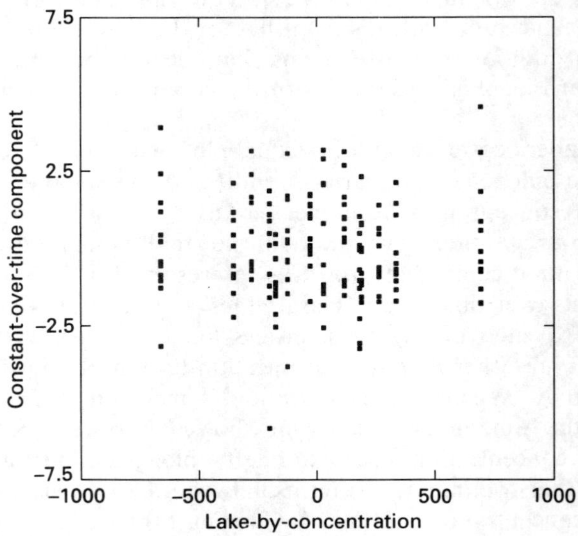

Fig. 9.6. A time-independent covariate plot for lake-by-concentration with the final model for the treated data, a model with the covariates lake type, age of larvae, feeding practice, concentration, lake-by-concentration, lake-by-feeding-practice, and log observation time.

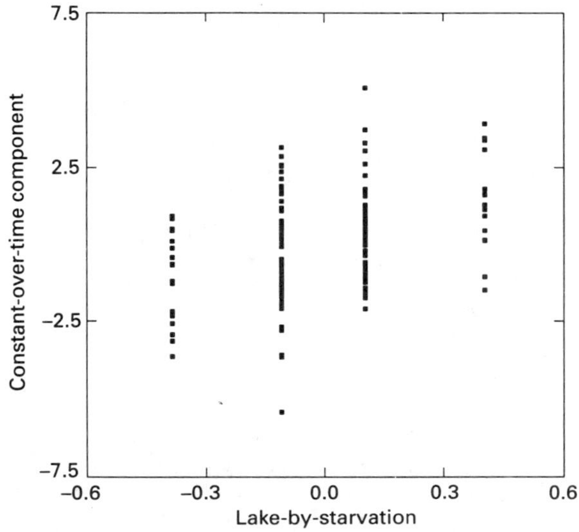

Fig. 9.7. A time-independent covariate plot for lake-by-starvation with the initial model for the treated data, but with log observation time replacing observation time.

to the slight suggestion given in the plots, examination of this term in the model indicates that it is significant at the 0.01 per cent level. We will see in the next section that this significance level is in fact overly small due to the presence of

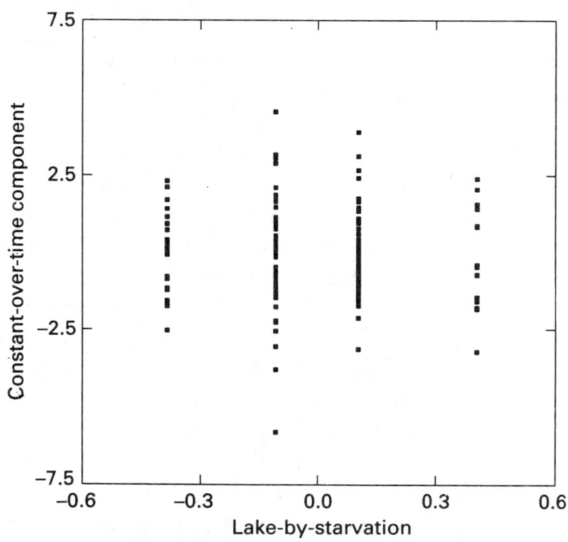

Fig. 9.8. A time-independent covariate plot for lake-by-starvation with the final model for the treated data.

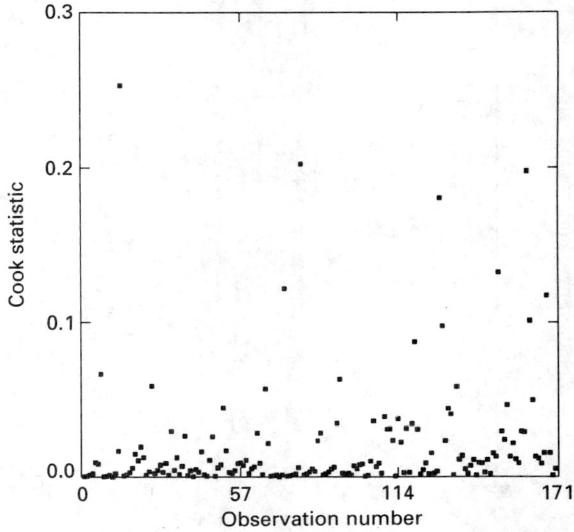

Fig. 9.9. A plot of the Cook statistic against observation number with the final model for the treated data.

extra-multinomial variation in the data. The plot for assessing the lake-by-feeding practice interaction term shows a stronger linear trend in residuals (Fig. 9.7), which disappears when that term is added to the model (Fig. 9.8). Plots that check for the need for interaction terms between time-independent and time-dependent covariates indicated that no such terms were required for either data set.

The next step was to examine the data for influential observations and outliers. A plot of the Cook statistic against observation number for each multinomial observation in the treated data set showed that there were no highly influential observations (Fig. 9.9). Further examination of three-dimensional plots showed, however, that there were associations among some of the observations with the larger values of the Cook statistic. In Fig. 9.10 is shown a plot of the Cook statistic for Lake Loken, broken down by age of larvae, feeding practice, and concentration, while Fig. 9.11 displays those for Lake Manitouwadge. The circles in these plots represent scaled values of the Cook statistic (times 15 plus 0.5, an *ad hoc* but effective choice). It can be seen from these plots that the observations for concentration 2200 at age 9 have some of the larger values of the Cook statistic. Plots of the observed logits of the cumulative probabilities against observation times (Figs. 9.12 and 9.13) show that, for concentration 2200, the mortalities for both lakes at age 9 are higher than those for age 13 and possibly age 17. This pattern led the toxicologists conducting the experiment to speculate that there was a non-monotone pattern in the LT_{50}s over age of larvae at this concentration (Munkittrick and Dixon 1989). Their results are based on a piecemeal analysis of the data, in which the

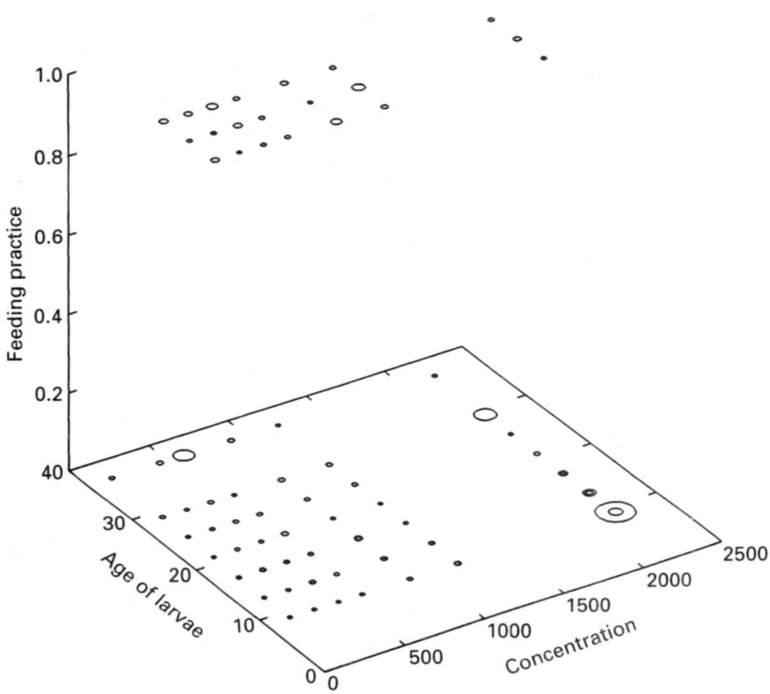

Fig. 9.10. A plot of the Cook statistic by age of larvae, concentration, and feeding practice for Loken Lake with the final model for the treated data. The circles represent the value of the Cook statistic scaled 15 times plus 0.5.

LT_{50}s were estimated separately for each treatment combination rather than from an overall model in which age of larvae is entered linearly, as we did in our analysis.

It should also be noted that their confidence intervals are estimated ignoring the correlation of observations over time and the possible overdispersion. In Table 9.1, the entries corresponding to the above-noted anomalies, other anomalies mentioned below, and the discrepancies between the replicate observations for ages 9–17 indicate that overdispersion is very probably present, making conclusions based on the assumption of independence quite suspect. Overdispersion provides a possible explanation for the observed non-monotone pattern over age at concentration 2200, a pattern which was not evident for any of the other treatment combinations. This suggests that the use of an overall model might be preferable to a piecemeal analysis of individual tanks. However, further investigation might be considered to be warranted to discover whether or not this phenomenon at concentration 2200 is real.

This data did exhibit a few other such non-monotone patterns, in particular for concentration. In Fig. 9.10 and 9.11 it is shown that, among the observations corresponding to the fed tanks at age 37, concentrations 450 and 600 have larger

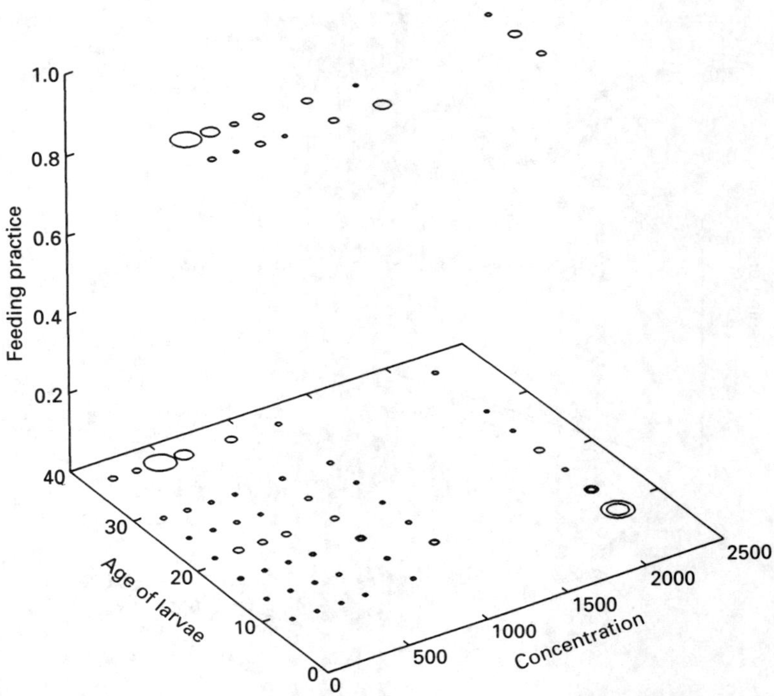

Fig. 9.11. A plot of the Cook statistic by age of larvae, concentration, and feeding practice for Lake Manigouwadge with the final model for the treated data. The circles represent the value of the Cook statistic scaled 15 times plus 0.5.

values of the Cook statistic. Further examination showed that mortality observations for Lake Manitouwadge at this age were higher for concentration 150 than those for concentration 450 and possibly 600 (Fig. 9.14). Additionally, the observations for Loken Lake at age 37 showed little difference between the mortalities for concentrations 600 and 1200 (Fig. 9.15). Another non-linearity is evident in Fig. 9.16, which shows that, for the starved tanks from Lake Manitouwadge at age 25, there is considerable overlap in the mortalities corresponding to concentrations 150–1200 corresponding to two more of the larger Cook statistic values apparent in Fig. 9.11. As discussed above, however, an increasing linear trend in mortalities over concentration fits the whole data set reasonably well and these non-increasing mortalities make little obvious sense biologically.

In Fig. 9.17 it is shown that in the control data set there is one possibly influential observation, number 13. Plots of a measure of coefficient sensitivity (change in estimated coefficient with single observation deletion; O'Hara Hines *et at*. 1992) indicate that observation number 13 influences the coefficient for the age of the larvae and, slightly, that for lake type. We removed observation number 13 (a tank which had lower mortalities at age 37 than that for the same

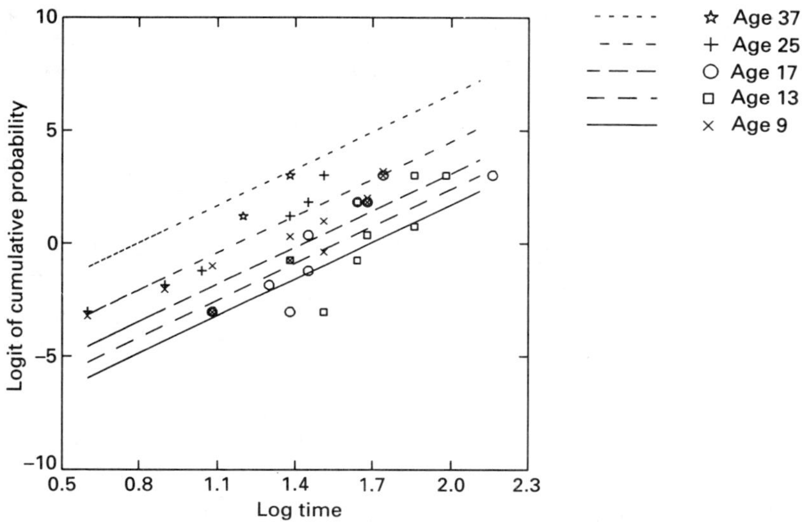

Fig. 9.12. A plot of the observed (point) and predicted (line) logits of cumulative mortalities against log observation time with the final model for the treated data: Loken Lake, concentration = 2200, fed.

lake, Lake Manitouwadge, at ages 21 and 29) and found that it lowered the predicted proportions by at most roughly 20 per cent for that same lake at age

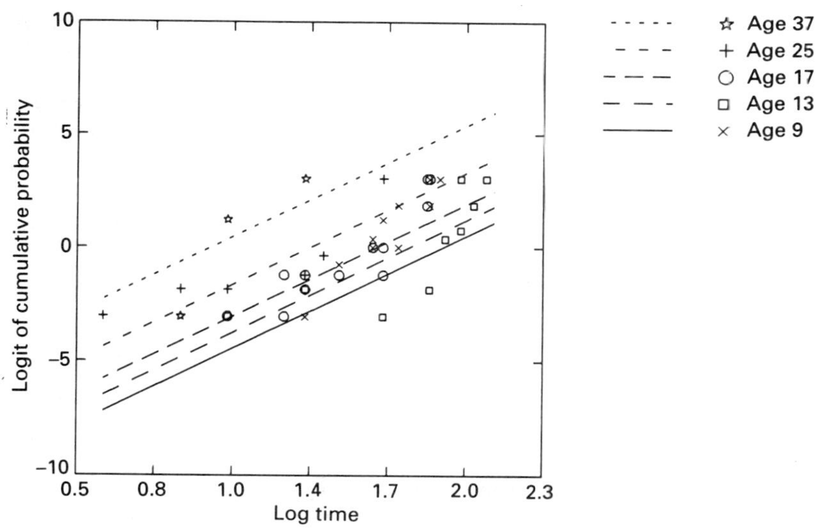

Fig. 9.13. A plot of the observed (point) and predicted (line) logits of cumulative mortalities against log observation time with the final model for the treated data: Lake Manitouwadge, concentration = 2200, fed.

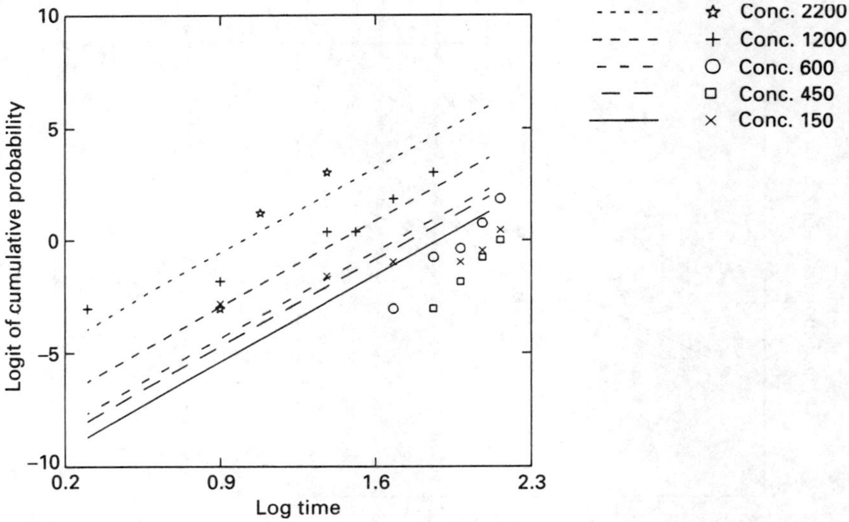

Fig. 9.14. A plot of the observed (point) and predicted (line) logits of cumulative mortalities against log observation time with the final model for the treated data: Lake Manitouwadge, age of larvae = 37, fed. Concentration is in μg Cu l^{-1}.

37. We also found that its removal had a negligible or very slight affect on estimated LT_{50}s, LC_{50}s, and their corresponding confidence intervals. Therefore, we decided to retain the observation in the data set. Finally, plots of the

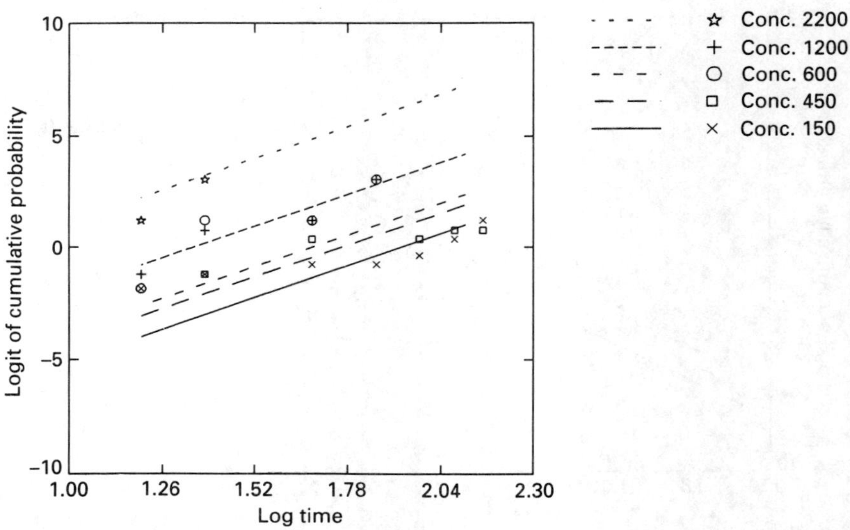

Fig. 9.15. A plot of the observed (point) and predicted (line) logits of cumulative mortalities against log observation time with the final model for the treated data: Loken Lake, age of larvae = 37, fed. Concentration is in μg Cu l^{-1}.

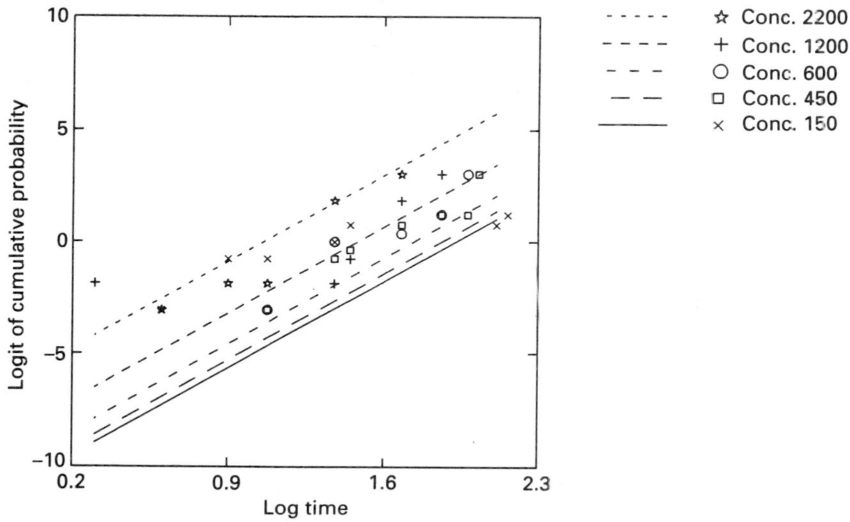

Fig. 9.16. A plot of the observed (point) and predicted (line) logits of cumulative mortalities against log observation time with the final model for the treated data: Lake Manitouwadge, age of larvae = 25, starved. Concentration is in μg Cu l^{-1}.

score residuals for each cell observation and the Pearson residuals for each multinomial observation indicated that there were no outliers in either data set.

At this point we felt that the models including effects for lake type, feeding practice, linear age of larvae, linear logged observation time plus linear concentration, lake-by-concentration, and lake-by-feeding practice for the treated data fitted the data sets fairly well. There was no longer any evidence of covariate misspecification and the data sets contained no outliers or highly influential observations. Yet there still remained strong evidence of lack of fit in both of the models. Assuming that proper randomization had been used in this designed experiment, we could attribute that lack of fit simply to overdispersion. (Some, hopefully small, part of this lack of fit is due to those few non-linearities discussed above. We should also note that the effect of the fed–starved condition may not be completely modelled, because we ignored the fact that the larvae were not fed over the 144 hours of tolerance testing. In addition, no matter how the fed–starved covariate is modelled, caution is advised when interpreting its effects because of its imbalance and censoring.)

The Pearson statistic divided by its degrees of freedom $M-q$, where M is the total number of non-redundant observations in the data set and q is the number of parameters in the fitted model, can be used as an indicator of overdispersion (McCullagh and Nelder 1989, Section 9.2). It has been shown for this type of data that when the covariates are correctly specified in the model, and when the multinomial distribution is used to generate the data, this overdispersion index has an expected value and a variance of approximately 1 and $2/(M-q)$, respectively (O'Hara Hines and Lawless 1993). The expectation of this index is

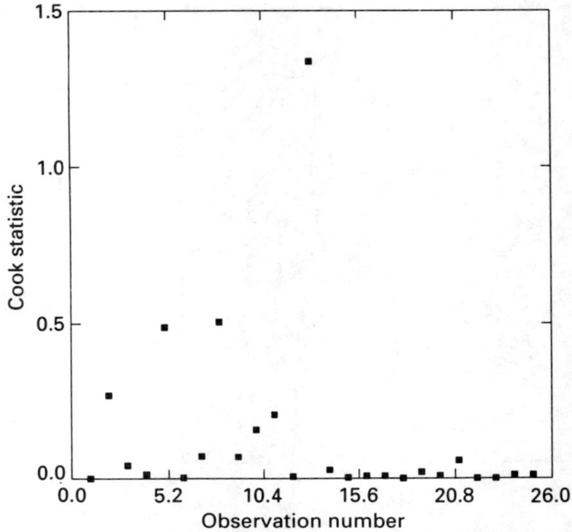

Fig. 9.17. A plot of the Cook statistic against observation number with the final model for the control data.

greater than 1 if overdispersion is present, if the mean specification of the model is incorrect, or both occur. The final fitted model for the control data had an overdispersion index of 3.0 with 87 degrees of freedom ($M = 92$, $q = 5$), while that for the treated data was 7.6 with 756 degrees of freedom ($M = 764$, $q = 8$). This, and the residual plots (Figs. 9.6 and 9.8), which failed to demonstrate the approximately unit variance expected under a multinomial model, indicated that overdispersion or extra-multinomial variation was present in the data.

9.3.3 *Analysis of overdispersion*

In studies in which groups of animals such as tanks of fish are the experimental units, it is not unusual to find that resulting proportions have extra-binomial or, in our case, extra-multinomial variation. This extra-multinomial variation or overdispersion, reflecting a correlation of observations within a tank, can be caused by the presence of tank-to-tank variation in addition to the treatment effects. Since overdispersion causes the observed effects of the covariates to appear excessively significant and estimated confidence intervals to be overly narrow, the toxicologist risks obtaining misleading information from the analysis unless it is taken into account. Williams (1982, 1988), Moore (1986, 1987), and Moore and Tsiatis (1991) have discussed moment methods for fitting data with extra-binomial variation. Liang and Zeger (1986), Zeger and Liang (1986), Prentice (1988), Zhao and Prentice (1990), Prentice and Zhao (1991), and Liang *et al.* (1992) have examined generalized estimating equations for regression parameter estimation and robust asymptotic covariance matrix estimation techniques. These can be applied to overdispersed multinomial data, as can some overdispersion models developed by O'Hara Hines and Lawless (1993), intended specifically for the type of grouped longitudinal mortality data that we are dealing with in this paper. One of the overdispersion models proposed by O'Hara Hines and Lawless (1993) allows for random shifts in the location of underlying response-time distribution, while another allows for random shifts both in the spread and in the location of the underlying response-time distribution. They also compared the resulting model-based asymptotic covariance estimators with the robust-asymptotic and Dirichlet-multinomial estimators. The Dirichlet-multinomial covariance structure was used by Petkau and Sitter (1989) in the analysis of a longitudinal fish mortality study in order to account for possible tank effects. The results of O'Hara Hines and Lawless (1993) indicate that, while the Dirichlet-multinomial covariance structure is not particularly suited to the type of grouped response time data that we are examining in this paper, the robust covariance estimators perform well on average, even when used in conjunction with the multinomial covariance structure. The robust covariance estimators, however, do prove more variable than the model-based estimators proposed by O'Hara Hines and Lawless. Breslow (1990) reaches a similar conclusion in the case of regression analysis of counts based on a Poisson model. An important point, noted by Breslow and deserving further study, is that hypothesis tests employing robust variance estimators have lower power, due to their larger variability, than ones using appropriate model-based variance estimators.

For the data being examined here, we used one of the overdispersion models developed in O'Hara Hines and Lawless (1993). The variance models presented in that paper are multivariate extensions of what is called Model III in Williams (1982). Since the covariate logged observation time is entered in a linear fashion in both the treated and control models, the most natural overdispersion model to use is one (such as Model 3 in O'Hara Hines and Lawless 1993) which allows for location shifts and scale changes in the underlying response-time distribution, thereby emulating simple tank effects. From Tables 9.2 and 9.3, we can see the changes in standard errors and significance levels for the covariates after accounting for overdispersion. In particular, once overdispersion was allowed for, the resulting significance level of the interaction term lake-by-concentration

Table 9.2. Coefficients (standard errors) for covariates in control model

Covariate	Adjusting for overdispersion: Before	After
Centred intercept	−1.911 (0.194)	−1.918 (0.291)
Lake type	1.373 (0.345)	1.219 (0.492)
Age of larvae	0.159 (0.024)	0.170 (0.033)
Feeding practice	1.378 (0.346)	1.302 (0.519)
Logged time	4.360 (0.542)	4.321 (0.923)

Table 9.3. Coefficients (standard errors) for covariates in treated model

Covariate	Adjusting for overdispersion	
	Before	After
Centred intercept	−1.261 (0.057)	−1.182 (0.109)
Lake type	0.203 (0.100)	0.172 (0.151)
Age of larvae ($\times 10^{-1}$)	1.860 (0.080)	1.748 (0.147)
Feeding practice	1.070 (0.119)	1.006 (0.192)
Concentration ($\times 10^{-3}$)	2.884 (0.106)	2.676 (0.239)
Lake by feeding practice	2.024 (0.236)	1.733 (0.376)
Lake by concentration ($\times 10^{-4}$)	−8.321 (1.489)	−7.223 (2.285)
Logged time	6.306 (0.199)	5.520 (0.593)

in the treated model indicated that it was not very important, in agreement with the impression given by the diagnostic plot (Fig. 9.5). We will also see below, when we examine estimated LT_{50}s and LC_{50}s and their corresponding confidence intervals that, in addition to the expected significance of concentration and log observation time, the age of the larvae also had a strong effect. Additionally, the fed larvae from Lake Manitouwadge showed a slightly greater tolerance to copper than those from Loken Lake; starvation, on the other hand, decreased the tolerance of the Lake Manitouwadge larvae compared to those from Loken Lake, which were apparently unaffected by starvation.

9.4 Adjusting for variable natural mortality

For experiments in which there is just a single measurement of natural mortality, Finney (1971) has outlined a method for adjusting for natural mortality. If the response due to natural mortality is considered to be independent of the response due to the toxicant, then the following probability statement relates the desired adjusted mortality (p), the observed mortality (p^*), and the natural mortality (c):

$$p^* = c + p(1 - c).$$

The adjusted mortality can then be written as

$$p = (p^* - c)/(1 - c) \tag{9.1}$$

and is commonly known as Abbott's formula (Finney 1971). This allows c to be included as an additional parameter in the model for p, with c and its standard error being estimated via maximum likelihood.

While we will also use eqn. (9.1) to adjust for natural mortality, we have to keep in mind for our study that c varies as a function of observation time and the other covariates used in the experiment. In particular, we assume a logistic response-time distribution for natural mortality the location and scale parameters of which depend on lake type, feeding practice, and age of larvae. Let the subscripts i, j, k, l, and t index lake type, age of larvae, feeding practice, concentration, and log observation time, respectively. Having previously fitted models for $\text{logit}(p^*_{ijklt})$ and $\text{logit}(c_{ijkt})$, we now want to estimate p_{ijklt}. More specifically, we want to estimate, for designated values of lake type, age of larvae, feeding practice, and log observation time, the concentration for which $p_{ijklt} = 0.5$ (i.e. the LC_{50} adjusted for natural mortality). Additionally, we want to estimate, for designated values of lake type, age of larvae, feeding practice, and concentration, the time for which $p_{ijklt} = 0.5$ (i.e. the LT_{50} adjusted for natural mortality). (Note that other quantiles can be obtained by replacing 0.5 in the equation $p_{ijklt} = 0.5$ by the desired fraction in a parallel formulation.)

Suppose first that we wish to estimate $LC_{50,\text{ADJ}}$ for a given lake type, age of larvae, feeding practice, and observation time. Let $\mathbf{x}_1$ be a $q_1 \times 1$ vector of the specified covariate values for lake type, age of larvae, feeding practice, and log observation time, with the value for concentration being replaced by the unknown quantity $LC_{50,\text{ADJ}}$, and let $\hat{\boldsymbol{\beta}}_1$ be the vector of estimated regression coefficients for the treated model with overdispersion. Furthermore, let $\mathbf{x}_2$ be a $q_2 \times 1$ vector containing the specified covariate values for lake type, age of larvae, feeding practice, and log observation time and let $\hat{\boldsymbol{\beta}}_2$ be the vector of estimated regression coefficients for the control model with overdispersion. Incorporating eqn. (9.1), we were able to develop, after some algebra, an estimating equation for the $LC_{50,\text{ADJ}}$:

$$m_{\text{CONC}}(LC_{50,\text{ADJ}}) = \mathbf{x}_1^{\mathrm{T}}\hat{\boldsymbol{\beta}}_1 - \text{logit}\left\{\tfrac{1}{2}\left(1 + \frac{\exp(\mathbf{x}_2^{\mathrm{T}}\hat{\boldsymbol{\beta}}_2)}{1+\exp(\mathbf{x}_2^{\mathrm{T}}\hat{\boldsymbol{\beta}}_2)}\right)\right\} = 0. \quad (9.2)$$

In contrast, if we are interested in estimating $LT_{50,\text{ADJ}}$, we now redefine $\mathbf{x}_1$ to be a $q_1 \times 1$ vector of the specified covariate values for lake type, age of larvae, feeding practice, and concentration, with the value for log observation time being replaced by the unknown quantity $\log LT_{50,\text{ADJ}}$ and redefine $\mathbf{x}_2$ to be a $q_2 \times 1$ vector containing the specified covariate values for lake type, age of larvae, and feeding practice, with the value for log observation time being replaced by the unknown quantity $\log LT_{50,\text{ADJ}}$. $\hat{\boldsymbol{\beta}}_1$ and $\hat{\boldsymbol{\beta}}_2$ are as defined in eqn. (9.2). Then the estimating equation developed for the $\log LT_{50,\text{ADJ}}$ is

$$m_{\text{CONC}}(\log LT_{50,\text{ADJ}}) = \mathbf{x}_1^{\mathrm{T}}\hat{\boldsymbol{\beta}}_1 - \text{logit}\left\{\tfrac{1}{2}\left(1 + \frac{\exp(\mathbf{x}_2^{\mathrm{T}}\hat{\boldsymbol{\beta}}_2)}{1+\exp(\mathbf{x}_2^{\mathrm{T}}\hat{\boldsymbol{\beta}}_2)}\right)\right\} = 0. \quad (9.3)$$

where, now, $\mathbf{x}_1$ and $\mathbf{x}_2$ both contain the quantity to be estimated, $\log LT_{50,\text{ADJ}}$.

The Newton–Raphson method can be used to solve eqns. (9.2) or (9.3). An initial estimate of the $LC_{50,\text{ADJ}}$ (or the $\log LT_{50,\text{ADJ}}$) can be obtained by using the first-order Taylor series expansion about $\mathbf{x}_2^{\mathrm{T}}\hat{\boldsymbol{\beta}}_2 = 0$,

$$\text{logit}\left\{\tfrac{1}{2}\left(1 + \frac{\exp(\mathbf{x}_2^{\mathrm{T}}\hat{\boldsymbol{\beta}}_2)}{1+\exp(\mathbf{x}_2^{\mathrm{T}}\hat{\boldsymbol{\beta}}_2)}\right)\right\} \approx \log(3) + \tfrac{2}{3}\,\mathbf{x}_2^{\mathrm{T}}\hat{\boldsymbol{\beta}}_2,$$

in eqn. (9.2) (or (9.3)) with the vector $\mathbf{x}_2$ defined appropriately.

The lower and upper values corresponding to a 95 per cent confidence interval for the estimated $LC_{50,ADJ}$ can be obtained by solving

$$m_{CONC}(LC_{50,ADJ}) \pm 2SE(m_{CONC}(LC_{50,ADJ})) = 0,$$

where

$$\begin{aligned}\mathrm{Var}(m_{CONC}(LC_{50,ADJ})) &= \mathbf{x}_1^T \mathrm{Cov}(\hat{\boldsymbol{\beta}}_1)\mathbf{x}_1 + \mathrm{Var}\left(\mathrm{logit}\left(\tfrac{1}{2}(1 + c_{ijkt})\right)\right) \\ &\approx \mathbf{x}_1^T \mathrm{Cov}(\hat{\boldsymbol{\beta}}_1)\mathbf{x}_1 + 4\frac{\mathbf{x}_2^T \mathrm{Cov}(\hat{\boldsymbol{\beta}}_2)\mathbf{x}_2}{\left(2 + \exp\left(-\mathbf{x}_2^T\hat{\boldsymbol{\beta}}_2\right)\right)^2},\end{aligned}$$

using a first order Taylor series expansion, and where the vectors $\mathbf{x}_1$ and $\mathbf{x}_2$ are as defined for eqn. (9.2). $\mathrm{Cov}(\hat{\boldsymbol{\beta}}_1)$ is the $q_1 \times q_1$ estimated overdispersed covariance matrix of the regression parameters for the treated model and $\mathrm{Cov}(\hat{\boldsymbol{\beta}}_2)$ is the $q_2 \times q_2$ estimated overdispersed covariance matrix of the regression parameters for the control model.

Similarly, confidence limits can be obtained for the estimated $\log LT_{50,ADJ}$.

In Tables 9.4 and 9.5 are shown estimated $LC_{50,ADJ}$s and $LT_{50,ADJ}$s and their corresponding 95 per cent confidence intervals for specified values of the other covariates. As mentioned before, it appears that age of the larvae and lake-by-feeding practice both affect the estimated $LC_{50,ADJ}$s and $LT_{50,ADJ}$s, and lake-by-concentration affects the estimated $LT_{50,ADJ}$s. In each case the adjustment used has assumed that the response due to the toxicant is independent of that due to natural mortality. The alternatives to that assumption, and their various implications, merit serious additional study.

Table 9.4. Estimated $LT_{50,ADJ}$s and 95 per cent confidence intervals (hours)

Lake[a]	Age	Feeding[b]	Concentration (μg Cu l^{-1})	$LT_{50,ADJ}$	Lower	Upper
L	13	F	1200	131	113	157
M	13	F	1200	174	144	242
L	13	F	2200	36	30	44
M	13	F	2200	61	50	77
L	29	F	1200	41	35	48
L	29	S	1200	42	33	57
M	29	F	1200	58	47	81
M	29	S	1200	30	19	41
L	29	F	2200	11	9	14
L	29	S	2200	11	8	14
M	29	F	2200	19	15	24
M	29	S	2200	9	6	12

[a] L = Loken Lake, M = Lake Manitouwadge.
[b] F = fed, S = starved.

Table 9.5. Estimated $LC_{50,ADJ}$s and 95 per cent confidence intervals (μg Cu l^{-1})

Lake[a]	Age	Feeding[b]	Concentration (μg Cu l^{-1})	$LT_{50,ADJ}$	Lower	Upper
L	13	F	96	1437	1329	1571
M	13	F	96	1750	1586	1973
L	13	F	144	1126	1014	1264
M	13	F	144	1367	1202	1584
L	29	F	96	612	478	753
L	29	S	96	746	516	994
M	29	F	96	860	623	1125
M	29	S	96	446	—	936
L	29	F	144	381	200	574
L	29	S	144	593	301	914
M	29	F	144	653	331	1014
M	29	S	144	312	—	901

[a] L = Loken Lake, M = Manitouwadge.
[b] F = fed, S = starved.
—, The value could not be estimated.

9.5 Summary

The analysis of grouped longitudinal mortality data presents a variety of challenges to the researcher: correlations among individuals in groups and among observations over time in the same group must be allowed for; adequacies of fitted models explored; and natural or control mortality adjusted for. Such issues concerned David Williams, and his influence is present in several of the techniques described in this chapter and elsewhere. The particular diagnostic tools used to check the goodness of fit of the control, and treated models fitted to the data sets are described further in O'Hara Hines *et al.* (1992); the method used to account for overdispersion is detailed in O'Hara Hines and Lawless (1993). Our intent here has been to describe and illustrate the use of a collection of analytical tools for studying grouped longitudinal mortality data sets, as well as to present a method for adjusting for natural mortality.

The approach used in this chapter has focused on relating a particular population's response to various independent variables, including time. A referee has questioned whether the results obtained by this approach are consistent with those from the simpler analyses that would result if, for example, cumulative mortality counts for, say, 144 hours only had been analyzed. While we agree wholeheartedly that models fitted should be assessed critically, we prefer to compare the model's predictions directly with the initial data rather than with summaries of the data such as conditional fitted models. While we recognize the intuitive attractiveness of the proposed conditional approach, we worry about the proper inferences from and our responses to an apparent mismatch between the two methods: Do we alter the time at which cumulative mortality was considered from 144 hours to some other time and try to model again? Do we worry if the form of conditional model which works well for one condition is inferior to another model under another condition? How do we reconcile models fitted under different conditions? Since the various diagnostic methods did not indicate any serious problems, we are comfortable with the multinomial models fitted over time, and recall that we have seen in Section 9.3 that piecemeal analyses can result in unexplainable anomalies. Fitting separate models for each observation time might be a more reasonable approach, however, when diagnostics indicate the impracticability of a single overall model.

The unified approach presented here has the obvious advantages that it provides a common model as the various covariates such as time vary, and it allows us to estimate a parameter of interest to toxicologists, the LT_{50}, which would not be possible if the data were analysed separately for each observation time. Additionally, the precision obtained for a given set of circumstances is enhanced by information obtained under different but similar circumstances. (Pack and Morgan (1990) and Kronlund (1988, unpublished Master's thesis, University of Guelph), for example, note a reduction in confidence interval width when unconditional fits are used rather than conditional ones.)

Acknowledgements

The authors thank Kelly Munkittrick of the Department of Fisheries and Oceans, Burlington, Ontario, Canada and George Dixon of the Department of Biology, University of Waterloo, Ontario, Canada for making the data available, and for some subsequent discussions.

References

Aranda-Ordaz, F. J. (1983). An extension of the proportional-hazards model for grouped data. *Biometrics*, **39**, 109–18.

Boyce, C. B. C. and Williams, D. A. (1967). The influence of exposure time on the susceptibility of *Australorbis glabratus* to *N*-tritylmorpholine. *Annals of Tropical Medicine and Parasitology*, **61**, 15–20.

Breslow, N. E. (1990). Tests of hypotheses in overdispersed Poisson regression and other quasi-likelihood models. *Journal of the American Statistical Association*, **85**, 565–71.

Cook, R. D. (1986). Assessment of local influence (with discussion). *Journal of the Royal Statistical Society, Series B*, **48**, 133–69.

Farewell, V. T. (1982). The use of mixture models for the analysis of survival data with long-term survivors. *Biometrics*, **38**, 1041–6.

Finkelstein, D. M. (1986). A proportional hazards model for interval-censored failure time data. *Biometrics*, **42**, 845–54.

Finney, D. J. (1971). *Probit analysis*, 3rd edn., Ch. 7. Cambridge University Press, Cambridge.

Green, P. J. (1984). Iteratively reweighted least squares for maximum likelihood estimation, and some robust and resistant alternatives (with discussion). *Journal of the Royal Statistical Society, Series B*, **46**, 149–92.

Landwehr, J. M., Pregibon, D., and Shoemaker, A. C. (1984). Graphical methods for assessing logistic regression models. *Journal of the American Statistical Association*, **79**, 61–83.

Lawless, J. F. (1982). *Statistical Models and Methods for Lifetime Data*, Section 7.3. John Wiley, New York.

Lesaffre, E. and Albert, A. (1989). Multiple-group logistic regression diagnostics. *Applied Statistics*, **38**, 425–40.

Liang, K.-Y. and Zeger, S. L. (1986). Longitudinal data analysis using generalized linear models. *Biometrika*, **73**, 13–22.

Liang, K.-Y. Zeger, S. L., and Qaqish, B. (1992). Multivariate regression analysis for categorical data (with discussion). *Journal of the Royal Statistical Society, Series B*, **54**, 3–40.

McCullagh, P. (1980). Regression models for ordinal data (with discussion). *Journal of the Royal Statistical Society, Series B*, **42**, 109–42.

McCullagh, P. and Nelder, J. A. (1989). *Generalized linear models*, 2nd edn., Ch. 5 and Section 9.2. Chapman and Hall, London.

Moore, D. F. (1986). Asymptotic properties of moment estimators for overdispersed counts and proportions. *Biometrika*, **73**, 583–8.

Moore, D. F. (1987). Modelling the extraneous variance in the presence of extra-binomial variation. *Applied Statistics*, **36**, 8–14.

Moore, D. F. and Tsiatis, A. (1991). Robust estimation of the variance in moment methods for extra-binomial and extra-poisson variation. *Biometrics*, **47**, 383–401.

Munkittrick, K. R. and Dixon, D. G. (1989). Effects of natural exposure to copper and zinc on egg size and larval copper tolerance in white sucker (*Catostomus commersoni*). *Ecotoxicology and Environmental Safety*, **18**, 15–26.

O'Hara Hines, R. J. and Carter, E. M. (1993). Improved added variable and partial residual plots for the detection of influential observations in generalized linear models. *Applied Statistics*, **42**, 3–20.

O'Hara Hines, R. J. and Hines, W. G. S. (1992). On selecting sample sizes and discrete observation times for longitudinal mortality studies. *Environmetrics*, **3**, 377–95.

O'Hara Hines, R. J. and Lawless, J. F. (1993). Modelling overdispersion in toxicological mortality data grouped over time. *Biometrics*, **49**, 107–21.

O'Hara Hines, R. J., Lawless, J. F., and Carter, E. M. (1992). Diagnostics for a multinomial generalized linear model, with applications to grouped toxicological mortality data. *Journal of the American Statistical Association*, **87**, 1059–69.

Pack, S. E. and Morgan, B. J. T. (1990). A mixture model for interval-censored time-to-response quantal assay data. *Biometrics*, **46**, 749–57.

Petkau, A. J. and Sitter, R. R. (1989). Models for quantal response experiments over time. *Biometrics*, **45**, 1299–307.

Pierce, D. A., Stewart, W. H., and Kopecky, K. J. (1979). Distribution-free regression analysis of grouped survival data. *Biometrics*, **35**, 785–93.

Pregibon, D. (1981). Logistic regression diagnostics. *Annals of Statistics*, **9**, 705–24.

Preisler, H. K. (1989). Analysis of a toxicological experiment using a generalized linear model with nested random effects. *International Statistical Review*, **57**, 145–59.

Prentice, R. L. (1988). Correlated binary regression with covariates specific to each binary observation. *Biometrics*, **44**, 1033–48.

Prentice, R. L. and Gloeckler, L. A. (1978). Regression analysis of grouped survival data with application to breast cancer. *Biometrics*, **34**, 57–67.

Prentice, R. L. and Zhao, L. P. (1991). Estimating equations for parameters in means and covariances of multivariate discrete and continuous responses. *Biometrics*, **47**, 825–39.

Tibshirani, R. J. and Ciampi, A. (1983). A family of proportional- and additive-hazards models for survival data. *Biometrics*, **39**, 141–7.

Williams, D. A. (1982). Extra-binomial variation in linear logistic models. *Applied Statistics*, **31**, 144–8.

Williams, D. A. (1986). Interval estimation of the median lethal dose. *Biometrics*, **42**, 641–5.

Williams, D. A. (1987). Generalized linear model diagnostics using the deviance and single case deletions. *Applied Statistics*, **36**, 181–91.

Williams, D. A. (1988). Extra-binomial variation in toxicology. Presented at the International Biometrics Conference meetings in Namur, Belgium.

Zeger, S. L. and Liang, K.-Y. (1986). Longitudinal data analysis for discrete and continuous outcomes. *Biometrics*, **44**, 1049–60.

Zhao, L. P. and Prentice, R. L. (1990). Correlated binary regression using a quadratic exponential model. *Biometrika*, **77**, 642–8.

10 Statistical evaluation of the fixed-dose procedure

A. WHITEHEAD AND R. N. CURNOW

10.1 Introduction

The generally accepted method for assessing the acute oral toxicity of a substance has, until recently, been the LD_{50} study. In such a study, groups of laboratory animals, often rats, are given a range of dose levels of the substance, with the dose levels chosen to span the 'expected' median lethal dose (LD_{50}). The internationally agreed guideline published by the Organization for Economic Co-operation and Development (OECD 1981) recommended that ten rats (five male and five female) be tested at each of a minimum of three dose levels. In 1987 the revised guideline (OECD 1987) reduced the recommended total number of animals to 20. In addition, the highest permitted test dose was reduced from 5000 mg/kg body weight to 2000 mg/kg body weight. From such a study it should be possible to estimate the LD_{50} and calculate a confidence interval, provided that mortality is seen at or below the highest test dose.

In the European Community the classification of substances according to their toxic hazard is based on the LD_{50} estimate. According to the Commission of the European Communities (1983), Council Directive 83/467/EEC, the classification is as follows: LD_{50} less than 25 mg/kg body weight, very toxic; 25–200, toxic; 200–2000, harmful; substances with an LD_{50} greater than 2000 mg/kg body weight are termed 'unclassified'.

The LD_{50} study has been criticized from both a scientific and ethical viewpoint (Zbinden and Flury-Roversi 1981), but it is still felt that some testing in animals is necessary in order to classify substances according to their toxic hazard. In 1984, the British Toxicology Society proposed a new type of study based on a fixed-dose procedure (FDP) (British Toxicology Society 1984). The intention was to rely on the observation of evident signs of toxicity at one of a series of fixed dose levels. It was claimed that the dose level at which toxic signs were detected could be used to classify substances rather than the LD_{50}. The lower and therefore sublethal doses prescribed by the procedure would tend to reduce the severity of toxic signs in addition to the reduction in mortality. In addition, it was felt that if the procedure was carefully conducted, the number of animals tested could be reduced to as few as ten.

The objective of this chapter is to present a statistical evaluation of the FDP. We attempt to find a suitable mathematical model to describe the procedure and investigate the effect of the starting dose on the toxic classification of a substance. The classification based on the FDP is compared with that based on the LD_{50}, and the results from an international validation study of the FDP (van den Heuvel *et al.* 1990) are compared with the results predicted from our mathematical model. The expected numbers of animals that will be tested, show toxic effects and die using the FDP are presented.

10.2 The fixed-dose procedure (FDP)

The version of the procedure that we have considered is described by van den Heuvel *et al.* (1990) and is as follows. Ten animals (five female and five male) are to be tested at each dose level that is investigated. The dose levels available to be used in the test are 5, 50, 500, or 2000 mg/kg body weight. The initial dose level chosen should be that which is judged likely to produce evident toxicity but

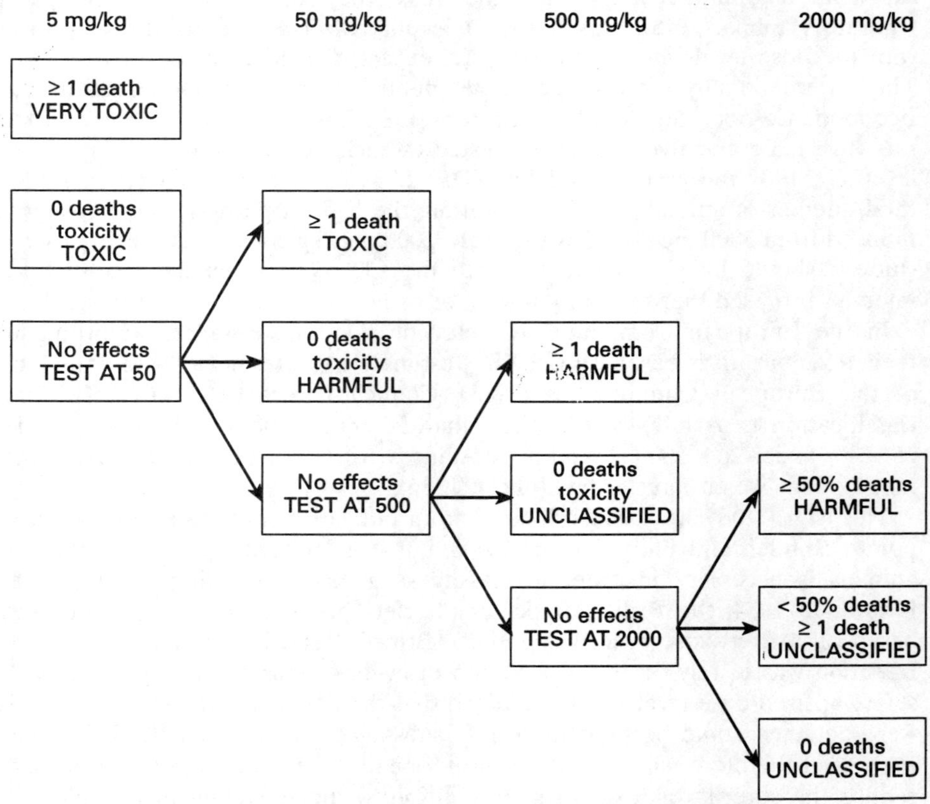

Fig. 10.1. FDP pathways from a starting dose of 5 mg/kg.

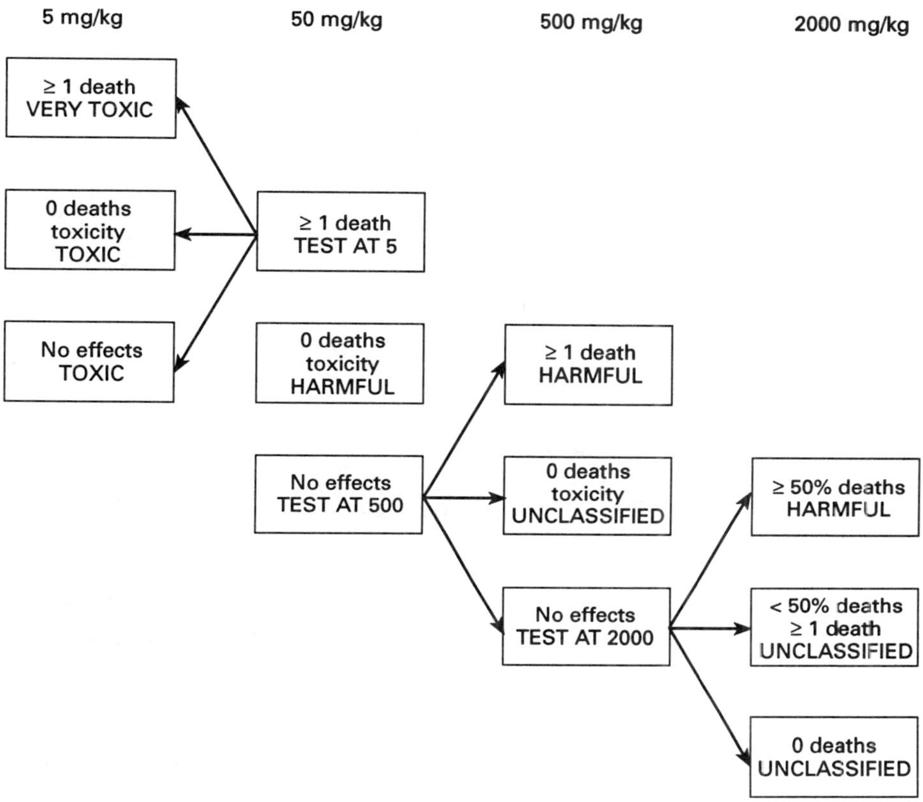

Fig. 10.2. FDP pathways from a starting dose of 50 mg/kg.

no mortality. When no information is available upon which to make such a judgement, an initial 'sighting' study should normally be carried out. Where evident toxicity does not result from administration of the chosen dose level, the substance should be re-tested at the next higher dose level. If a severe toxic reaction occurs requiring a humane kill, or if death occurs, the substance should be retested at the next lower dose level. Evident toxicity is a general term describing clear signs of compound-related toxicity, but not such as to cause very severe pain, distress or mortality.

In Figs. 10.1–10.4 are shown, for the four possible starting doses, the possible routes that would be taken by the toxicologist, based on the results of the tests at the dose levels used. Also included are the toxic classifications based on the results. For each of the dose levels, 5, 50, and 500 mg/kg body weight, there are three outcomes, which result in different actions regarding the substance (i.e. one or more deaths; no deaths but one or more animals suffering toxicity; no deaths and no toxicity). However, if the substance is tested at 2000 mg/kg, the three outcomes resulting in different actions are (50 per cent or more deaths; at least one death but less than 50 per cent mortality; no mortality). This does lead to one inconsistency for substances tested at 500 mg/kg; if the result is no

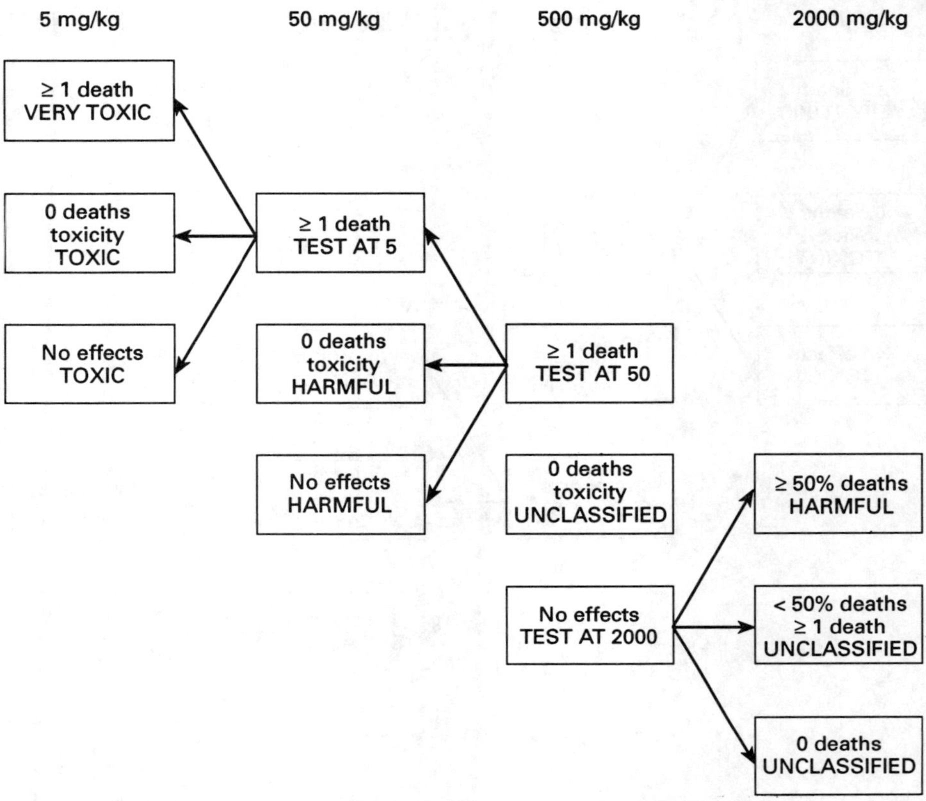

Fig. 10.3. FDP pathways from a starting dose of 500 mg/kg.

deaths and some toxicity, the substance would be unclassified; however, if at 500 there were no deaths or toxicity, the substance may be classified as harmful when tested at 2000, albeit only in the unlikely event that 50 per cent or more of the animals die at that dose.

10.3 Modelling the FDP

At each dose level tested, results will be available from ten animals. Each animal can be categorized into one of three groups (i.e. dead; showing signs of toxicity; unaffected) provided that there is reasonable agreement about what constitutes a toxic sign. In order to model the FDP we need dose–response relationships for death and for death or toxicity. Inevitably, there is a lack of data on the dose–response relationship for toxicity, but if death can be considered as an extreme form of toxicity it is perhaps not unreasonable to propose parallel sigmoid-shaped curves for toxicity and death, as illustrated in Fig. 10.5, and this is what has been assumed. Let $p_1(x)$, $p_2(x)$ and $p_3(x)$ denote the respective probabilities that an animal dies, remains alive but shows signs of

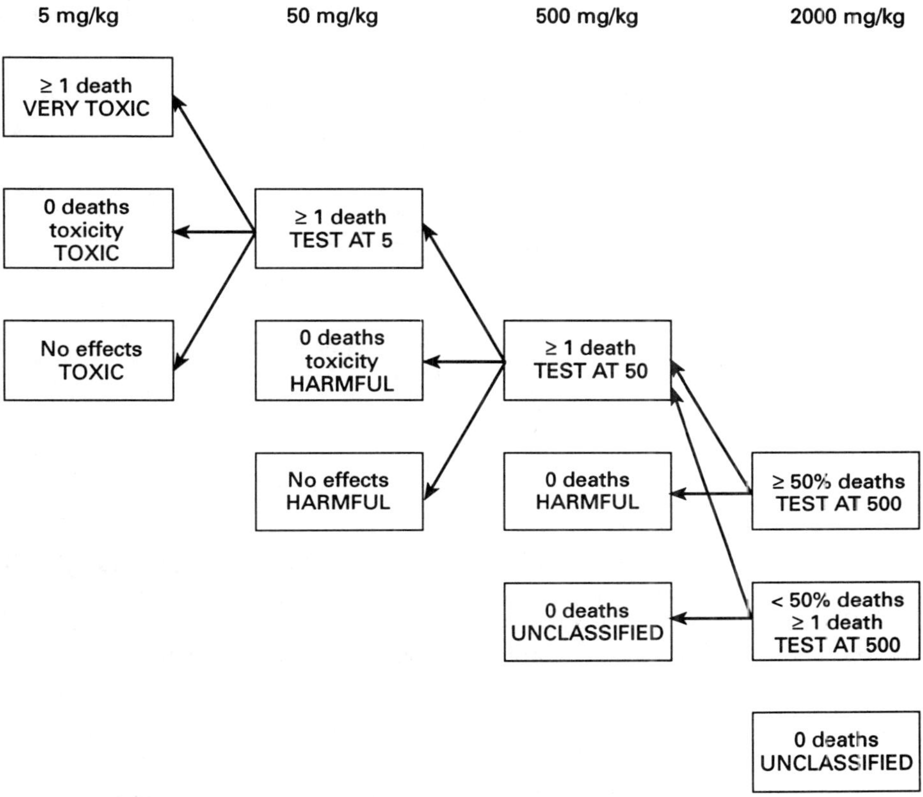

Fig. 10.4. FDP pathways from a starting dose of 2000 mg/kg.

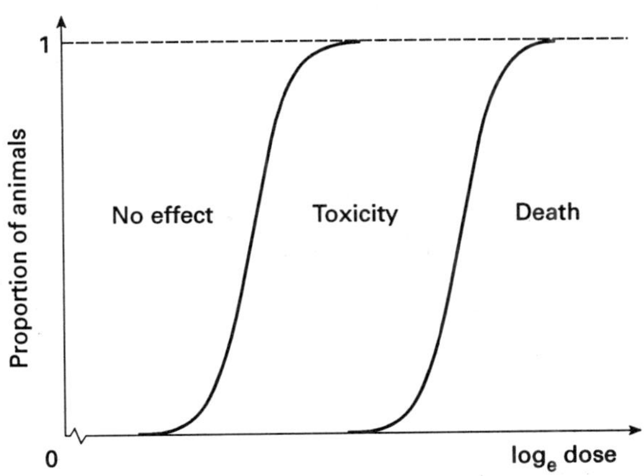

Fig. 10.5. Dose–response relationships for death and for toxicity or death: the proportion of animals showing an effect against $\log_e$ dose.

toxicity, and is unaffected by dose x of a substance. The dose–response relationships can then be expressed in the form

$$\text{logit}(p_1(x)) = \alpha + \beta \log_e x, \tag{10.1}$$

$$\text{logit}(p_1(x) + p_2(x)) = \alpha' + \beta \log_e x, \tag{10.2}$$

where

$$\text{logit}(p_1(x)) = \log_e\left[\frac{p_1(x)}{1 - p_1(x)}\right]$$

and

$$\text{logit}(p_1(x) + p_2(x)) = \log_e\left[\frac{p_1(x) + p_2(x)}{1 - p_1(x) - p_2(x)}\right]$$

$$= \log_e\left[\frac{1 - p_3(x)}{p_3(x)}\right].$$

Each particular substance has three parameters associated with it, namely α, α', and β. We can, however, reassign the parameters in terms of β, the $LD_{50}(l)$, and the factor (R) by which the dose needs to be increased in order to equate eqns. (10.1) and (10.2). (R would be a relative potency if eqns. (10.1) and (10.2) represented two different substances: see Fig. 10.6.) We note that

$$\log_e l = -\frac{\alpha}{\beta} \quad \text{and} \quad \log_e R = \frac{(\alpha' - \alpha)}{\beta}.$$

Consequently, for a substance with a given slope, LD_{50}, and R, the probability of getting a particular outcome from a test of ten animals at a fixed dose, x, can be calculated. There are five such probabilities that need to be calculated:

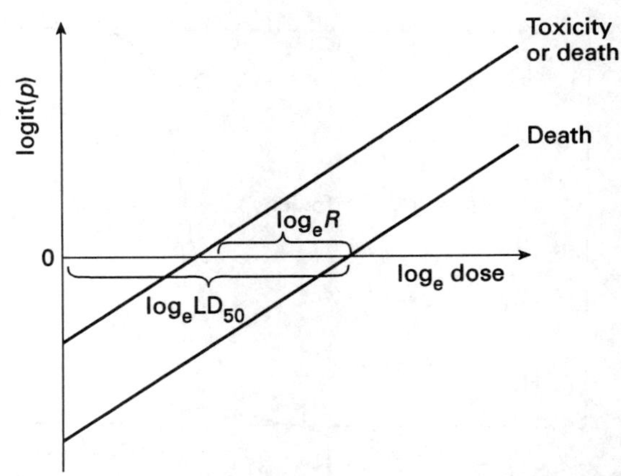

Fig. 10.6. Dose–response relationships for death and for toxicity or death: the proportion of animals showing an effect (logit transformation) against $\log_e$ dose.

1. $P(\geqslant 1 \text{ death}) = 1 - (1 - p_1(x))^{10} = d(x)$.
2. $P(\geqslant 50 \text{ per cent deaths}) = \sum_{j=5}^{10} \begin{bmatrix} 10 \\ j \end{bmatrix} p_1(x)^j (1 - p_1(x))^{10-j} = d_1(x)$.
3. $P(< 50 \text{ per cent deaths, but } \geqslant 1 \text{ death}) = \sum_{j=1}^{4} \begin{bmatrix} 10 \\ j \end{bmatrix} p_1(x)^j (1 - p_1(x))^{10-j} = d_2(x)$.
4. $P(\text{no effects}) = (p_3(x))^{10} = n(x)$.
5. $P(\text{some toxicity, no deaths}) = 1 - d(x) - n(x) = t(x)$.

The probabilities of following particular routes (Figs. 10.1–10.4) through the FDP can be calculated in terms of $d(x)$, $d_1(x)$, $d_2(x)$, $n(x)$, and $t(x)$.

The probability that a substance will be classified as very toxic, toxic, harmful, or unclassified will depend on the starting dose, as shown in Table 10.1. For substances that are likely to produce toxic effects but no mortality at two or more of the fixed dose levels, that starting dose will be important to the toxic classification. These substances will be characterized by shallow slopes and/or a high value of R. Classification probabilities were calculated for each of the four starting doses using R equal to 50, for a range of slopes from 1 to 15 in steps of 0.25 and a range of LD_{50} values from 4 to 8100 ($\log_e LD_{50}$ from 1.4 to 9 in steps

Table 10.1. Classification probabilities for each starting dose in the FDP

Classification	Starting dose (mg/kg body weight)	Probability of classification
Very toxic	5	$d(5)$
	50	$d(50) \times d(5)$
	500	$d(500) \times d(50) \times d(5)$
	2000	$d(2000) \times d(500) \times d(50) \times d(5)$
Toxic	5	$t(5) + n(5) \times d(50)$
	50	$d(50) \times (1 - d(5))$
	500	$d(500) \times d(50) \times (1 - d(5))$
	2000	$d(2000) \times d(500) \times d(50) \times (1 - d(5))$
Harmful	5	$n(5) \times (t(50) + n(50) \times d(500) + n(50) \times n(500) \times d_1(2000))$
	50	$t(50) + n(50) \times d(500) + n(50) \times n(500) \times d_1(2000)$
	500	$d(500) \times (1 - d(50)) + n(500) \times d_1(2000)$
	2000	$d(2000) \times d(500) \times (1 - d(50)) + d_1(2000) \times (1 - d(500)$
Unclassified	5	$n(5) \times n(50) \times [t(500) + n(500) \times (1 - d_1(2000))]$
	50	$n(50) \times [t(500 + n(500) \times (1 - d_1(2000))]$
	500	$t(500) + n(500) \times (1 - d_1(2000))$
	2000	$(1 - d(2000)) + d_2(2000) \times (1 - d(500))$

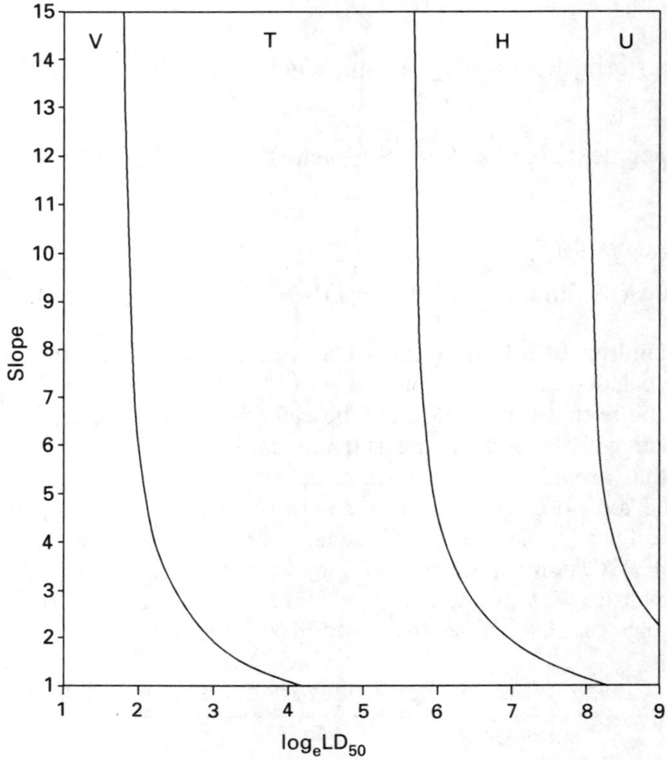

Fig. 10.7. Toxic classification with the highest probability for $R = 50$; starting dose = 5 mg/kg. V = very toxic, T = toxic, H = harmful, U = unclassified.

of 0.1). The classification with the highest probability was recorded for each set of values and freehand curves drawn where the classification with the highest probability changed (see Figs. 10.7–10.10 for each starting dose separately).

Generally speaking, the higher the starting dose used the more likely it is that the substance will be classified as less toxic, although if the dose of 2000 mg/kg body weight is used this may not be the case. It is thought, therefore, that companies will choose the highest dose expected to give toxicity with only a small chance of mortality. In reality, the toxicologist will have prior information about a substance, either because it is similar to other tested compounds or from earlier work with the substance. The next stage is to try to incorporate this into our model.

10.4 Choice of starting dose

We shall assume that we have information about a substance equivalent to having carried out the sighting study recommended for use in the international

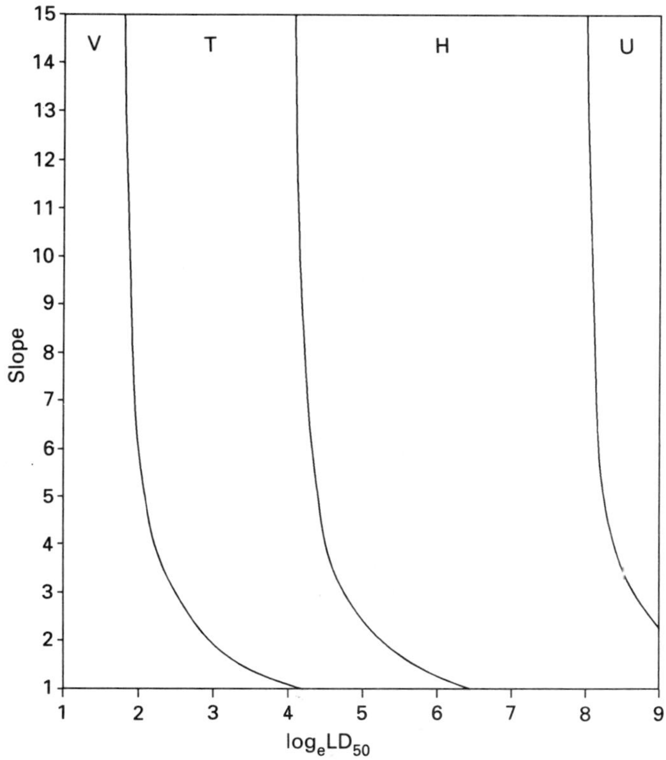

Fig. 10.8. Toxic classification with the highest probability for $R = 50$; starting dose = 50 mg/kg. V = very toxic, T = toxic, H = harmful, U = unclassified.

validation study of the FDP. Major toxicological laboratories in 11 countries were involved in this study. Each laboratory was asked to conduct the FDP on the same 20 substances, which included industrial chemicals and pesticides spanning the full range from very toxic to relatively innocuous. The study was to be conducted 'blind', in that laboratories had no indications as to the toxicity of a test substance. It was, therefore, suggested that before the main test a sighting study be carried out in order to select the starting dose for the main test.

The sighting study consisted of taking three groups of one male and one female rat. One pair received 5, one pair 50, and one pair 500 mg of the test substance per kg of body weight. The dose level that resulted in evident toxicity but no mortality was identified. If evident toxicity was not seen at 500 mg/kg body weight, the dose to be used in the main test was 2000 mg/kg body weight.

There are six possible results from the two animals at one particular dose level (Table 10.2), giving a total of $6^3 = 216$ different sets of results taking all three doses into consideration. We can associate every possible outcome from the sighting study with a starting dose for the FDP, and this is shown in Table 10.3.

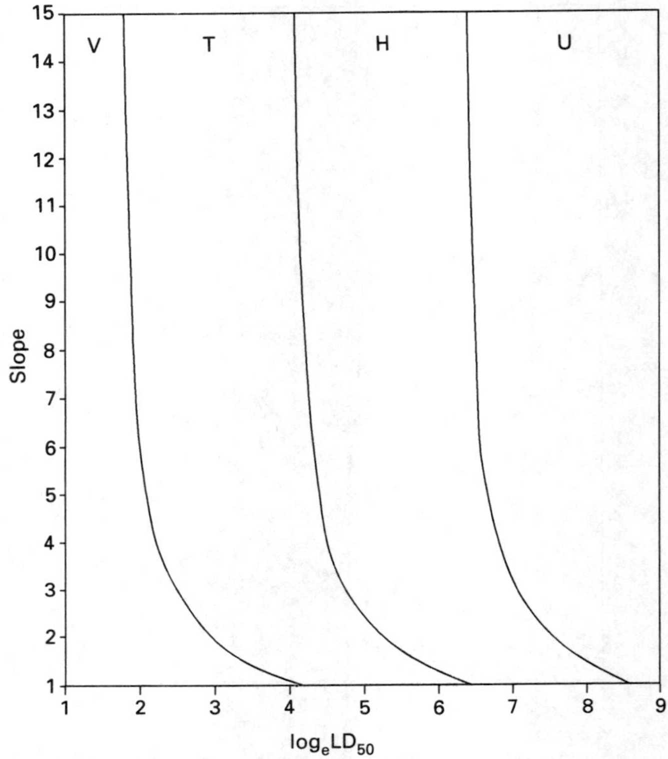

Fig. 10.9. Toxic classification with the highest probability for R = 50; starting dose = 500 mg/kg. V = very toxic, T = toxic, H = harmful, U = unclassified.

Thus, the probability that the starting dose for a substance is 5, 50, 500, or 2000 mg/kg can be calculated as follows:

$$P(\text{choose } 5) = 1 - [1 - p_1(5)]^2 + [1 - p_1(5)]^2\{1 - [1 - p_1(50)]^2\},$$

$$P(\text{choose } 500) = [1 - p_1(5)]^2[1 - p_1(50)]^2\{[1 - p_1(500)]^2 - [p_3(500)]^2\},$$

$$P(\text{choose } 2000) = [p_3(5)]^2[p_3(50)]^2[p_3(500)]^2,$$

$$P(\text{choose } 50) = 1 - P(\text{choose } 5) - P(\text{choose } 500) - P(\text{choose } 2000).$$

Assuming that the sighting study is not an integral part of the FDP but just provides the starting dose for the procedure, we can calculate the probability that a substance is classified as very toxic by the FDP as follows:

$$P(\text{classify very toxic}) = \sum_{x=5,50,500,2000} [P(\text{classify very toxic given starting dose } x) \times P(\text{choose starting dose } x)].$$

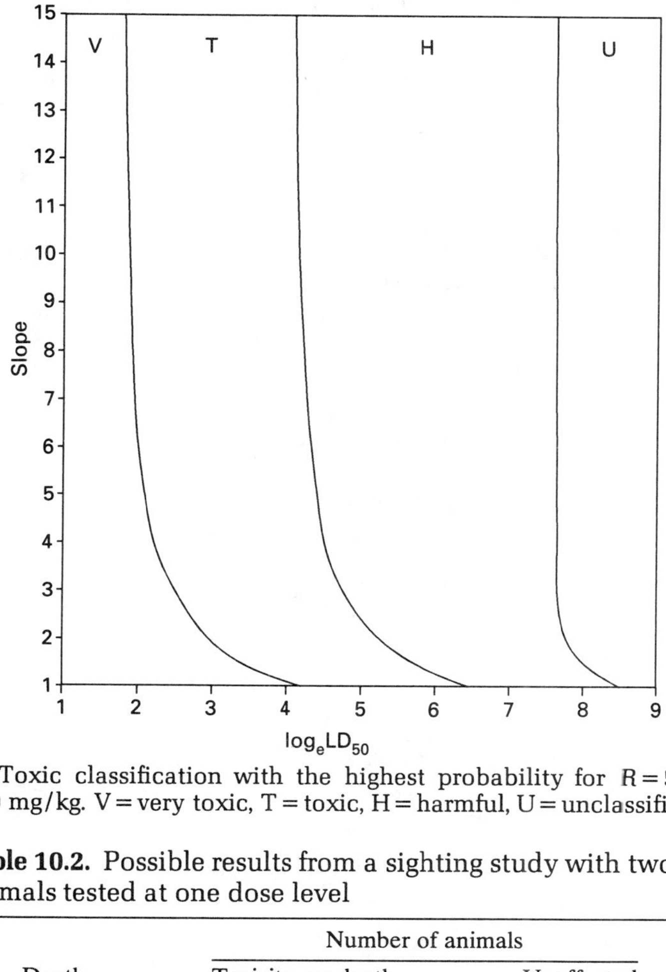

Fig. 10.10. Toxic classification with the highest probability for $R = 50$; starting dose = 2000 mg/kg. V = very toxic, T = toxic, H = harmful, U = unclassified.

Table 10.2. Possible results from a sighting study with two animals tested at one dose level

	Number of animals	
Death	Toxicity, no death	Unaffected
2	0	0
1	1	0
1	0	1
0	2	0
0	1	1
0	0	2

The probabilities that a substance is classified as toxic, harmful, or unclassified are calculated in a similar fashion.

The classification probabilities were calculated for the FDP, using the above formula, with R equal to 50, and the ranges of slopes and LD_{50} values previously defined. The classification with the highest probability is presented in

Table 10.3. Choice of starting dose for the FDP based on results from a sighting study

Results for sighting study	Choice of dose (mg/kg body weight)
Any mortal at 5[a] No mortality at 5, but mortality at 50	5
No mortality at 5 or 50, but mortality at 500 Toxicity at 5, no effects at 50 or 500 No mortality at 5, toxicity at 50, no effects at 500	50
No mortality at 5 or 50, toxicity at 500	500
No effects at 5, 50 and 500	2000

[a] Units throughout are mg/kg body weight.

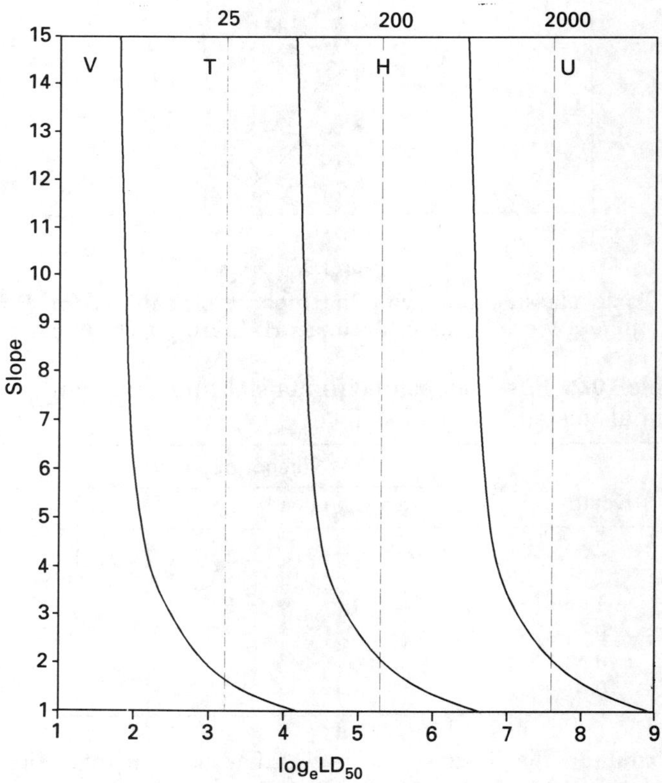

Fig. 10.11. Toxic classification with the highest probability for $R = 50$; starting dose chosen from sighting study. V = very toxic, T = toxic, H = harmful, U = unclassified. The vertical dashed lines are placed at LD_{50} values of 25, 200, and 2000 mg/kg body weight.

Fig. 10.11 for comparison with Figs. 10.7–10.10. For substances with low LD_{50} values there would be a high probability that the results from the sighting study would indicate a starting dose of 5 mg/kg. Consequently, the left-hand side of Fig. 10.11 will agree quite well with Fig. 10.7. As the LD_{50} increases, the results from the sighting study will be more likely to indicate a starting dose of 50 mg/kg and then 500 mg/kg and finally 2000 mg/kg. Consequently, moving to the right in Fig. 10.11, the most likely classification will first of all agree with Fig. 10.7, then Fig. 10.8, then Fig. 10.9, and finally Fig. 10.10.

10.5 Toxic classification of substances

For any values of the slope, LD_{50}, and R, we can calculate the probability that a substance with those properties will be classified into each of the four toxic classifications. This is assuming that a sighting study is performed to find the starting dose for the FDP and using the proposed mathematical model. These classification probabilities were calculated for the ranges of slopes and LD_{50} values as previously defined and for a range of values of R from 5 to 100. The classification with the highest probability did not alter very much as R changed from 5 to 100; Fig. 10.11 therefore represents how the classification alters with slope and LD_{50}. For slopes greater than about 6, the most likely classification changes from very toxic to toxic, from toxic to harmful and from harmful to unclassified for LD_{50} values of approximately 7.5, 75, and 750 mg/kg body weight, respectively. The boundaries for the toxic classification based on the LD_{50} estimate are at 25, 200, and 2000 mg/kg body weight and are represented by dashed lines. Generally, the FDP is likely to classify substances as the same as, or less toxic than, the LD_{50} classification. However, as the slope becomes shallower then the substance is more likely to be given a higher toxic classification for a given LD_{50}. Obviously, if an LD_{50} test and an FDP were carried out on a compound, it would be possible for the LD_{50} classification to be less toxic than, the same as or more toxic than the FDP classification because of the biological variability associated with both studies; what we are presenting here is the most likely outcome.

To obtain closer agreement between the FDP and the LD_{50} classification for substances with slopes greater than 3, it would be necessary to increase the fixed dose levels. In order to explore the effect of increasing these dose levels, classification probabilities were calculated for five sets of fixed dose levels: these were 7.5, 75, 750, and 3000; 10, 100, 1000, and 4000; 15, 150, 1500, and 6000; 20, 200, 2000, and 8000; and 25, 250, 2500, and 10,000 mg/kg body weight. By setting the fixed doses at 15, 150, 1500, and 6000 mg/kg body weight there would be good agreement between the FDP classification and the LD_{50} classification for substances and slopes of greater than about 6. However, the FDP could classify substances with smaller slopes as more toxic than the LD_{50} classification. A series of 57 substances consecutively subjected to a routine LD_{50} test had a median slope of 6.1, with the minimum being 2.4. By changing the fixed doses to 10, 100, 1000, and 4000 mg/kg body weight, the FDP would be unlikely to classify substances as more toxic than the LD_{50} classification for substances with slopes greater than 3, but would be more likely to classify substances as less toxic than the LD_{50} classification. To obtain closer agreement between the FDP and the LD_{50} classification, it would therefore be necessary to increase the fixed doses to between two and three times the current levels. However, there would never be complete agreement because the FDP allocates a more severe toxic classification to substances with a shallow slope than for substances with the same LD_{50} and a steep slope. Any change to the fixed dose levels would require careful consideration: for example, increasing the highest dose level to between 4000 and 6000 mg/kg might create ethical problems, as well as problems in administering the dose.

Close to the boundaries of classification, the probability that a substance is classified into an adjacent classification becomes higher and in Fig. 10.12 are shown the areas in which the probability of classification into one of the other groups is greater than or equal to 0.1. Clearly, at slopes lower than 3 there will be more disagreement between laboratories.

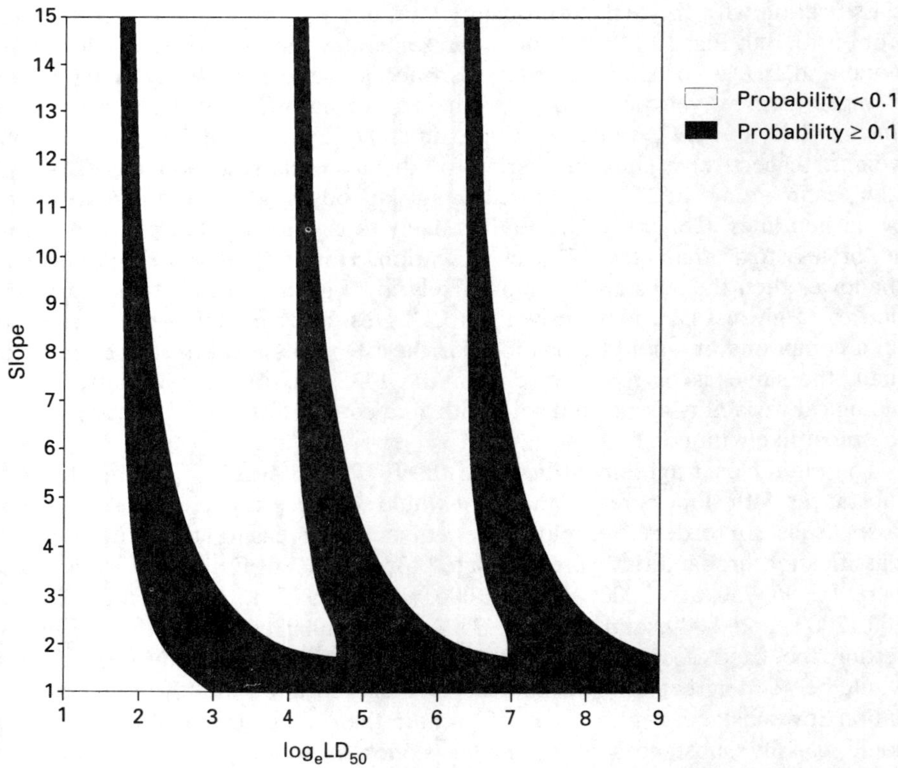

Fig. 10.12. The probability of classification into one of the toxic categories, excluding the category with the highest probability; $R = 50$, starting dose chosen from sighting study.

10.6 Expected numbers of animals to be tested, found dead, and suffering toxicity

For each starting dose we can calculate the expected number of animals required in the fixed dose procedure and also the expected number of deaths and number of animals suffering toxicity (Table 10.4). These are obtained from the outcome probabilities $d(x)$, $t(x)$, and $n(x)$. For example, the expected number of animals to be used when the starting dose is 5 mg/kg is given by

$$\begin{aligned}
&\text{E(number of animals tested given starting dose 5)} \\
&\quad = 10 + 10 \times P(\text{no effects at dose 5}) \\
&\qquad + 10 \times P(\text{no effects at 5 and at 50}) + 10 \times P(\text{no effects at 5, 50, and 500}) \\
&\quad = 10 + 10 \times n(5) + 10 \times n(50) \times n(5) + 10 \times n(500) \times n(50) \times n(5).
\end{aligned}$$

The expected number of deaths is obtained by multiplying the number of animals tested at dose x (i.e. 10) by the probability that an animal dies at dose x

Table 10.4. Expected numbers of animals to be used, found dead, and suffering toxicity for each starting dose

Starting dose (mg/kg body weight)	Expected numbers
Animals to be used	
5	$10 \times (1 + n(5) + n(5) \times n(50) + n(5) \times n(50) \times n(500))$
50	$10 \times (1 + d(50) + n(50) + n(50) \times n(500))$
500	$10 \times (1 + d(500) + d(500) \times d(50) + n(500))$
2000	$10 \times (1 + d(2000) + d(2000) \times d(500) + d(2000) \times d(500) \times d(50))$
Deaths	
5	$10 \times (p_1(5) + n(5) \times p_1(50) + n(5) \times n(50) \times p_1(500)$ $+ n(5) \times n(50) \times n(500) \times p_1(2000))$
50	$10 \times (p_1(50) + d(50) \times p_1(5) + n(50) \times p_1(500)$ $+ n(50) \times n(500) \times p_1(2000))$
500	$10 \times (p_1(500) + d(500) \times p_1(50) + d(500) \times d(50) \times p_1(5)$ $+ n(500) \times p_1(2000))$
2000	$10 \times (p_1(2000) + d(2000) \times p_1(500) + d(2000) \times d(500) \times p_1(50)$ $+ d(2000) \times d(500) \times d(50) \times p_1(5))$
Animals suffering toxicity	
5	$10 \times (p_2(5) + n(5) \times p_2(50) + n(5) \times n(50) \times p_2(500)$ $+ n(5) \times n(50) \times n(500) \times p_2(2000))$
50	$10 \times (p_2(50) + d(50) \times p_2(5) + n(50) \times p_2(500)$ $+ n(50) \times n(500) \times p_2(2000))$
500	$10 \times (p_2(500) + d(500) \times p_2(50) + d(500) \times d(50) \times p_2(5)$ $+ n(500) \times p_2(2000))$
2000	$10 \times (p_2(2000) + d(2000) \times p_2(500) + d(2000) \times d(500) \times p_2(50)$ $+ d(2000) \times d(500) \times d(50) \times p_2(5))$

(i.e. $p_1(x)$). Similarly, the expected number of animals suffering toxicity is obtained by multiplying the number of animals tested at dose x (i.e. 10) by the probability that an animal suffers toxicity at dose x (i.e. $p_2(x)$). These expected numbers depend on the starting dose and, in a similar way to the toxic classification probabilities, we can calculate the expected numbers assuming that a sighting study has been carried out, but excluding those animals from the calculation. For example, the expected number of animals required to test a particular substance is given by

$$\begin{aligned} &\text{E(number of animals tested)} \\ &= \sum_{x=5,50,500,2000} [\text{E(number tested given starting dose } x) \\ &\qquad \times P(\text{choose starting dose } x)]. \end{aligned}$$

The expected number of animals to be tested, assuming that a sighting study has been carried out but excluding those animals from the calculation, was calculated for the ranges of slopes, LD_{50} values, and values of R as previously defined. The results are shown in Fig. 10.13 for $R = 50$. It can be seen that more

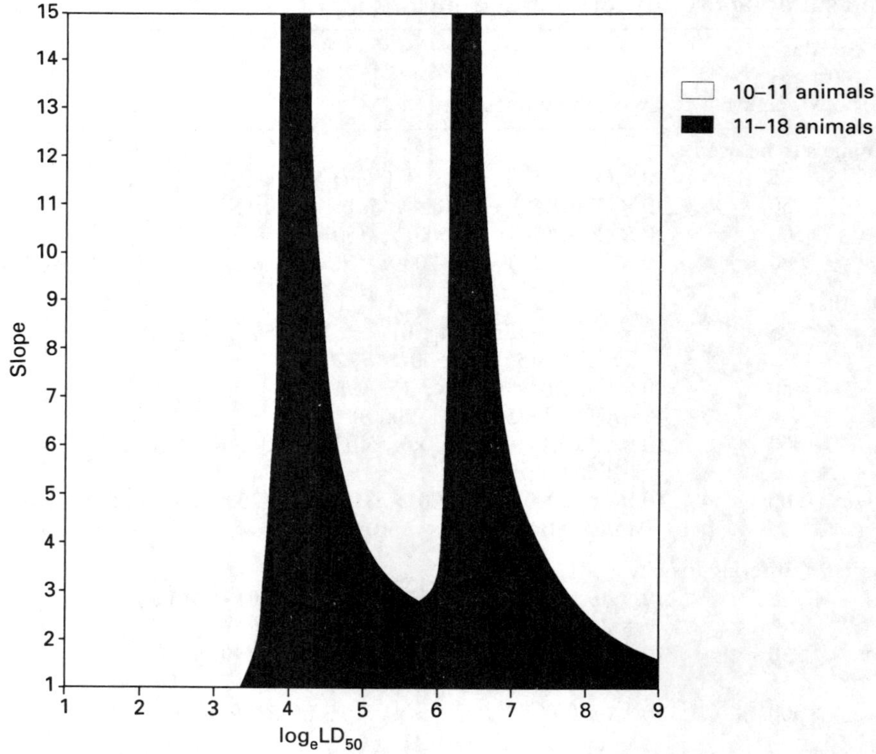

Fig. 10.13. The expected number of animals tested; $R = 50$, starting dose chosen from sighting study.

animals are required for substances with an LD_{50} close to the boundaries of classification toxic/harmful and harmful/unclassified, and for substances with shallow slopes. This is not the case for the very toxic/toxic boundary. For substances with low LD_{50} values there would be a high probability that the results from the sighting study would indicate a starting dose of 5 mg/kg. If either toxicity or death occurred at 5 mg/kg, the classification would be based on only ten animals. For the remaining substances, the expected number lies between 10 and 11 animals compared with the fixed value of 30 for the LD_{50} test. As R changes from 10 to 100, the expected numbers do not change very much. As R decreases from 10, more animals are required around the boundaries of classification and the size of these boundary regions increases. The absolute maximum number of animals required by the FDP will be 40, corresponding to the unlikely use of all four dose levels.

The expected number of deaths is also relatively insensitive to values of R between 10 and 100. Apart from substances that will be classified as very toxic, the expected number of deaths lies between 0 and 2. The LD_{50} test would generally result in about 50 per cent mortality (i.e. 15 deaths). As R decreases from 10, the expected number of deaths increases close to the boundaries of classification toxic/harmful and harmful/unclassified. The expected number of animals showing signs of toxicity is very dependent on the value of R and consequently no one choice of R can represent the general picture.

10.7 Testing the model

We compared the results from our mathematical model with the results from the international validation study. There were eight substances for which a slope and LD_{50} estimate were available (Table 10.5). It should be noted that the slopes quoted from the study were obtained by fitting a probit transformation with $\log_{10}$ dose. In our model we have used a logit transformation with $\log_e$ dose, and consequently the slopes have been multiplied by $\pi/\sqrt{3}/\log_e 10 = 0.79$.

The results from the individual laboratories on the numbers of animals that died and showed signs of toxicity at the various doses in the FDP were made

Table 10.5. Substances used in international validation study

Substance	Slope	LD_{50} (mg/kg)	R
A. Nicotine	2.4	70	64.7
B. Sodium pentachlorophenate	5.8	348	2.6
D. 2-Chloroethyl alcohol	8.4	60	6.1
E. Sodium arsenite	6.0	42	4.9
F. Phenyl mercury acetate	5.8	37	3.7
H. Fentin hydroxide	5.9	110	54.4
J. Acetanilide	5.5	1959	37.8
X. Resorcinol	6.3	510	4.1

Table 10.6. Starting dose chosen by laboratories in international validation study

Substance[a]	Number of laboratories choosing dose (mg/kg) of: 5	50	500	2000	Total
A	18	8	0	0	26
B	1	20	3	2	26
D	10	16	0	0	26
E	21	5	0	0	26
F	21	5	0	0	26
H	5	21	0	0	26
J	0	1	23	2	26
X	0	20	4	2	26

[a] Substances as in Table 10.5.

available to us. The dose–response relationships represented by eqns. (10.1) and (10.2) are known in mathematical terms as a 'proportional odds model', from which R can be estimated (McCullagh 1980). An estimate of R was calculated for each of the eight compounds using PROC LOGISTIC in SAS (SAS Technical Report 1990) (Table 10.5), resulting in values from 2.6 to 64.7. For each compound the estimates of the slope, LD_{50}, and R were used to calculate the outcome probabilities $d(x)$, $t(x)$, and $n(x)$ for $x = 5$, 50, 500, and 2000 mg/kg and, from these, the classification probabilities for each starting dose. In Table 10.6 are shown the starting doses chosen by the 26 laboratories in the study. The expected number of laboratories that would classify the compound as very toxic was calculated as

$$\text{E(number of laboratories classifying compound as very toxic)}$$
$$= \sum_{x=5,50,500,2000} [P(\text{classify very toxic given starting dose } x)$$
$$\times \text{number of laboratories choosing starting dose } x].$$

The expected numbers of laboratories that would classify the compound as toxic, harmful, or unclassified were calculated in a similar manner. These expected numbers were compared with the observed classifications from the laboratories. The results are shown in Table 10.7 and the substances plotted on the classification grid in Fig. 10.14.

There is very good agreement between the observed and expected classifications by the FDP. For substances A, B, E, F, and X, good agreement would be expected with the LD_{50} classification because these substances lie in the areas where the two classification systems agree. A change in the starting dose would also have a very small effect on the probabilities of classification into the different toxic groups for these five substances. Substance D lies on the border of the toxic/harmful categories of the FDP, and it is not surprising to find both

Table 10.7. Comparison of the classification allocated to the test substances by the FDP [observed (Obs.) and expected (Exp.)] and by the LD_{50} test

		FDP							
		Number of laboratories classifying substances as:							
	LD_{50} test	Very toxic		Toxic		Harmful		Unclassified	
Substance[a]	classification	Obs.	Exp.	Obs.	Exp.	Obs.	Exp.	Obs.	Exp.
A	Toxic	—	0.5	23	25.3	3	0.2	—	0.0
B	Harmful	—	0.0	1	0.0	25	26.0	—	0.0
D	Toxic	—	0.0	19	22.4	7	3.6	—	0.0
E	Toxic	—	0.0	25	26.0	1	0.0	—	0.0
F	Toxic	2	0.0	24	26.0	—	0.0	—	0.0
H	Toxic	—	0.0	8	6.9	17	19.1	1	0.0
J	Harmful	—	0.0	—	0.0	4	2.5	22	23.5
X	Harmful	—	0.0	—	0.0	25	26.0	1	0.0

[a] Substances as in Table 10.5.

observed and expected results showing this feature. A change in the starting dose for D would have a very small effect on the probabilities of classification into the different toxic groups. Substance J lies in the unclassified category of the FDP, but is just into the harmful category of the LD_{50} classification. The starting dose is extremely important to the classification of this substance: a starting dose of 500 would give the probability of an unclassified category of nearly 1, whereas a starting dose of 2000 would give this probability a value of 0.31. Of the 26 laboratories, 22 put J into the unclassified category. Substance H falls into the harmful category of the FDP but the toxic category of the LD_{50} classification. Again, the starting dose is extremely important to the classification of this substance: if the starting dose is 5, the probability of a toxic classification is close to 1, whereas for the other three starting doses this probability is equal to 0.09. Of the 26 laboratories, 17 put H into the harmful category. The numbers were too small to obtain an accurate picture of the extent to which observed and expected classifications agreed for a particular starting dose.

Using estimates of the slope, LD_{50}, and R, and the starting doses chosen by laboratories, the expected numbers of animals used, found dead, or showing signs of toxicity per fixed dose test performed by these laboratories were calculated. For example, the expected number of animals used by the laboratories is given by

$$\text{E(number of animals tested)} = \sum_{x=5,50,500,2000} [\text{E(number tested given starting dose } x) \times \text{proportion of laboratories choosing starting dose } x].$$

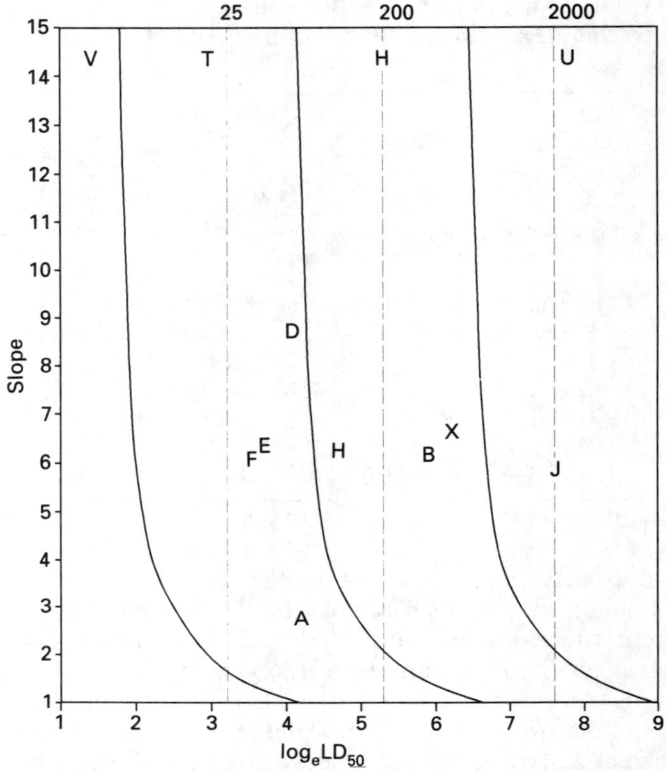

Fig. 10.14. The position of the substances tested in the international validation study on the toxic classification grid for $R = 50$; starting dose chosen from sighting study. V = very toxic, T = toxic, H = harmful, U = unclassified.

These are compared with the observed numbers in Table 10.8, showing reasonably good agreement.

10.8 Conclusions

Our mathematical description of the procedure predicted results that agreed very well with the observed classifications from the laboratories taking part in the international validation study. We have shown that the starting dose can affect the toxic classification of a substance and that, for substances H and J, the probabilities of classification into the four toxic classifications are very dependent on the starting dose.

There is one inconsistency in the FDP when the substance is tested at 500 mg/kg body weight. If the result is no deaths and some toxicity, the substance would be unclassified, whereas if at 500 there were no deaths or toxicity, the

Table 10.8. Average numbers of rats tested, dead, and suffering toxicity in a FDP: observed (Obs.) compared with expected (Exp.)

Substance[a]	Average number tested		Average number dead		Average number suffering toxicity	
	Obs.	Exp.	Obs.	Exp.	Obs.	Exp
A	13.65	13.00	1.12	0.98	10.12	11.76
B	17.88	20.88	7.27	9.42	3.56	1.11
D	17.50	19.01	3.27	1.77	6.72	8.13
E	16.54	17.40	4.12	5.47	5.00	2.31
F	16.00	18.71	5.42	7.43	4.36	1.46
H	15.00	10.73	1.50	0.08	9.12	10.64
J	12.50	10.82	1.00	0.41	10.92	10.17
X	14.23	20.52	5.62	5.34	4.28	5.21

[a] Substances as in Table 10.5.

substance tested at 2000 may be classified as harmful, albeit only in the unlikely event that 50 per cent or more of the animals die at that dose.

Our model for the FDP assumed parallel dose–response relationships for death and toxicity or death. In order to determine whether or not this assumption is realistic, studies would need to be conducted in which the dose levels of a substance are chosen to span the median lethal dose and the median dose for producing evident toxicity; these data are unlikely to be available from past LD_{50} studies.

The FDP is likely to classify substances as the same or less toxic than the LD_{50} procedure. For slopes greater than about 6, the most likely classification changes from very toxic to toxic, from toxic to harmful and from harmful to unclassified for LD_{50} values of approximately 7.5, 75, and 750 mg/kg body weight, respectively. For lower slopes, a more conservative classification results, which is entirely appropriate when the unpredictability inherent in a low slope is considered. To obtain closer agreement between the FDP and the LD_{50} classification it would be necessary to increase the fixed doses to between two and three times the current level. There would, however, never be complete agreement because of the desirable conservative property of the FDP for substances with low slopes. Any change to the fixed dose levels would require careful consideration: it may not be optimal, desirable, or practical to increase all dose levels by a factor of two or three.

Calculation of the expected numbers of animals to be tested and found dead showed that, in general, the FDP would require considerably fewer animals and cause fewer deaths than the LD_{50} test.

Additional information is available from an FDP that is not used in the classification process. For example, a finding of one animal with toxic signs and nine unaffected carries the same weight as that of ten animals with toxic signs. One way in which the information could be used is in the calculation of an approximate median toxic dose.

Acknowledgements

We should like to thank Mr Michael Russell-Yarde, whose work for his MSc dissertation formed the starting point for this study, and Mr Keith Freeman and Mr Colin Bishop for assistance with the computer programming. We should like to thank Professor Tony Dayan, Department of Toxicology, St Bartholomew's Hospital Medical College, for his helpful discussions and access to data.

References

British Toxicology Society (1984). Special report: a new approach to the classification of substances and preparations on the basis of their acute toxicity. *Human Toxicology*, **3**, 85–92.

Commission of the European Communities (1983). Council Directive 83/467/EEC amending for the fifth time Council Directive 67/548/EEC on the approximation of laws, regulations and administrative provisions relating to the classification, packaging and labelling of dangerous substances: Annex III. *Official Journal of the European Communities* (L257), 13–33.

McCullagh, P. (1980). Regression models for ordinal data. *Journal of the Royal Statistical Society B*, **42**, 109–42.

OECD (1981). *Guidelines for the testing of chemical substances—no. 401: acute oral toxicity*. OECD, Paris.

OECD (1987). *Guidelines for the testing of chemical substances—no. 401 (1987): acute oral toxicity*. OECD, Paris.

SAS Technical Report (1990). *P-200 SAS/STAT software: CALIS and LOGISTIC procedures, release 6.04*. SAS Institute Inc., Cary, North Carolina, USA.

van den Heuvel, M. J., Clark, D. G., Fielder, R. J., Koundakjian, P. P., Oliver, G. J. A., Pelling, D., Tomlinson, N. J., and Walker, A. P. (1990). The international validation of a fixed-dose procedure as an alternative to the classical LD_{50} test. *Food and Chemical Toxicology*, **28**, 469–82.

Zbinden, G. and Flury-Roversi, M. (1981). Significance of the LD_{50} test for the toxicology evaluation of chemical substances. *Archives of Toxicology*, **47**, 79–99.

PART IV

GENERAL APPLICATIONS

11 Statistical analysis of overdispersed multinomial data from developmental toxicity studies

DANIEL KREWSKI, YILIANG ZHU, AND KAREN FUNG

11.1 Introduction

Toxic chemicals present in the human environment may induce developmental anomalies in the offspring of exposed parents, particularly as a consequence of maternal exposure. In addition to epidemiological evidence of adverse effects on fetal development, laboratory experiments in small mammalian species represent a major source of data on developmental toxicity. Laboratory studies afford a greater level of control than is possible in observational studies of human populations, and can be conducted in advance of human exposure. This chapter discusses statistical methods for analysing overdispersed multinomial data arising from laboratory studies of developmental toxicity.

11.1.1 Developmental toxicity data

The objective of developmental toxicity studies is to investigate the potential of the test agent to cause structural abnormalities, prenatal death, growth alterations, or functional deficits (Environmental Protection Agency 1991). Test animals are selected on the basis of species, strain, age, weight, and health status. Typically, groups of 20–30 pregnant females are exposed to one of 4–5 doses, including an unexposed control, in a critical period during gestation: days 6–16, 6–15, and 6–19 in rats, mice, and rabbits respectively (cf. International Life Sciences Institute 1989). The highest dose is chosen to produce minimal maternal toxicity, and not more than 10 per cent mortality (Environmental Protection Agency 1991). Routes of exposure are chosen with respect to major human exposure conditions.

Upon examining the uterine contents of pregnant animals just prior to term or at parturition, multiple indicators of developmental toxicity are recorded for each litter. These include the number of implantation sites per dam, the number of resorptions, the number of fetal deaths, the number of live offspring, and the number of malformed live births. For live births, fetal weight and specific types of malformation are also recorded. Although each end-point has traditionally been analysed separately, joint analyses of these correlated end-points are desirable. Ryan *et al.* (1991), Catalano and Ryan (1992), and Chen (1993*a*) considered joint analysis of fetal malformation and fetal weight. Catalano *et al.* (1993) proposed a multivariate dose–response model for fetal death, fetal weight, and malformation. Ryan (1992), Chen and Li (1994), Krewski and Zhu (1994, 1995), and Zhu *et al.* (1994) discussed joint dose–response modelling of the incidences of prenatal death and fetal malformation. In this chapter, we focus on multivariate analyses of fetal malformation and prenatal death (including both early resorptions and late fetal deaths). We also discuss the estimation of benchmark doses for risk assessment on the basis of multivariate dose–response models.

Consider an experiment in which n_i pregnant animals are exposed at dose level d_i $(i = 1, \ldots, t)$, with $d_1 = 0$ being that of the control group. For the jth litter (dam) in the ith dose group, let $(y_{ij}, r_{ij}, s_{ij}, m_{ij})$ denote the numbers of malformed fetuses (of a specific or unspecified type of malformation, depending on the objective of the analysis), prenatal deaths, live births, and the number of implants respectively. When there is no ambiguity, the subscripts (ij) will be suppressed for convenience. Since exposure to the test agent takes place after implantation, the number of implants is not expected to be dose-related, and is hence an ancillary statistic containing no information with respect to the dose–response relationship. Consequently, it is natural to conduct statistical analyses after conditioning on the observed implantation number m. For joint analysis of the malformation rate y/s and the prenatal death rate r/m, the responses $(y, r, s-y)$, given the number of implants m, represent trinomial counts obtained by classifying each implant into one of the three mutually exclusive categories: malformed, dead, or normal (Fig. 11.1). Due to both

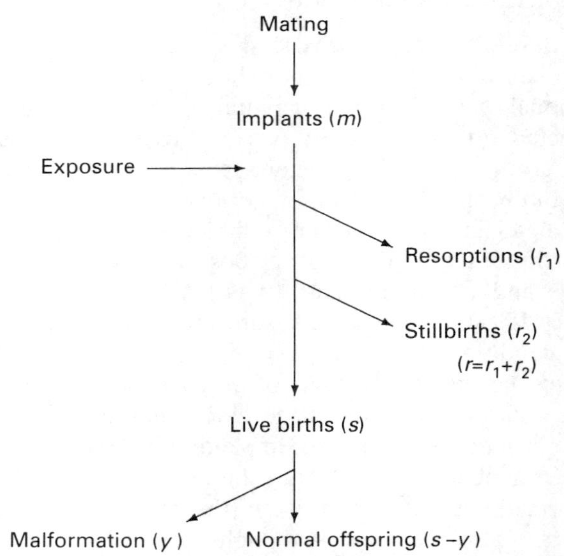

Fig. 11.1. A schematic representation of a developmental toxicity experiment.

genetic similarity and comparable exposures received by fetuses within the same litter, the binary responses on these fetuses are usually correlated. This intra-litter correlation, often called the *litter effect*, induces extra-multinomial variation in the data, and must be taken into account in statistical analyses. Although we focus on statistical analysis of the trinomial responses $(y, r, s - y)$, the methods described in this chapter are readily applicable to higher-dimensional categorical data (such as those obtained by the disaggregation of resorptions and late fetal deaths), and can be extended to the case in which categories may not be mutually exclusive (e.g. multiple malformations in live fetuses).

11.1.2 *Two examples*

Throughout this chapter, we will use data from two experiments conducted under the US National Toxicology Program to illustrate the statistical methods to be discussed. The first experiment involves 28, 32, 26, and 31 pregnant rabbits exposed to ethylene glycol diethyl ether (EGDE) at dose levels of 0, 25, 50, and 100 mg/kg/day respectively (Table 11.1). The second study involves 28, 28, 29, and 27 female rats exposed to ethylene glycol (EG) at dose levels of 0, 1250, 2500, and 5000 mg/kg/day respectively (Table 11.2). In these two tables, the observations $(y, r, m)_k$ within each dose group are arranged according to the number of implants, with the subscript k indicating the number of litters from which identical responses were observed. In the experiment on EGDE, for example, the occurrence of malformations of any type or prenatal death is clearly dose-related: the incidence of malformations increased from about 7 per cent in controls to about 55 per cent in the highest dose group; the proportion of implants resulting in either resorption or stillbirth increased from about 12 per cent in controls to nearly 36 per cent in the highest dose group.

11.1.3 *A brief review*

Given the constraint $s + r = m$, the joint probability $\mathbf{P}(y, r, m)$ of observing m implants, among which there are s live fetuses, y malformed live fetuses, and r prenatal deaths, may be factored as

$$\mathbf{P}(y, r, m) = \mathbf{P}(y, r \mid m)\mathbf{P}(m). \tag{11.1}$$

Since the random variable m is an ancillary statistic providing no information about developmental toxicity, statistical inference may be based on the conditional distribution of y and r:

$$\mathbf{P}(y, r \mid m) = \mathbf{P}(y \mid s, m)\mathbf{P}(r \mid m), \tag{11.2}$$

given m. Here, the conditional probability $\mathbf{P}(y \mid s, m)$ characterizes the fetal malformation rate, conditioning on both the number of implants m and live births s. The conditional probability $\mathbf{P}(r \mid m)$ reflects the prenatal death rate.

Chen *et al.* (1991) used a Dirichlet-trinomial distribution for $\mathbf{P}(y, r \mid m)$ to

Table 11.1. Developmental toxicity data[a] in rabbits exposed to ethylene glycol diethyl ether (EGDE)

Dose (mg/kg/day)			
0	25	50	100
$(0,0,2)_2$	$(0,0,3)$	$(0,0,2)_2$	$(0,0,2)$
$(0,3,3)$	$(0,0,4)$	$(0,0,3)$	$(1,0,2)$
$(1,0,3)$	$(0,0,5)_4$	$(1,1,4)$	$(0,0,3)_2$
$(0,0,5)$	$(0,0,6)_2$	$(0,0,5)$	$(3,1,4)$
$(0,1,5)$	$(0,1,6)$	$(1,0,5)$	$(0,5,5)$
$(4,0,5)$	$(0,4,6)$	$(1,0,6)$	$(3,0,5)$
$(0,0,6)$	$(0,0,7)$	$(1,1,6)$	$(1,4,6)$
$(0,1,6)$	$(0,7,7)$	$(0,0,7)$	$(2,1,6)$
$(0,0,7)_2$	$(1,0,7)$	$(1,1,7)$	$(2,2,6)$
$(0,0,8)_3$	$(0,0,8)_2$	$(2,1,7)$	$(1,5,7)$
$(0,1,8)$	$(0,8,8)$	$(0,0,8)$	$(5,2,7)$
$(0,4,9)$	$(0,0,9)_2$	$(0,8,8)$	$(2,3,8)$
$(2,2,9)$	$(0,1,9)$	$(1,1,8)$	$(3,3,8)$
$(0,0,9)$	$(1,2,9)$	$(0,0,9)$	$(4,1,8)_2$
$(0,0,10)_3$	$(0,0,10)$	$(1,1,9)$	$(5,1,8)$
$(0,8,10)$	$(1,0,10)_2$	$(0,0,10)$	$(7,1,8)$
$(1,0,10)$	$(1,2,10)$	$(1,0,10)$	$(4,0,9)$
$(1,4,10)$	$(3,0,10)$	$(2,0,10)$	$(4,5,9)$
$(0,0,11)$	$(3,1,10)$	$(1,0,11)$	$(5,0,9)$
$(0,0,12)$	$(0,1,11)$	$(1,2,11)$	$(7,2,9)$
$(5,1,12)$	$(0,0,12)$	$(2,0,12)$	$(0,0,10)$
$(0,1,13)$	$(0,2,12)_2$	$(5,2,13)$	$(0,10,10)$
	$(1,1,13)$	$(1,7,14)$	$(2,4,10)$
	$(2,1,13)$	$(2,2,14)$	$(3,0,10)$
		$(0,3,15)$	$(4,6,11)$
			$(6,0,11)$
			$(0,12,12)$
			$(5,7,12)$
			$(1,11,13)$

[a] Observations $(y, r, m)_k$ represent y malformations and r deaths among m implants in a litter; the subscript k denotes the multiplicity of litters producing the same response.

develop likelihood ratio tests for dose effects on the malformation and prenatal death rates. The Dirichlet-multinomial distribution can be derived as a Dirichlet mixture of multinomial distributions, and provides a means of characterizing extra-multinomial variation induced by positive intra-litter correlation. Ryan (1992) considered simultaneous dose–response modelling of y/s and r/m using quasi-likelihood methods. In this latter analysis, the covariance function of the data was assumed to be proportional to the trinomial covariance function with the same proportionality constant across dose groups. Following Ryan (1992), Zhu *et al.* (1994) and Krewski and Zhu (1994) discussed the use of generalized

Table 11.2. Developmental toxicity data[a] in rats exposed to ethylene glycol (EG)

Dose (mg/kg/day)			
0	1250	2500	5000
$(0,0,12)_2$	$(1,0,11)$	$(0,0,1)$	$(4,2,6)$
$(0,2,12)$	$(2,1,11)$	$(3,0,6)$	$(5,1,6)$
$(0,0,13)_4$	$(0,0,12)_4$	$(2,1,9)$	$(2,0,10)$
$(0,2,13)$	$(0,1,12)$	$(1,0,10)$	$(9,2,11)$
$(2,0,13)$	$(1,0,12)$	$(4,1,11)$	$(0,12,12)$
$(0,0,14)_4$	$(1,1,12)$	$(0,0,12)$	$(1,11,12)$
$(0,2,14)_2$	$(4,1,12)$	$(0,1,12)_2$	$(6,4,12)$
$(3,1,14)$	$(0,0,13)$	$(2,3,12)$	$(8,1,12)$
$(0,0,15)_4$	$(0,1,13)$	$(4,1,12)$	$(10,0,12)_2$
$(0,1,15)_2$	$(0,2,13)$	$(7,0,12)$	$(10,3,13)$
$(0,2,15)_2$	$(0,0,14)_2$	$(9,2,12)$	$(3,2,14)$
$(0,0,16)$	$(0,1,14)$	$(0,0,13)$	$(9,3,14)$
$(0,1,16)$	$(1,2,14)$	$(0,1,13)$	$(10,3,14)$
$(0,0,17)$	$(2,0,14)$	$(1,0,13)$	$(11,3,14)$
$(0,3,17)$	$(0,0,15)$	$(1,1,13)$	$(12,2,14)$
	$(0,1,15)_2$	$(5,0,13)$	$(0,0,15)$
	$(0,3,15)$	$(7,0,13)$	$(3,0,15)$
	$(1,0,15)$	$(2,1,14)$	$(12,0,15)$
	$(2,0,15)$	$(3,3,14)$	$(13,1,15)$
	$(3,2,15)$	$(9,0,14)$	$(13,2,15)$
	$(3,7,15)$	$(1,0,15)$	$(1,2,16)$
	$(0,1,17)$	$(3,1,15)$	$(8,3,16)$
	$(0,0,18)$	$(9,3,15)$	$(10,2,16)$
		$(0,2,16)$	$(7,2,17)$
		$(4,0,16)$	$(17,0,17)$
		$(0,1,17)_2$	$(3,15,18)$
		$(9,0,17)$	

[a] Observations $(y, r, m)_k$ represent y malformations and r deaths among m implants in a litter; the subscript k denotes the multiplicity of litters producing the same response.

estimating equations (GEEs) in conjunction with an extended Dirichlet-multinomial covariance function allowing for negative intra-litter correlation for modelling developmental toxicity data. Krewski and Zhu (1995) further proposed a simple data transformation that allows the mean and covariance of the transformed data to be approximated by those of a multinomial distribution, hence permitting the use of standard methods for analysing multinomial data. Chen and Li (1994) also discussed joint dose–response modelling of fetal malformation and prenatal death data using quasi-likelihood methods. Lefkopoulou *et al.* (1989) used quasi-likelihood methods in conjunction with generalized linear models for the analysis of multiple fetal malformations.

Historically, statistical analysis of developmental toxicity data has focused on individual end-points such as the rate y/s of a particular malformation. Rai and Van Ryzin (1985) based their analysis on the marginal distribution

$$\mathbf{P}(y, s) = \int \mathbf{P}(y, s, m)\,\mathrm{d}\mathbf{P}(m) = \mathbf{P}(y \mid s)\mathbf{P}(s). \tag{11.3}$$

These authors used a Poisson distribution to describe the marginal distribution $\mathbf{P}(s)$ of litter size. However, empirical results reported by Williams (1987) and Krewski and Zhu (1994*a*) indicate that $\mathbf{P}(s)$ can exhibit both underdispersion and overdispersion relative to Poisson variation. Moreover, due to the constraint $r + s = m$, the conditional model $\mathbf{P}(r \mid m)$ in eqn. (11.2) is preferred to the marginal model $\mathbf{P}(s)$ in making inferences about the prenatal death rate.

The beta-binomial model has been widely assumed for the conditional distribution

$$\mathbf{P}(y \mid s) \tag{11.4}$$

in the analysis of fetal malformation data (cf. Williams 1975; Crowder 1978; Paul 1982; Kupper *et al.* 1986; Chen and Kodell 1989; Kodell *et al.* 1991). The beta-binomial distribution is preferred to the binomial distribution because of the presence of extra-binomial variation in the data. In a recent simulation study, Carr and Portier (1993) considered the estimation of the slope of the dose–response curve based on an exponential (complementary-log) or extreme-value dose–response model under the beta-binomial distribution. Their results confirm that quasi-likelihood estimation generally provides accurate estimates of the model parameter when the number of litters per dose group is moderately large. On the other hand, maximum likelihood estimates based on the beta-binomial distribution with equal intra-litter correlation across dose groups are typically biased when the true correlation increases with dose (Kupper *et al.* 1986). Carr and Portier (1993) also showed that the variance estimates for the slope obtained using quasi-likelihood, bootstrap, or jackknife methods are generally close to the true variance. Alternative distributions for correlated binary data allowing extra-binomial variation have also been proposed by Altham (1978), Kupper and Haseman (1978), and Paul (1987). One drawback of inferences based solely on eqn. (11.4) is that since s is not an ancillary statistic, conditioning on s will result in some loss of information.

In the presence of extra-binomial variation, the Cochran–Armitage test for trend (Cochran 1954; Armitage 1955) with binary data cannot be used because the type I error rate exceeds the nominal value (Portier and Hoel 1984). However, other tests have been proposed for use with correlated binary data. Lefkopoulou *et al.* (1989) proposed a generalized score statistic based on GEEs with a logistic dose–response model and the variance $\mathrm{Var}(y \mid s) = s\pi(1 - \pi)\phi$, where the inflation factor ϕ to the binomial variance is constant across treatment groups. Ryan (1994) modified this statistic using a moment estimate of ϕ based on Pearson's chi-squared statistic. Rao and Scott (1992) suggested the use of the Cochran–Armitage test following the application of a simple transformation of the data. This transformation is based on the concept of design effects widely used in survey sampling. Fung *et al.* (1994) conducted an extensive simulation study of the small sample properties of these and related tests for trend. It was found that these tests yield type I error rates close to the nominal level in the presence of the intra-litter correlation, although the test proposed by Lefkopoulou *et al.* (1989) appears to be somewhat conservative under certain conditions. In another simulation study, Chen (1993*b*) found that the type I error of Wald type tests for trend is more likely to exceed the nominal level than that of score tests when the intra-litter correlation of the underlying beta-binomial distribution increases with dose. However, Carr and Portier (1993) found that the Wald type tests based on quasi-likelihood estimation are often more powerful than the likelihood ratio tests based on beta-binomial distributions in this case. Moreover, statistical methods based on quasi-likelihood appear somewhat robust against slight departures from the beta-binomial distribution.

11.1.4 *Organization*

This chapter is concerned with the statistical analyses of overdispersed multinomial data from developmental toxicity studies. Statistical methods for modeling extra-multinomial variation are discussed in Section 11.2. Emphasis is placed on an extended Dirichlet-multinomial mean-covariance structure and a simple data transformation that allows the mean and covariance of the transformed data to be approximated by those of the multinomial distribution. Dose–response models for trinomial data are described in Section 11.3. Generalized score tests for trend are presented in Section 11.4. The use of GEEs for fitting dose–response models is described in Section 11.5. Estimation of benchmark doses for risk assessment is discussed in Section 11.6. Our conclusions are presented in Section 11.7.

11.2 Overdispersed multinomial data

11.2.1 *Dirichlet-multinomial distribution*

The Dirichlet-multinomial distribution (cf. Johnson and Kotz 1969, p. 308) may be used to describe the extra-multinomial variation exhibited in multinomial data from developmental toxicity studies. In the present context, the Dirichlet-multinomial distribution may be derived by assuming that the response probability of each implant within a litter varies according to a Dirichlet distribution and, given this probability, that the total of the binary responses of all implants within a litter follows a multinomial distribution. A useful property of the Dirichlet-multinomial distribution is its collapsibility, inherited from the multinomial and Dirichlet distributions. Specifically, when a group of categories are collapsed, the original Dirichlet-multinomial distribution factors into a product of two lower-dimensional Dirichlet-multinomial distributions, one conditional on the total counts in the collapsed group and the other marginal with one category being the union of the collapsed categories. Any number of groups can be collapsed in this manner.

Let π_1 be the probability of observing at least one of several specific types of malformation in a live fetus, let π_2 be the probability of a prenatal death, and let ϕ be the correlation coefficient for the binary indicators of prenatal death within the same litter. Chen *et al.* (1991) used the Dirichlet-trinomial distribution

$$\begin{aligned}
&\mathbf{P}(y, r \mid m; \pi_1, \pi_2, \phi) \\
&\quad = \binom{m}{y, r, s-y} \frac{\Gamma[(1-\phi)/\phi]}{\Gamma[m+(1-\phi)/\phi]} \\
&\quad \times \frac{\Gamma[y+\pi_1(1-\pi_2)(1-\phi)/\phi]}{\Gamma[\pi_1(1-\pi_2)(1-\phi)/\phi]} \frac{\Gamma[s-y+(1-\pi_1)(1-\pi_2)(1-\phi)/\phi]}{\Gamma[(1-\pi_1)(1-\pi_2)(1-\phi)/\phi]} \\
&\quad \times \frac{\Gamma[r+\pi_2(1-\phi)/\phi]}{\Gamma[\pi_2(1-\phi)/\phi]} \qquad (11.5)
\end{aligned}$$

for joint analysis of the malformation rate y/s and the prenatal death rate r/m, where $\Gamma(\cdot)$ denotes the gamma function. Letting $\mu_2 \equiv \pi_2$ and μ_1 denote the probability of a malformed fetus unconditional on whether or not it is a live birth, it follows that $\mu_1 = \pi_1(1-\pi_2)$. Although the Dirichlet-trinomial distribution is defined only for $\phi \geqslant 0$, the probability function eqn. (11.5) remains valid for negative values of ϕ provided that

$$\phi \geqslant \max\left\{-\frac{\mu_k}{m-1-\mu_k}; \qquad k=1,2,3; \quad m \geqslant 2\right\}, \qquad (11.6)$$

where $\mu_3 = 1-\mu_1-\mu_2$. This result follows from the arguments given by Prentice (1986) for the beta-binomial distribution, and can be easily extended to higher-dimensional cases. Moreover, the Dirichlet-trinomial distribution $\mathbf{P}(y, r \mid m; \pi_1, \pi_2, \phi)$ can be expressed as a product of two beta-binomial distributions $\mathbf{P}(y \mid s, m; \pi_1, \rho)$ and $\mathbf{P}(r \mid m; \pi_2, \phi)$, reflecting the distributions of the fetal malformation rate y/s and the prenatal death rate r/m respectively. Here, $\rho = \phi(\phi\pi_2 + 1 - \pi_2)^{-1}$ is the correlation coefficient between binary indicators of malformations among live births within the same litter.

11.2.2 *Dirichlet-multinomial covariance*

Although useful in the analysis of multinomial developmental toxicity data, the specification of a Dirichlet-multinomial distribution for $\mathbf{P}(y, r \mid m)$ can be avoided by moment-based methods such as GEEs. The score tests and GEEs discussed in this chapter require specification of only the first two moments for the data. Letting $z = (y, r)^{\mathrm{T}}$, Zhu *et al.* (1994) assume that

$$\mathrm{E}(z \mid m) = m\mu = m\begin{pmatrix} \mu_1 \\ \mu_2 \end{pmatrix} = m\begin{pmatrix} \pi_1(1-\pi_2) \\ \pi_2 \end{pmatrix} \tag{11.7}$$

and

$$\mathbf{Cov}(z \mid m) = m[1+(m-1)\phi](1-\pi_2)\begin{pmatrix} \pi_1[1-\pi_1(1-\pi_2)] & -\pi_1\pi_2 \\ -\pi_1\pi_2 & \pi_2 \end{pmatrix}. \tag{11.8}$$

The covariance function in eqn. (11.8) corresponds to that of a trinomial distribution when $\phi = 0$, and to a Dirichlet-trinomial distribution when $0 < \phi \leqslant 1$. It corresponds to an extended Dirichlet-trinomial distribution when eqn. (11.6) holds. We may also permit $-(m-1)^{-1} < \phi < 0$ to allow for moderate underdispersion. Although we have not attempted further to characterize the distributions that have moments of the form (11.7) and (11.8), it is possible that these moments span a broad class of distributions. In the univariate case for example, the mean-covariance structure given in eqns. (11.7) and (11.8) with appropriate reparametrization encompasses the correlated-binomial models of Altham (1978), Kupper and Haseman (1978), and Paul (1987). Because of the upper bound $\phi \leqslant 1$, however, the extended Dirichlet-trinomial covariance function may not be able to describe extreme overdispersion. Since the degree of overdispersion in developmental toxicity data is likely to increase with dose (Williams 1988; Krewski and Zhu 1994*a*), we may postulate a unique value of ϕ for each dose group (Kupper *et al.* 1986; Zhu *et al.* 1994). Alternatively, it is possible to model the intra-litter correlation ϕ as a smooth function of dose (Prentice 1986; Moore 1987; Williams 1988), although the choice of a simple parametric function to describe the dependence of ϕ on dose may not always be clear.

11.2.3 Rao–Scott transformation

Rao and Scott (1992) proposed a simple transformation for correlated binary data which, after the transformation, permits the use of standard methods for uncorrelated data. Krewski and Zhu (1995) extended the Rao–Scott transformation to the case of correlated multinomial data. The Rao–Scott transformation has several advantages over direct analysis of the original correlated data. First, since the transformation does not require specification of the covariance function, it may enjoy a certain degree of robustness. Second, since the first two moments of the transformed data can be approximated by those of the multinomial distribution, standard methods associated with the multinomial distribution are readily applicable. For example, chi-squared statistics may be used as a measure of goodness of fit. Third, analysis of the transformed data is computationally simpler than analysis of the original data. In an analysis of 11 experiments conducted under the US National Toxicology Program, Krewski and Zhu

(1995) found that dose–response models fitted after applying the Rao–Scott transformation were practically equivalent to models fitted to the original data using the Dirichlet-trinomial covariance function.

We now describe the Rao–Scott transformation. Suppose that the response probabilities $\mu_i = (\mu_{i1}, \mu_{i2})^{\mathrm{T}}$ for fetuses from the jth litter in the ith dose group are constant within the dose group, with expected numbers of deaths and malformed fetuses

$$\mathrm{E}(\mathbf{z}_{ij} \mid m_{ij}) = m_{ij}(\mu_{i1}, \mu_{i2})^{\mathrm{T}} = m_{ij}\,\mu_i$$

given the number of implants m_{ij}, where $\mathbf{z}_{ij} = (y_{ij}, r_{ij})^{\mathrm{T}}$. Let $\mathbf{z}_{i\cdot} = \Sigma_{j=1}^{n_i} \mathbf{z}_{ij} = (y_{i\cdot}, r_{i\cdot})^{\mathrm{T}}$, $m_{i\cdot} = \Sigma_{j=1}^{n_i} m_{ij}$, and write

$$\mathrm{Var}(\mathbf{z}_{i\cdot}) = \sum_{j=1}^{n_i} m_{ij}\mathbf{V}_{ij} = m_{i\cdot}\mathbf{V}_i,$$

where the dependence of $\mathbf{V}_i$ on m_{ij} is suppressed for notational simplicity. The special case in which $\mathbf{V}_i$ is equal to

$$\mathbf{V}_0(\mu_i) = \mathrm{diag}(\mu_i) - \mu_i\,\mu_i^{\mathrm{T}} \tag{11.9}$$

corresponds to the multinomial covariance function. When intra-litter correlation is ignored, the Pearson chi-squared statistic for the ith dose group is given by

$$\begin{aligned} X_i^2 &= \frac{(y_{i\cdot} - m_{i\cdot}\mu_{i1})^2}{m_{i\cdot}\mu_{i1}} + \frac{(r_{i\cdot} - m_{i\cdot}\mu_{i2})^2}{m_{i\cdot}\mu_{i2}} + \frac{(s_{i\cdot} - y_{i\cdot} - m_{i\cdot}\mu_{i3})^2}{m_{i\cdot}\mu_{i3}} \\ &= m_{i\cdot}(\hat{\mu}_i - \mu_i)^{\mathrm{T}}[\mathbf{V}_0(\mu_i)]^{-1}(\hat{\mu}_i - \mu_i), \end{aligned} \tag{11.10}$$

where $\mu_{i3} = 1 - \mu_{i1} - \mu_{i2}$ and $\hat{\mu}_i = \mathbf{z}_{i\cdot}/m_{i\cdot}$. When μ_i and $m_{i\cdot}\mathbf{V}_i$ correspond to the true mean and covariance function respectively, standard arguments (cf. Rao and Scott 1981) yield the large sample approximation

$$X_i^2 = \lambda_{i1}Z_1^2 + \lambda_{i2}Z_2^2 + O_p(n_i^{-1/2}). \tag{11.11}$$

Here, Z_k^2 $(k = 1, 2)$ are independent chi-squared variates, each with one degree of freedom. The positive eigenvalues λ_{i1} and λ_{i2} of $[\mathbf{V}_0(\mu_i)]^{-1}\mathbf{V}_i$ have been called *generalized design effects* by Rao and Scott (1981), and represent a multivariate ratio of $\mathbf{V}_i$ to $\mathbf{V}_0(\mu_i)$.

After dividing X_i^2 by the average design effects $\bar{\lambda}_i = (\lambda_{i1} + \lambda_{i2})/2$, we have $\mathrm{E}(X_i^2/\bar{\lambda}_i) \approx \mathrm{E}(\chi_2^2) = 2$. If the λ_{ik} $(k = 1, 2)$ differ only slightly, we have $\mathrm{Var}(X_i^2/\bar{\lambda}_i) \approx 4(1 + \rho^2) \approx \mathrm{Var}(\chi_2^2)$, where $\rho = (\lambda_{i1} - \lambda_{i2})/(\lambda_{i1} + \lambda_{i2})$ is the coefficient of variation for the λ_{ik}. If the λ_{ik} are identical in limit as $n_i \to \infty$, we have

$$X_i^2/\bar{\lambda}_i = \chi_2^2 + O_p(n_i^{-1/2}).$$

This is the case when, for example, $\mathrm{Var}(\mathbf{z}_{ij}) = m_{ij}h_{ij}^{-1}\mathbf{V}_0(\mu_i)$, where h_{ij} is a positive, real-valued function. (Note that the Dirichlet-multinomial covariance function corresponds to $h^{-1}=[1+(m-1)\phi]$.) Since scaling X_i^2 by $\bar{\lambda}_i$ is equivalent to scaling $\mathbf{z}_{ij}$ and m_{ij}, eqn. (11.11) suggests the simple data transformation

$$\tilde{\mathbf{z}}_{ij}=\mathbf{z}_{ij}/\bar{\lambda}_i, \tag{11.12}$$

with $\tilde{m}_{ij}=m_{ij}/\bar{\lambda}_i$. With moderately large samples, the mean and covariance of the transformed data are given by

$$\mathbf{E}\left(\tilde{\mathbf{z}}_{ij}\mid \tilde{m}_{ij}\right)=\tilde{m}_{ij}\,\mu_i+O(n_i^{-1/2})$$

and

$$\operatorname{Var}\left(\tilde{\mathbf{z}}_{ij}\mid \tilde{m}_{ij}\right)=\tilde{m}_{ij}\left[\operatorname{diag}(\mu_i)-\mu_i\,\mu_i^{\mathrm{T}}\right]+O(n_i^{-1/2}).$$

Therefore, they can be approximated by the mean and covariance of the multinomial distribution.

To use the transformation we need to estimate $\bar{\lambda}_i$. Notice that

$$\bar{\lambda}_i=\tfrac{1}{2}\operatorname{trace}\left[\mathbf{V}_0^{-1}(\mu_i)\mathbf{V}_i\right]+O(n_i^{-1/2})=\tfrac{1}{2}\left(\frac{v_{i11}}{\mu_{i1}}+\frac{v_{i22}}{\mu_{i2}}+\frac{v_{i33}}{\mu_{i3}}\right)+O(n_i^{-1/2}), \tag{11.13}$$

where $m_{i\cdot}v_{ikk}$ $(k=1,2,3)$ are the variances of $y_{i\cdot}$, $r_{i\cdot}$, and $s_{i\cdot}-y_{i\cdot}$ given $m_{i\cdot}$ respectively. It follows that estimates of $\bar{\lambda}_i$ may be obtained by using estimates of v_{ikk} and μ_{ik} in eqn. (11.13). For example, the response probabilities μ_{i1}, μ_{i2} and μ_{i3} may be estimated by $\hat{\mu}_{i1}=y_{i\cdot}/m_{i\cdot}$, $\hat{\mu}_{i2}=r_{i\cdot}/m_{i\cdot}$, and $\hat{\mu}_{i3}=1-\hat{\mu}_{i1}-\hat{\mu}_{i2}$, respectively. The sample variances

$$\hat{v}_{i11}=\frac{n_i}{(n_i-1)m_{i\cdot}}\sum_{j=1}^{n_i}(y_{ij}-m_{ij}\,\hat{\mu}_{i1})^2,\qquad \hat{v}_{i22}=\frac{n_i}{(n_i-1)m_{i\cdot}}\sum_{j=1}^{n_i}(r_{ij}-m_{ij}\,\hat{\mu}_{i2})^2$$

and

$$\hat{v}_{i33}=\frac{n_i}{(n_i-1)m_{i\cdot}}\sum_{j=1}^{n_i}(s_{ij}-y_{ij}-m_{ij}\,\hat{\mu}_{i3})^2$$

of the three component responses may be used to estimate v_{ikk} $(k=1,2,3)$. Values of $\bar{\lambda}_i$ greater or less than unity indicate overdispersion or underdispersion respectively relative to trinomial variation.

11.3 Dose–response models

Although biologically based dose–response models for developmental toxicity are not well developed (Gaylor and Razzaghi 1992), statistical models for the response probabilities π_1 and π_2 are available. For example, any non-decreasing cumulative distribution function $F(a+b\eta(d_i))$ which depends linearly on the dose d_i through a monotone function $\eta(d)$ may be used for dose–response modelling. Commonly used dose–response models include the probit model $F(x) = \Phi(x)$, the linear logistic model $F(x) = (1 + \exp(-x))^{-1}$, and the extreme value model $F(x) = 1 - \exp(\exp(x))$. Krewski and Van Ryzin (1981) noted that the extreme value model can be reparametrized to the Weibull model discussed below.

Motivated by single-hit kinetics, Rai and Van Ryzin (1985) proposed the model

$$P(d \mid s) = [1 - \exp\{-(a + bd)\}]\exp(-sd)$$

to describe the probability $P(d \mid s)$ of a fetal malformation at dose d, incorporating litter size s as a covariate to account for extra-binomial variation in the data. Kodell *et al.* (1991) proposed a Weibull model incorporating both a threshold dose and litter size. Using likelihood ratio tests based on the beta-binomial distribution, these latter authors found that the inclusion of litter size s did not significantly improve the goodness of fit of the model.

Lefkopoulou *et al.* (1989) used linear logistic models to jointly model data on multiple malformations. Catalano and Ryan (1992) suggested a probit model for fetal malformations, conditioning on fetal weight. Ryan (1992) and Krewski and Zhu (1995) considered jointly fitting the Weibull models

$$\pi_1(d) = 1 - \exp\{-(a_1 + b_1 d^{\gamma_1})\} \quad \text{and} \quad \pi_2(d) = 1 - \exp\{-(a_2 + b_2 d^{\gamma_2})\} \tag{11.14, 11.15}$$

to the data on fetal malformation and prenatal death respectively. Given π_1 and π_2, the probability of an implant being either dead or resorbed, or developing a malformation, is given by

$$\pi_3(d) = 1 - [1 - \pi_1(d)][1 - \pi_2(d)]. \tag{11.16}$$

Although one may include the number of implants m as a covariate in these models, a previous analysis of data from 11 developmental studies provided no evidence that the implant number m is a predictor of the probability of fetal malformation or death (Krewski and Zhu 1994). However, in another analysis of a large-scale study of the developmental toxicity of the herbicide 2,4,5-trichlorophenoxyacetic acid, implant number did appear to be related to the response probabilities π_1 and π_2 (Zhu *et al.* 1994). Kupper *et al.* (1986) and Allen *et al.* (1994*b*) also considered the use of litter size s as a covariate of dose–response modelling.

Notice that the proportions $1 - \exp(-a_k)$ $(k = 1, 2)$ are the population average probabilities of an anomaly occurring spontaneously in the absence of exposure to the test agent. The constraints $a_k \geqslant 0$ and $b_k \geqslant 0$ ensure that $0 \leqslant \lambda_k \leqslant 1$. The Weibull parameter γ_k determines the shape of the dose–response curve. For $\gamma_k < 1$ the curve is concave; for $\gamma_k > 1$ the curve is convex when $d < \{(1 - \gamma_k^{-1})b_k^{-1}\}^{1/\gamma_k}$ and concave when $d > \{(1 - \gamma_k^{-1})b_k^{-1}\}^{1/\gamma_k}$. If dose is scaled to be in the range of $[0, 1]$, the inflection point is a strictly increasing function of γ_k, and approaches 1 as $\gamma_k \to \infty$. Although the Weibull models may not be suitable for use with data that are incompatible with these properties, they are sufficiently flexible to describe the dose–response relationships observed in a number of developmental toxicity studies conducted under the US National Toxicology Program (Krewski and Zhu 1994, 1995). For purposes of model fitting, the two sets of parameters $\theta_k = (a_k, b_k, \gamma_k)^{\mathrm{T}}$ involved in π_k $(k = 1, 2)$ may be regarded as functionally independent.

11.4 Generalized score tests for trend

Generalized score functions (GSFs) for the unknown parameters are defined here in analogy with quasi-score functions. For developmental toxicity data (y, r, s) given m, the parameter vector θ involved in the dose–response models discussed in Section 11.3 can be written as $\theta = (\psi^{\mathrm{T}}, \lambda^{\mathrm{T}})^{\mathrm{T}}$, where $\psi = (b_1, b_2)^{\mathrm{T}}$ denotes the parameters of interest characterizing the slope of the dose–response curves, and λ denotes the remaining parameters. In the case of a generalized linear model ($\eta(d) \equiv d$), for example, $\psi = (b_1, b_2)^{\mathrm{T}}$ and $\lambda = (a_1, a_2)^{\mathrm{T}}$, where (a_k, b_k) are the parameters involved in the model π_k $(k = 1, 2)$. The composite null hypothesis of no dose effect can be generally formulated as

$$\mathrm{H}_0 : \psi = (b_1, b_2)^{\mathrm{T}} = (0, 0)^{\mathrm{T}}, \tag{11.17}$$

or, equivalently,

$$\mathrm{H}_0 : \mu_i = \mu_0 \qquad (i = 1, \ldots, t),$$

with the nuisance parameters λ unspecified. The generalized score tests of the null hypothesis H_0 to be discussed here are similar in spirit to Neyman's $C(\alpha)$ tests (Neyman 1959). Moreover, they are based on the GSFs for ψ after being orthogonalized with respect to the GSFs for the nuisance parameters λ. The nuisance parameters involved in the orthogonalized scores are replaced by their estimates under H_0. Further theoretical motivation for such tests will be reported separately. Similar methods have been considered by Basawa (1991).

11.4.1 *Orthogonalized score statistics*

The GSFs for ψ and λ are given by

$$\mathbf{g}_\psi = \sum_{i=1}^{t} \sum_{j=1}^{n_i} m_{ij} \mathbf{D}_{i\psi}^{\mathrm{T}} \mathbf{V}_{ij}^{-1} (\mathbf{z}_{ij} - m_{ij} \mu_i) \tag{11.18}$$

and

$$\mathbf{g}_\lambda = \sum_{i=1}^{t} \sum_{j=1}^{n_i} m_{ij} \mathbf{D}_{i\lambda}^{\mathrm{T}} \mathbf{V}_{ij}^{-1} (\mathbf{z}_{ij} - m_{ij} \mu_i) \tag{11.19}$$

respectively, where $\mathbf{D}_{i\psi} = \partial \mu_i / \partial \psi^{\mathrm{T}}$, $\mathbf{D}_{i\lambda} = \partial \mu_i / \partial \lambda^{\mathrm{T}}$, $\mu_i = (\mu_{i1}, \mu_{i2})^{\mathrm{T}}$, and $\mathbf{V}_{ij}$ is the covariance function. Because $\mathbf{g}_\psi$ and $\mathbf{g}_\lambda$ are correlated and may involve the entire parameter vector θ, we orthogonalize $\mathbf{g}_\psi$ locally with respect to $\mathbf{g}_\lambda$ in the sense of Cox and Reid (1987). Since the distributions of the orthogonalized score functions are asymptotically independent, inferences about ψ based on the orthogonalized score for ψ will be independent of the nuisance parameters λ. Specifically, the locally orthogonalized GSFs for λ are given by

$$\mathbf{g}_{\psi\cdot\lambda} = \mathbf{g}_{\psi} - \mathbf{\Sigma}_{\psi\lambda}\mathbf{\Sigma}_{\lambda\lambda}^{-1}\mathbf{g}_{\lambda} = \sum_{i=1}^{t}\sum_{j=1}^{n_i} m_{ij}\mathbf{D}_{i\psi\cdot\lambda}^{\mathrm{T}}\mathbf{V}_{ij}^{-1}(\mathbf{z}_{ij} - m_{ij}\mu_i), \tag{11.20}$$

where $\mathbf{\Sigma}_{\psi\lambda} = \mathbf{Cov}(\mathbf{g}_{\psi}, \mathbf{g}_{\lambda})$, $\mathbf{\Sigma}_{\lambda\lambda} = \mathbf{Cov}(\mathbf{g}_{\lambda}, \mathbf{g}_{\lambda})$, and

$$\mathbf{D}_{i\psi\cdot\lambda}^{\mathrm{T}} = \mathbf{D}_{i\psi}^{\mathrm{T}} - \Sigma_{\psi\lambda}\Sigma_{\lambda\lambda}^{-1}\mathbf{D}_{i\lambda}^{\mathrm{T}}.$$

One may view $\mathbf{D}_{i\psi\cdot\lambda}$ as the residual design matrix after projecting $\mathbf{D}_{i\psi}$ on to the linear space spanned by the row vectors of $\mathbf{D}_{i\lambda}$.

The generalized score statistic is then given by

$$T_2 = \mathbf{g}_{\psi\cdot\lambda}^{\mathrm{T}}\mathbf{\Sigma}_{\psi\cdot\lambda}^{-1}\mathbf{g}_{\psi\cdot\lambda}, \tag{11.21}$$

where

$$\mathbf{\Sigma}_{\psi\cdot\lambda} = \mathbf{Cov}(\mathbf{g}_{\psi\cdot\lambda}, \mathbf{g}_{\psi\cdot\lambda}) = \mathbf{\Sigma}_{\psi\psi} - \mathbf{\Sigma}_{\psi\lambda}\mathbf{\Sigma}_{\lambda\lambda}^{-1}\mathbf{\Sigma}_{\lambda\psi}.$$

The unspecified value of λ involved in T_2 needs to be estimated in order to use T_2 as a test statistic. Consistent estimates of λ can be obtained by setting the GSF $\mathbf{g}_{\lambda}$ to zero and solving the resulting estimating equations under H_0 with respect to λ. Under the null hypothesis H_0, we than have

$$T_2 = \chi_2^2 + O_p(n^{-1/2}),$$

where $n = \Sigma_i$ and χ_2^2 is a chi-squared variate with $2 = \dim(\psi)$ degrees of freedom. Large values of T_2 indicate departures from the null hypothesis.

Since GSFs depend on the specification of dose–response models for π_1 and π_2 and the covariance function $\mathbf{V}_{ij}$, the generalized score statistic T_2 is generally model-dependent. Although we may consider any reasonable dose–response models to construct generalized score statistics, there are several reasons for focusing on the generalized linear dose–response models (excluding the Weibull model) discussed in Section 11.3. First, under the null hypothesis the generalized scores for ψ are identical (up to a proportionality constant) with respect to all generalized linear dose–response models. Thus, the generalized score statistic is unique within this class of generalized linear models, and in this sense possesses a certain non-parametric property (Cox 1958). Second, generalized score tests based on a specific generalized linear model are likely to be reasonably powerful for detecting monotone increasing dose-related effects, even if the true dose–response relationship may not be well described by this model. This robustness has been demonstrated in a related context by Tarone and Gart (1980). Third, the use of a non-linear dose–response model is generally more complicated. Under the Weibull models in eqns. (11.14) and (11.15), for example, the nuisance parameters γ_1 and γ_2 cannot be estimated under H_0 because of their non-indentifiability with respect to b_1 and b_2.

11.4.2 *A class of test statistics*

We will exploit the non-parametric property of the generalized score statistic within the class of generalized linear dose–response models, and derive a broad family of test statistics on the basis of the logistic models

$$\mu_{ik} = \mu_k(d_i) = \exp(a_k + b_k d_i)/[1 + \exp(a_1 + b_1 d_i) + \exp(a_2 + b_2 d_i)] \quad (11.22)$$

$(k = 1, 2)$. It follows from eqn. (11.7) that

$$\pi_1(d_i) = \mu_{i1}/(1 - \mu_{i2}) = [1 + \exp(-a_1 - b_1 d_i)]^{-1}$$

with $\pi_2 = \mu_2$. For simplicity, we consider the covariance function

$$\mathbf{V}_{ij} = \operatorname{Var}(\mathbf{z}_{ij}) = m_{ij} h_{ij}^{-1} \mathbf{V}(\mu_i), \quad (11.23)$$

where $h_{ij} = h(m_{ij}, \mu_i)$ is a positive real-valued function and $\mathbf{V}(\mu_i)$ may be unspecified.

Under the null hypothesis H_0: $\mu_i = \mu_0 = (\mu_{01}, \mu_{02})^{\mathrm{T}}$ and the covariance function in eqn. (11.23), we have

$$T_2 = \frac{1}{\sum_{i=1}^{t}\sum_{j=1}^{n_i}(d_i - \bar{d})^2 m_{ij} h_{ij}} \left\{ \sum_{i=1}^{t}\sum_{j=1}^{n_i}(d_i - \bar{d}) h_{ij} \mathbf{z}_{ij}^{\mathrm{T}} \right\} \times [\mathbf{V}(\hat{\mu}_0)]^{-1} \left\{ \sum_{i=1}^{t}\sum_{j=1}^{n_i}(d_i - \bar{d}) h_{ij} \mathbf{z}_{ij} \right\}, \quad (11.24)$$

where

$$\bar{d} = \sum_{i=1}^{t}\sum_{j=1}^{n_i} d_i m_{ij} h_{ij} \Big/ \left[\sum_{i=1}^{t}\sum_{j=1}^{n_i} m_{ij} h_{ij} \right].$$

The nuisance parameters μ_0 (a one-to one transformation of λ) are estimated by

$$\hat{\mu}_0 = \sum_{i=1}^{t}\sum_{j=1}^{n_i} h_{ij} \mathbf{z}_{ij} \Big/ \left[\sum_{i=1}^{t}\sum m_{ij} h_{ij} \right].$$

Letting $\mathbf{V}(\hat{\mu}_0) = \operatorname{diag}(\hat{\mu}_0) - \hat{\mu}_0 \hat{\mu}_0^{\mathrm{T}}$, we have

$$T_2 = \frac{1}{\sum_{i=1}^{t}\sum_{j=1}^{n_i}(d_i - \bar{d})^2 h_{ij} m_{ij}} \left\{ \frac{\left[\sum_{i=1}^{t}\sum_{j=1}^{n_i}(d_i - \bar{d}) h_{ij} y_{ij}\right]^2}{\hat{\mu}_{01}} + \frac{\left[\sum_{i=1}^{t}\sum_{j=1}^{n_i}(d_i - \bar{d}) h_{ij} r_{ij}\right]^2}{\hat{\mu}_{02}} + \frac{\left[\sum_{i=1}^{t}\sum_{j=1}^{n_i}(d_i - \bar{d}) h_{ij} (s_{ij} - y_{ij})\right]^2}{\hat{\mu}_{03}} \right\},$$

where $\hat{\mu}_{03} = 1 - \hat{\mu}_{01} - \hat{\mu}_{02}$. Choosing $h_{ij} = 1$, we obtain a multinomial version of the Cochran–Armitage trend test, which is applicable after applying the Rao–Scott transformation. This family of generalized score tests can be extended in straightforward fashion to the case of multiple binary responses. For example, the tests of Lefkopoulou *et al.* (1989) and Lefkopoulou and Ryan (1996) can be derived using our method with appropriate empirical covariance functions.

In the case of a univariate outcome such as the malformation rate y/s, a family of the generalized score statistics T_1 is easily obtained. This family of test statistics encompasses trend tests proposed previously in the literature for correlated binary data. Taking the square-root of T_1, we have

$$Z = \sqrt{T_1} = \frac{\left\{ \sum_{i=1}^{t} \sum_{j=1}^{n_i} (d_i - \bar{d}) V_{ij}^{-1} s_{ij} y_{ij} \right\}}{\left\{ \left[\sum_{i=1}^{t} \sum_{j=1}^{n_i} (d_i - \bar{d})^2 s_{ij}^2 V_{ij}^{-1} \right]^{1/2} \right\}}. \tag{11.25}$$

Substituting $s_{ij}\hat{\pi}_{10}(1 - \hat{\pi}_{10})$ for V_{ij} yields the Cochran–Armitage test. Replacing $\mathbf{V}_{ij}$ with $\hat{\phi} s_{ij}\hat{\pi}_{10}(1 - \hat{\pi}_{10})$, with the moment estimate $\hat{\phi}$, gives the test proposed by Ryan (1994). Any reasonable sample-based estimate of $\mathbf{V}_{ij}$ may also be used. The test statistic of Lefkopoulou *et al.* (1989) may be obtained by first assuming $V_{ij} = s_{ij}\mathbf{V}$, and then replacing $s_{i\cdot}\mathbf{V}$ in the denominator by the sample estimate

$$\hat{V}_{i\cdot} = \sum_{j=1}^{n_i} (y_{ij} - s_{ij}\hat{\pi}_{10})^2.$$

Finally, estimating V_{ij} by

$$\bar{\lambda} s_{ij}\hat{\pi}_{10}(1 - \hat{\pi}_{10}),$$

with $\bar{\lambda}$ being the estimated design effect pooled across dose groups, yields the test statistic suggested by Rao and Scott (1992).

11.4.3 Applications

The application of the generalized score tests are illustrated using the data sets EG and EGDE. Test statistics for the univariate outcome y/s, r/m, and $(y + r)/m$ are given in Table 11.3. For each outcome, test statistics based on the extended beta-binomial variance (BB), the generalized linear model variance (GLM), and Rao–Scott transformation (RS) are computed. The corresponding multivariate statistics based on the multivariate responses (y, r) are given in Table 11.4, using the Dirichlet-trinomial (DT) covariance function as an extension of the beta-binomial variance.

The observed values of these three test statistics for both the univariate and multivariate responses are highly significant for both data sets. Although a

Table 11.3. Generalized score statistics for trend based on univariate data[a]

End-point	Compound	Test statistics[b] BB	GLM	RS
Fetal malformation	EG	8.23	7.93	11.42
	EGDE	6.93	6.90	8.51
Prenatal death	EG	3.93	3.85	3.49
	EGDE	3.04	3.63	3.45
Overall toxicity	EG	8.16	8.10	11.46
	EGDE	6.01	6.56	7.23

[a] Square root of the score statistics are used, which follow the standard normal distribution.
[b] BB, beta-binomial variance function; GLM variance function of generalized linear model; RS, binomial variance applied to transformed data.

Table 11.4. Generalized score statistics for trend in overall toxicity based on multivariate data[a]

Compound	Test statistics[b] DT	GLM	RS
EG	89.27	88.86	143.93
EGDE	47.33	53.35	55.83

[a] All statistics follow a chi-squared distribution with two degrees of freedom.
[b] DT, Dirichlet-trinomial covariance function; GLM, covariance function of generalized linear model; RS, trinomial covariance applied to transformed data.

preliminary simulation study of these univariate statistics with a general correlation structure indicates that they are comparable in terms of type I and type II error, further investigation of the behaviour of the multivariate statistics with different variance structures would be helpful. *A priori*, we would expect multivariate tests based on the trinomial data to be more sensitive than univariate tests based on binomial data.

11.5 Fitting dose–response models

The method of generalized estimating equations (GEEs) (Liang and Zeger 1986; Liang *et al.* 1992) has been widely used in analysing multivariate data for which the underlying distribution is difficult to specify. GEEs are not only flexible in terms of distributional assumptions; they are often computationally simpler than maximum likelihood estimation. With the specification of a working covariance function when the true covariance is unknown, GEEs still yield consistent and asymptotically normally distributed estimator under mild regularity conditions, although efficiency may decrease. GEEs include quasi-likelihood and likelihood equations as special cases. Williams (1982) used quasi-likelihood methods to fit a linear logistic model to the fetal malformation rate y/s. Whereas Williams (1982), Ryan (1992), and Krewski and Zhu (1994) used the moment method based on Pearson's chi-squared statistics, Zhu *et al.* (1994) and Krewski and Zhu (1995) used quadratic GEEs to estimate the overdispersion parameters.

11.5.1 *Generalized estimating equations*

Given dose–response models $\mu(d_i; \theta) = \mu_i = (\mu_{i1}, \mu_{i2})^{\mathrm{T}}$, the GEEs for estimating the unknown parameters $\theta = (\theta_1^{\mathrm{T}}, \theta_2^{\mathrm{T}})^{\mathrm{T}} = (a_1, b_1, \gamma_1, a_2, b_2, \gamma_2)^{\mathrm{T}}$ are given by

$$\sum_{i=1}^{t} \sum_{j=1}^{n_i} m_{ij} \mathbf{D}_{1i}^{\mathrm{T}} \mathbf{W}_{1ij}^{-1} (\mathbf{z}_{ij} - m_{ij} \mu_i) = \mathbf{0}, \tag{11.26}$$

where $\mathbf{D}_{1i} = \partial \mu_i / \partial \theta^{\mathrm{T}}$ and $\mathbf{W}_{1ij}$ are 'working covariance' or weight matrices, preferably chosen to approximate the actual covariance matrix of $\mathbf{z}_{ij}$ in order to achieve high efficiency. When the working covariance matrices involve additional parameters such as the intra-litter correlation coefficients $\{\phi_i\}$ in eqn. (11.8), these parameters need to be estimated using another set of equations.

To fit the Weibull models (11.14) and (11.15), we set $\mathbf{W}_{1ij}$ equal to the Dirichlet-trinomial covariance given in eqn. (11.8). Equations (11.26) then simplify to two separate sets of equations,

$$\sum_{i=1}^{t} \sum_{j=1}^{n_i} \frac{1}{1 + (m_{ij} - 1)\phi_i} \frac{1}{\pi_{1i}(1 - \pi_{i1})} \frac{\partial \pi_{i1}}{\partial \theta_1} (y_{ij} - s_{ij} \pi_{i1}) = \mathbf{0} \tag{11.27}$$

and

$$\sum_{i=1}^{t} \sum_{j=1}^{n_i} \frac{1}{1 + (m_{ij} - 1)\phi_i} \frac{1}{\pi_{i2}(1 - \pi_{i2})} \frac{\partial \pi_{i2}}{\partial \theta_2} (r_{ij} - m_{ij} \pi_{i2}) = \mathbf{0}, \tag{11.28}$$

involving θ_1 and θ_2 respectively.

To estimate the intra-litter correlation coefficients $\{\theta_i\}$, the multivariate Pearson squared residuals $(\mathbf{z}_{ij} - m_{ij} \mu_i)^{\mathrm{T}} \mathbf{W}_{1ij}^{-1} (\mathbf{z}_{ij} - m_{ij} \mu_i)$ can be used to construct another set of equations that are quadratic in the $\mathbf{z}_{ij}$. Letting

$$Q_{ij} = m_{ij}\{1 + (m_{ij} - 1)\phi_i\} \pi_{i1}(1 - \pi_{i1}) \pi_{i2}(1 - \pi_{i2}) (\mathbf{z}_{ij} - m_{ij} \mu_i)^{\mathrm{T}}$$
$$\times \mathbf{W}_{1ij}^{-1} (\mathbf{z}_{ij} - m_{ij} \mu_i),$$

$$\sigma_{ij} = \mathrm{E}(Q_{ij}) = 2 m_{ij}\{1 + (m_{ij} - 1)\phi_i\} \pi_{i1}(1 - \pi_{i1}) \pi_{i2}(1 - \pi_{i2}),$$

and $\mathbf{D}_{2ij} = \partial \sigma_{ij} / \partial \phi_i$, we have the quadratic GEEs for $\{\phi_i\}$,

$$\sum_{j=1}^{n_i} \mathbf{D}_{2ij}^{\mathrm{T}} \mathbf{W}_{2ij}^{-1} (Q_{ij} - \sigma_{ij}) = 0 \tag{11.29}$$

$(i = 1, \ldots, t)$. Equations (29) reduce to the usual Pearson moment equations,

$$\sum_{j=1}^{n_i} (z_{ij} - m_{ij} \mu_i)^{\mathrm{T}} \mathbf{W}_{1ij}^{-1} (z_{ij} - m_{ij} \mu_i) = 2 n_i,$$

if we choose $\mathbf{W}_{2ij} = \mathbf{D}_{2ij}\sigma_{ij}/2$. In practice, the Pearson moment equations given above would be multiplied by a factor of $1 - p(2n)^{-1}$ where $n = \sum_i n_i$, to adjust for the simultaneous estimation of p regression parameters in the dose–response models. In what follows, we set $\mathbf{W}_{2ij} = \sigma_{ij}^2$ for convenience, as the third and fourth moments of $\mathbf{z}_{ij}$ are unknown. The use of the quadratic estimating equations of the form (11.29) is equivalent to generalized least squares estimation when the weights $\mathbf{W}_{2ij}$ are evaluated at a fixed value of ϕ_i. They can be viewed as a multivariate version of a class of regression equations based on absolute residuals (Davidian and Carroll 1987, eqn. 4.1). Joint estimation of the mean and correlation parameters based on GEEs has also been discussed by Zhao and Prentice (1990) and Prentice and Zhao (1991).

The parameter estimates $\hat{\theta}_1$, $\hat{\theta}_2$, and $\{\hat{\phi}_i\}$ are obtained by iteratively solving eqns. (11.27), (11.28), and (11.29) until convergence. At each iteration, eqns. (11.27) and (11.28) are solved for θ_1 and θ_2 respectively with $\{\phi_i\}$ fixed at $\{\hat{\phi}_i\}$; eqns. (11.29) are solved for $\{\phi_i\}$ with θ_1 and θ_2 fixed at $\hat{\theta}_1$ and $\hat{\theta}_2$ respectively. For the transformed data $(\tilde{y}, \tilde{r}\}$ obtained using the Rao–Scott transformation, we simply set $\phi_i = 0$ and solve just eqns. (11.27) and (11.28) for θ_1 and θ_2.

11.5.2 *Large sample properties of parameter estimates*

Under mild regularity conditions, estimators of the unknown model parameters using the GEEs in eqns. (11.27)–(11.29) are consistent and normally distributed as each $n_i \to \infty$ at comparable rates (cf. Zhu *et al.* 1994). The covariance matrix of $(\hat{\theta}^{\mathrm{T}}, \hat{\phi}_1, \ldots, \hat{\phi}_t)^{\mathrm{T}}$ may be estimated by

$$\begin{pmatrix} \boldsymbol{\Delta}_{11} & \mathbf{0} \\ \boldsymbol{\Delta}_{21} & \boldsymbol{\Delta}_{22} \end{pmatrix}^{-1} \begin{pmatrix} \mathbf{V}_{11} & \mathbf{V}_{12} \\ \mathbf{V}_{21} & \mathbf{V}_{22} \end{pmatrix} \begin{pmatrix} \boldsymbol{\Delta}_{11} & \mathbf{0} \\ \boldsymbol{\Delta}_{21} & \boldsymbol{\Delta}_{22} \end{pmatrix}^{-\mathrm{T}},$$

where

$$\boldsymbol{\Delta}_{11} = \sum_{i=1}^{t} \sum_{j=1}^{n_i} m_{ij}^2 \mathbf{D}_{1i}^{\mathrm{T}} \mathbf{W}_{1ij}^{-1} \mathbf{D}_{1i},$$

$$\boldsymbol{\Delta}_{21} = \begin{pmatrix} \sum_{j=1}^{n_1} \mathbf{D}_{21j}^{\mathrm{T}} \mathbf{W}_{21j}^{-1} \delta_{1j} \\ \vdots \\ \sum_{j=1}^{n_t} \mathbf{D}_{2tj}^{\mathrm{T}} \mathbf{W}_{2tj}^{-1} \delta_{tj} \end{pmatrix},$$

and

$$\boldsymbol{\Delta}_{22} = \mathrm{diag}\left(\sum_{j=1}^{n_i} \mathbf{D}_{2ij}^{\mathrm{T}} \mathbf{W}_{2ij}^{-1} \mathbf{D}_{2ij};\ i = 1, \ldots, t \right),$$

with $\delta_{ij} = \mathrm{E}(\partial(Q_{ij} - \sigma_{ij})/\partial\theta^{\mathrm{T}})$. The high order moments involved in the $\mathbf{V}$

matrix can be replaced by the corresponding sample moments to guard against misspecification, giving

$$\mathbf{V}_{11} = \sum_{i=1}^{t} \sum_{j=1}^{n_i} m_{ij}^2 \mathbf{D}_{1i}^{\mathrm{T}} \mathbf{W}_{1ij}^{-1} (\mathbf{z}_{ij} - m_{ij}\mu_i)(\mathbf{z}_{ij} - m_{ij}\mu_i)^{\mathrm{T}} \mathbf{W}_{1ij}^{-1} \mathbf{D}_{1i},$$

$$\mathbf{V}_{12} = \begin{pmatrix} \sum_{j=1}^{n_1} m_{ij} \mathbf{D}_{11}^{\mathrm{T}} \mathbf{W}_{11j}^{-1} (\mathbf{z}_{1j} - m_{1j}\mu_1)(Q_{1j} - \sigma_{1j}) \mathbf{W}_{21j}^{-1} \mathbf{D}_{21j} \\ \vdots \\ \sum_{j=1}^{n_t} m_{ij} \mathbf{D}_{1t}^{\mathrm{T}} \mathbf{W}_{1tj}^{-1} (\mathbf{z}_{tj} - m_{tj}\mu_t)(Q_{tj} - \sigma_{tj}) \mathbf{W}_{2tj}^{-1} \mathbf{D}_{2tj} \end{pmatrix}$$

and

$$\mathbf{V}_{22} = \mathrm{diag}\left(\sum_{j=1}^{n_i} \mathbf{D}_{2ij}^{\mathrm{T}} \mathbf{W}_{2ij}^{-1} (Q_{ij} - \sigma_{ij}) \mathbf{W}_{2ij}^{-1} \mathbf{D}_{2ij};\ i = 1, \ldots, t \right),$$

so-called 'sandwich estimates' (Liang and Zeger 1986; Moore and Tsiatis 1991). Here, all quantities in the covariance estimate are evaluated at $\hat{\theta}$ and $\{\hat{\phi}_i\}$. Under the Dirichlet-trinomial covariance function with the observed moments in $\mathbf{V}_{11}$ replaced by their expectation, we have $\mathbf{\Delta}_{11} = \mathbf{V}_{11}$. Therefore, the asymptotic covariance matrix for $\hat{\theta}$ reduces to $\mathbf{\Delta}_{11}^{-1}$, which is block-diagonal with the two diagonal blocks corresponding to $\hat{\theta}_1$ and $\hat{\theta}_2$. This implies that $\hat{\theta}_1$ and $\hat{\theta}_2$ are asymptotically independent, a result also seen from the fact that the two sets of eqns. (11.27) and (11.28) are uncorrelated. Since the dispersion parameters $\{\phi_i\}$ are only involved in the weight matrices $\mathbf{W}_{1ij}$, estimation of the $\{\phi_i\}$ only affects the efficiency of $\hat{\theta}_1$ and $\hat{\theta}_2$. Ignoring terms of order $O(n^{-1})$, the variance of $\hat{\phi}_i$ is given by

$$\mathrm{Var}(\hat{\phi}_i) = \left\{ \sum_{j=1}^{n_i} \mathbf{D}_{2ij}^{\mathrm{T}} \mathbf{W}_{2ij}^{-1} (Q_{ij} - \sigma_{ij})^2 \mathbf{W}_{2ij}^{-1} \mathbf{D}_{2ij} \right\} \left\{ \sum_{j=1}^{n_i} \mathbf{D}_{2ij}^{\mathrm{T}} \mathbf{W}_{2ij}^{-1} \mathbf{D}_{2ij} \right\}^{-2},$$

where θ and $\{\phi_i\}$ are replaced by $\hat{\theta}$ and $\{\hat{\phi}_i\}$ respectively. This variance estimate corresponds to ignoring the correlation between the quadratic GEEs (11.29) for ϕ_i and the GEEs (11.27) and (11.28) for θ.

11.5.3 *Applications*

The methods for model fitting described in this section can be illustrated using the EGDE and EG data. In particular, the Weibull models can be fitted to both the original data assuming a Dirichlet-trinomial covariance function (DT) and the transformed data after applying the Rao–Scott transformation (RS). The estimated design effects $\bar{\lambda}_i$ $(i = 1, 2, 3, 4)$ are 3.61, 2.85, 2.39, and 3.60 for the

Table 11.5. Estimates of the parameters of Weibull dose–response models fitted to the original (DT) and transformed (RS) data[a] (standard error in parentheses)

Parameter		EGDE		EG	
		DT	RS	DT	RS[b]
Fetal malformation	a_1	0.063 (0.027)	0.065 (0.026)	0.013 (0.008)	0.013 (0.008)
	b_1	0.696 (0.151)	0.742 (0.173)	1.228 (0.218)	1.188 (0.219)
	γ_1	3.368 (1.143)	3.384 (1.117)	2.233 (0.282)	2.214 (0.289)
Prenatal death	a_2	0.133 (0.036)	0.129 (0.034)	0.055 (0.013)	0.056 (0.013)
	b_2	0.272 (0.088)	0.324 (0.098)	0.183 (0.069)	0.178 (0.071)
	γ_2	3.334 (3.092)	3.334 (2.592)	3.718 (2.841)	3.711 (2.984)
Intra-litter correlation	ϕ_1	0.435 (0.163)		0.068 (0.067)	
	ϕ_2	0.262 (0.147)		0.094 (0.077)	
	ϕ_3	0.160 (0.105)		0.139 (0.042)	
	ϕ_4	0.299 (0.072)		0.416 (0.113)	

[a] Highest dose scaled to unity.
[b] DT, estimates based on GEEs with the extended Dirichlet-trinomial covariance; RS, estimates based on GEEs with multinomial covariance function after applying the Rao–Scott transformation.

EGDE data, and 1.96, 2.23, 2.82, and 6.69 for the EG data. The estimates of the parameters based on these two methods are comparable, as are the associated standard errors (Table 11.5). The fitted models are shown in Fig. 11.2, where the dotted and solid lines represent the models fitted using the DT and RS methods respectively. Each circle represents the number of identical proportions observed in individual litters, with the radius of the circle being proportional to the number of litters represented. A cross denotes the average response rate in a single dose group. The Weibull models based on both the DT and RS methods appear to fit the data reasonably well.

For the transformed data, standard methods may be used to check model fit. The Pearson chi-squared statistics applied to the total counts $(\tilde{y}_{i\cdot}, \tilde{r}_{i\cdot})$ given $\tilde{m}_{i\cdot}$ are $X^2 = 0.20$ $(p = 0.90)$ and $X^2 = 0.80$ $(p = 0.67)$, each with two degrees of freedom, for the EGDE and EG data respectively.

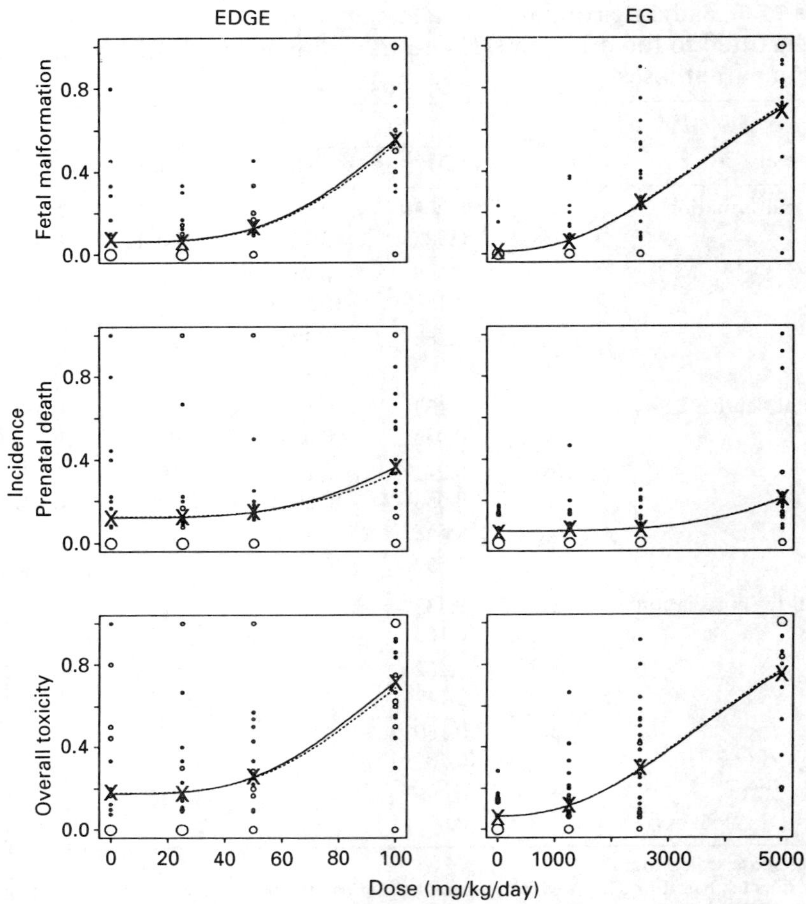

Fig. 11.2. Dose–response models for fetal malformations, prenatal death, and overall toxicity.

11.6 Benchmark dose for risk assessment

An established dose–response relationship provides a useful basis for quantitative risk assessment. At present, human exposure guidelines for developmental toxicants are largely based on the no-observed-adverse-effect-level (NOAEL) derived from laboratory studies. A NOAEL is defined as the highest experimental dose that failed to induce a significant increase in risk in comparison with unexposed controls. A reference dose (RfD) is then obtained by dividing the NOAEL by a suitable uncertainty factor (UF) allowing for difference in susceptibility between animals and humans, and for heterogeneity within the human population. The resulting RfD is then used as a guideline for human exposure. Where a NOAEL is not established, a lowest-observed-adverse-effect-level (LOAEL) is used instead in a similar fashion. Guidelines on the magnitude of the UF to be used in specific cases are given by Barnes and Dourson (1988).

The NOAEL is subject to several limitations (Gaylor 1983, 1989; Kimmel and Gaylor 1988). Restricted to be one of the experimental doses, the NOAEL fails to properly take sample size into account (smaller and less sensitive experiments lead to higher NOAELs than larger studies), and largely ignores the shape of the dose–response curve. Although no explicit statement of risk is made at doses at or above the NOAEL, Gaylor (1992) has shown that the observed risk associated with the NOAEL exceeded 1 per cent in about one quarter of the cases in a series of 120 developmental toxicity experiments. Leisenring and Ryan (1992) found that the NOAEL may identify a dose level associated with unacceptably high risk with a relatively high probability. Consequently, the US Environmental Protection Agency (1991) is considering the use of the benchmark dose (BMD) proposed by Crump (1984) as the basis for derivation of the RfD for developmental toxicity. Ryan (1993) also suggested developing potency measure of developmental toxicity on the basis of benchmark doses.

The BMD was originally defined as the lower confidence limit on the effective dose ED_α that induces $\alpha \times 100$ per cent increase in risk (Crump 1984). In particular, the ED_α may be defined as the solution d_α to the equation

$$\frac{\pi(d_\alpha) - \pi(0)}{1 - \pi(0)} = \alpha,$$

where $\pi(d)$ represents an appropriate dose–response model for a particular end-point. Crump (1984) and Chen and Kodell (1989) discussed the estimation of BMD based on a dose–response model for a single end-point. Allen *et al.* (1994*a*, *b*) and Faustman *et al.* (1994) compared the BMDs with the NOAELs using data from a large database and several dose–response models. On average, they found that the BMD at 5 per cent level of excess risk was similar to the NOAEL. Ryan (1992) and Krewski and Zhu (1994*a*, *b*) used joint dose–response models to estimate the BMDs.

Under the Weibull models (11.14) and (11.15) for the rates of fetal malformation and prenatal death, the ED_α is given by

$$d_\alpha = \left(\frac{-\log(1-\alpha)}{b} \right)^{1/\gamma}, \tag{11.30}$$

where the subscript $k = 1, 2$ for the parameters (b, γ) is suppressed for simplicity of notation. An estimate $\hat{d}_\alpha$ of d_α is obtained by evaluating eqn. (11.30) at $(\hat{b}, \hat{\gamma})$. The variance of $\hat{d}_\alpha$ can be approximated by

$$\mathrm{Var}(\hat{d}_\alpha) = \gamma^{-2} d_\alpha^2 \mathbf{C}_1^{\mathrm{T}} \boldsymbol{\Omega}_1 \mathbf{C}_1 \tag{11.31}$$

using the δ-method, with the unknown parameters involved replaced by $(\hat{b}, \hat{\gamma})$. Here, $\boldsymbol{\Omega}_1$ is the covariance matrix of the estimates $(\hat{b}, \hat{\gamma})^{\mathrm{T}}$ and

$$\mathbf{C}_1 = (b^{-1}, \gamma^{-1} \log[-b^{-1} \log(1-\alpha)])^{\mathrm{T}}.$$

The ED_α for overall toxicity based on eqn. (11.16) is obtained as the solution to the equation

$$b_1 d_\alpha^{\gamma_1} + b_2 d_\alpha^{\gamma_2} = -\log(1-\alpha).$$

The variance of $\hat{d}_\alpha$ based on the δ-method is given by

$$\mathrm{Var}(\hat{d}_\alpha) = \left[b_1\gamma_1 d_\alpha^{\gamma_1 - 1} + b_2\gamma_2 d_\alpha^{\gamma_2 - 1}\right]^{-2} \mathbf{C}_2^{\mathrm{T}}\mathbf{\Omega}_2\mathbf{C}_2, \tag{11.32}$$

where $\mathbf{\Omega}_2$ is the covariance matrix of the estimates $(\hat{b}_1, \hat{\gamma}_1, \hat{b}_2, \hat{\gamma}_2)^{\mathrm{T}}$ and

$$\mathbf{C}_2 = (d_\alpha^{\gamma_1}, b_1 d_\alpha^{\gamma_1}\log d_\alpha, d_\alpha^{\gamma_2}, b_2 d_\alpha^{\gamma_2}\log d_\alpha)^{\mathrm{T}}.$$

The ED_α for overall toxicity is a more sensitive indicator of developmental toxicity than the EDs for fetal malformation or prenatal death. This is because the former is always below the minimum of the latter two (Ryan 1992; Krewski and Zhu 1994*a*), and approximates to the minimum when a strong dose–response relationship is absent for either malformation or death. Moreover, estimates of the ED_α for overall toxicity based on a joint analysis of the prenatal death rate r/m and the fetal malformation rate y/s are expected to be more efficient than estimates based on a direct analysis of the combined rate $(y+r)/m$ (Ryan 1992).

Estimates of ED_{05}'s along with their standard errors for prenatal death, fetal malformation, and overall toxicity based on the Weibull models for the EGDE and EG data are given in Table 11.6. In these examples, the estimates based on Rao–Scott transformation (RS) or GEEs in conjunction with the Dirichlet-trinomial covariance (DT) are comparable. Since EG has less of an effect on the prenatal death rate than on the fetal malformation rate, the ED_{05} for overall toxicity is close to that for fetal malformations.

11.7 Conclusions

In this chapter, we have discussed the statistical analyses of developmental toxicity data, focusing on recent developments in multivariate dose–response

Table 11.6. Estimates of the ED_{05} (mg/kg/day) based on Weibull dose–response models fitted to the original (DT) and transformed (RS) data[a] (standard error in parentheses)

	Malformations		Prenatal death		Overall toxicity	
Compound	RS	DT	RS	DT	RS	DT
EGDE	45.40 (11.56)	46.11 (11.97)	57.54 (25.63)	60.62 (29.58)	40.63 (12.12)	41.70 (13.18)
EG	1209.21 (171.52)	1206.20 (166.77)	3576.57 (1005.22)	3550.64 (966.95)	1199.68 (170.98)	1198.68 (166.04)

[a] DT, estimates based on GEEs with Dirichlet-trinomial covariance; RS, estimates based on GEEs with multinomial covariance after applying the Rao–Scott transformation.

modelling and trend tests for fetal malformation and prenatal death. Conditional on the number of implants per litter, joint analyses are generally more efficient than separate analysis of a single end-point. The extra-multinomial variation associated with litter effects may be characterized using a specified covariance function such as the extended Dirichlet-multinomial covariance. Alternatively, the Rao–Scott transformation based on the concept of generalized design effects may be used so that the transformed data can be approximated by the multinomial mean and covariance.

Generalized score functions were used to obtain a class of statistics associated with generalized linear dose–response models for testing increasing trend in developmental toxicity. This family of statistics includes many other tests previously proposed in the literature. Further investigation of the small sample properties of these generalized score tests under various conditions would be useful.

Weibull dose–response models considered by several authors appear to be sufficiently flexible to describe the dose–response relationships exhibited in a number of developmental toxicity studies. The GEEs employed for model fitting are not only flexible in terms of relaxed distributional assumptions, but also computationally simpler than maximum likelihood estimation based on the Dirichlet-multinomial distribution. The estimates of the model parameters based on GEEs are reasonably efficient relative to maximum likelihood estimates, although estimates of the intra-litter correlation coefficients based on the quadratic GEEs are inefficient (Zhu *et al.* 1994). Improved methods for estimating the dispersion parameters are desirable, since the estimates of these parameters are used to calculate the BMD, defined as the lower confidence limits on the ED_α. Here, we have used $\alpha = 0.05$ in calculation relating to the BMD.

The joint Weibull dose–response models discussed here can be used to estimate the benchmark doses of developmental toxicants. The BMD is currently receiving serious consideration as an alternative to the NOAEL/UF approach to establishing reference doses which serve as human exposure guidelines. The BMD based on the multivariate model for overall toxicity provides a sensitive indicator of risk in that it is less than or equal to the minimum of the BMDs for fetal malformation and prenatal death.

References

Allen, B., Kavlock, R., Kimmel, C., and Faustman, E. (1994*a*). Dose response assessments for developmental toxicity: II. Comparison of generic benchmark dose estimates with NOAELs. *Fundamental and Applied Toxicology*, **23**, 487–95.

Allen, B., Kavlock, R., Kimmel, C., and Faustman, E. (1994*b*). Dose response assessments for developmental toxicity: III. Statistical models. *Fundamental and Applied Toxicology*, **23**, 496–509.

Altham, P. M. E. (1978). Two generalizations of the binomial distribution. *Applied Statistics*, **27**, 162–7.

Armitage, P. (1955). Tests for linear trends in proportions and frequencies. *Biometrics*, **11**, 375–86.

Barnes, D. G. and Dourson, M. (1988). Reference dose (RfD): description and use in health risk assessment. *Regulatory Toxicology and Pharmacology*, **8**, 471–87.

Basawa, I. V. (1991). Generalized score tests for composite hypothesis. In *Estimating functions* (ed. V. P. Godambe), pp. 121–32. Oxford University Press.

Carr, G. and Portier, C. (1993). An evaluation of some methods for fitting dose–response models to quantal-response developmental toxicology data. *Biometrics*, **49**, 779–91.

Catalano, P. J. and Ryan, L (1992). Bivariate latent variable models for clustered discrete and continuous outcomes. *Journal of the American Statistical Association*, **87**, 651–8.

Catalano, P. J., Scharfstein, D. O., Ryan, L., Kimmel, C., and Kimmel, G. (1993). Statistical model for fetal death, fetal weight, and malformation in developmental toxicity studies. *Teratology*, **47**, 281–90.

Chen, J. J. (1993*a*). A malformation incidence dose–response model incorporating fetal weight and/or litter size as covariates. *Risk Analysis*, **14**, 559–64.

Chen, J. J. (1993*b*). Trend test for overdispersed proportions. *Biometrical Journal*, **35**, 949–58.

Chen, J. J. and Kodell, R. L. (1989). Quantitative risk assessment for teratological effects. *Journal of the American Statistical Association*, **84**, 966–71.

Chen, J. J. and Li, L. A. (1994). Dose-response modeling of trinomial responses from developmental experiments. *Statistical Sinica*, **4**, 265–74.

Chen, J. J., Kodell, R. L., Howe, R. B., and Gaylor, D. W. (1991). Analysis of trinomial responses from reproductive and developmental toxicity experiments. *Biometrics*, **47**, 1049–58.

Cochran, W. G. (1954). Some methods for strengthening the common χ^2 tests. *Biometrics*, **10**, 417–51.

Cox, D. R. (1958). The regression analysis of binary sequences (with discussion). *Journal of the Royal Statistical Society, Series B*, **20**, 215–42.

Cox, D. R. and Reid, N. (1987). Parameter orthogonality and approximate conditional inference (with discussion). *Journal of the Royal Statistical Society, Series B*, **49**, 1–39.

Crowder, M. J. (1978). Beta-binomial Anova for proportion. *Applied Statistics*, **27**, 34–37.

Crump, K. S. (1984). A new method for determining allowable daily intakes. *Fundamental and Applied Toxicology*, **4**, 854–71

Davidian, M. and Carroll, R. J. (1987). Variance function estimation. *Journal of the American Statistical Association*, **82**, 1079–91.

Environmental Protection Agency (1991). Guidelines for developmental toxicity risk assessment. *Federal Register*, **56**, 63 797–63 826

Faustman, E. M., Allen, B., Kavlock, R., and Kimmel, C. (1994). Dose response assessments for developmental toxicity: I. Characterization of data base and determination of NOAELs. *Fundamental and Applied Toxicology*, **23**, 478–86.

Fung, K. Y., Krewski, D., Rao, J. N. K., and Scott, A. J. (1994). Tests for trend in developmental toxicity experiments with correlated binary data. *Risk Analysis*, **14**, 621–30.

Gaylor, D. W. (1983). The use of safety factors in controlling risk. *Journal of Toxicology and Environmental Health*, **11**, 329–36.

Gaylor, D. W. (1989). Quantitative risk analysis for quantal reproductive and developmental effects. *Environmental Health Perspectives*, **79**, 243–6.

Gaylor, D. W. (1992). Incidence of developmental defects at the no observed adverse effect level (NOAEL). *Regulatory Toxicology and Pharmacology*, **15**, 151–60.

Gaylor, D. W. and Razzaghi, M. (1992). Process of building biologically based dose–response models for developmental defects. *Teratology*, **46**, 573–81.

Johnson, N. L. and Kotz, S. (1969). *Discrete distributions*. John Wiley, New York.

International Life Sciences Institute (1989). Interpretation and extrapolation of reproductive data to establish human safety standards. In *Current issues in toxicology*, pp. 1–133. Springer-Verlag, New York.

Kimmel, C. A. and Gaylor, D. W. (1988). Issues in qualitative and quantitative risk analysis for developmental toxicology. *Risk Analysis*, **8**, 15–20.

Kodell, R. L., Howe, R. B., Chen, J. J., and Gaylor, D. W. (1991). Mathematical modeling of reproductive and developmental toxic effects for quantitative risk assessment. *Risk Analysis*, **11**, 583–90.

Krewski, D. and Van Ryzin, J. (1981). Dose response models for quantal response toxicity data. In *Statistics and Related Topics* (eds. M. Csorgo, D. A. Dawson, J. N. K. Rao, and E. Saleh), pp. 201–31. North Holland, Amsterdam

Krewski, D. and Zhu, Y. (1994). Applications of multinomial dose–response models in developmental toxicity risk assessment. *Risk Analysis*, **14**, 595–609.

Krewski, D. and Zhu, Y. (1995). A simple data transformation for estimating benchmark dose in developmental toxicity experiments. *Risk Analysis*, **15**, 29–39.

Kupper, L. L. and Haseman, J. K. (1978). The use of a correlated binomial model for the analysis of certain toxicological experiments. *Biometrics*, **34**, 69–76.

Kupper, L. L., Portier, C., Hogan, M. D., and Yamamoto, E. (1986). The impact of litter effects on dose–response modeling in teratology. *Biometrics*, **42**, 85–98.

Lefkopoulou, M. and Ryan, L. (1996). Global tests for multiple binary outcomes, submitted for publication.

Lefkopoulou, M., Moore, D., and Ryan, L. (1989). The analysis of multiple correlated binary outcomes: application to rodent teratology experiments. *Journal of the American Statistical Association*, **84**, 810–15.

Leisenring, W. and Ryan, L. (1992). Statistical properties of the NOAEL. *Regulatory Toxicology and Pharmacology*, **15**, 161–71.

Liang, K.-Y. and Zeger, S. (1986). Longitudinal data analysis using generalized linear models. *Biometrika*, **73**, 13–22.

Liang, K.-Y., Zeger, S., and Qaqish, B. (1992). Multivariate regression analysis for categorical data. *Journal of the Royal Statistical Society, Series B*, **54**, 3–40.

Moore, D. F. (1987). Modelling the extraneous variation in the presence of extra-binomial variation. *Applied Statistics*, **36**, 8–14.

Moore, D. F. and Tsiatis, A. (1991). Robust estimation of the variance in moment methods for extra-binomial and extra-Poisson variation. *Biometrics*, **47**, 383–401.

Neyman, J. (1959). Optimal asymptotic tests of composite hypothesis. In *Probability and statistics* (ed. U. Grenander), pp. 213–34. John Wiley, New York.

Paul, S. R. (1982). Analysis of proportions of affected foetuses in teratological studies. *Biometrics*, **38**, 361–70.

Paul, S. R. (1987). On the beta-correlated binomial (bcb) distribution—a three parameter generalization of the binomial distribution. *Communication in Statistics—Theory and Methods*, **16**, 1473–8.

Portier, C. and Hoel, D. (1984). Type I error of trend tests in proportions and the design of cancer screens. *Communications in Statistics—Theory and Methods*, **13**, 1–14.

Prentice, R. L. (1986). Binary regression using an extended beta-binomial distribution, with discussion of correlation induced by covariate measurement errors. *Journal of the American Statistical Association*, **81**, 321–7.

Prentice, R. L. and Zhao, L. P. (1991). Estimating equations for parameters in means and covariances of multivariate discrete and continuous responses. *Biometrics*, **47**, 825–39.

Rai, K. and Van Ryzin, J. (1985). A dose–response model for teratological experiments involving quantal responses. *Biometrics*, **41**, 1–9.

Rao, J. N. K. and Scott, A. (1981). The analysis of categorical data from complex sample surveys: chi-squared tests for goodness of fit and independence in two-way tables. *Journal of the American Statistical Association*, **76**, 221–9.

Rao, J. N. K. and Scott, A. (1992). A simple method for analysis of clustered binary data. *Biometrics*, **48**, 577–85.

Ryan, L. (1992). Quantitative risk assessment for developmental toxicity. *Biometrics*, **48**, 163–74.

Ryan, L. (1993). Potency measures for developmental toxicity. *Environmetrics*, **4**, 507–18.

Ryan, L., Catalano, P., Kimmel, C. A., and Kimmel, G. L. (1991). Relationship between fetal weight and malformation in developmental toxicity studies. *Teratology*, **44**, 215–23.

Tarone, R. E. and Gart, J. J. (1980). On the robustness of combined tests for trends in proportions. *Journal of the American Statistical Association*, **75**, 110–16.

Williams, D. A. (1975). The analysis of binary responses from toxicological experiments involving reproduction and teratogenicity. *Biometrics*, **31**, 949–52.

Williams, D. A. (1982). Extra-binomial variation in logistic linear models. *Applied Statistics*, **31**, 144–8.

Williams, D. A. (1987). Dose–response models for teratological experiments. *Biometrics*, **43**, 1013–16.

Williams, D. A. (1988). Estimation bias using the beta-binomial distribution in teratology. *Biometrics*, **44**, 305–9.

Zhao, L. P. and Prentice, R. L. (1990). Correlated binary regression using a quadratic exponential model. *Biometrika*, **77**, 642–8.

Zhu, Y., Krewski, D., and Ross, W. H. (1994). Multinomial dose–response models for correlated multinomial data from developmental toxicity studies. *Applied Statistics*, **44**, 583–98.

12 Trend tests for clustered data

MYRTO LEFKOPOULOU, ANDREA ROTNITZKY, AND LOUISE RYAN

12.1 Introduction

Tests for trend are often applied to toxicological data in order to assess dose effects. In this chapter, we consider the problem of testing for trend in the context of clustered binary data. Here, traditional trend tests, such as the Cochran–Armitage test, will tend to have inflated type I error probabilities, because they do not account for the extra-binomial variation induced by clustering. Our work is motivated by the analysis of developmental toxicity studies, in which the offspring of exposed and control rodents are examined for defects. The clustering of offspring is responsible for the well-known litter effect that has been widely discussed by Williams (1975, 1982, 1987) and many others.

Several authors have explored likelihood-based approaches to characterizing clustered binary data (Williams 1975; Altham 1978; Kupper and Haseman 1978; Haseman and Kupper 1979; Ochi and Prentice 1984). Williams (1982) was one of the first to apply moment-based estimation techniques in this area. Moore (1986) studied the theoretical properties of the models proposed by Williams. Liang and Zeger (1986) generalized these moment-based approaches using the concept of Generalized Estimating Equations (GEE) to analyse multivariate binary data with extra-binomial variation. Since that time, GEEs have become very popular as a tool for analysing developmental toxicity data. While these methods provide a means of model fitting, they require sophisticated software, and are often inaccessible to the average scientist. A need exists for computationally simple tests for trend in the context of clustered binary outcomes.

Recently, Rao and Scott (1992) proposed a series of easily computed test statistics based on the concept of effective sample size. They proposed adjusting the sample size and binomial counts by an appropriate factor accounting for over- (or under-) dispersion and then applying the usual binomial methods on the transformed data. Fung *et al.* (1994) compare this test with several others that have been recently proposed for the analysis of cluster binary data. Piegorsch (1993, 1994) suggests the use of rank-based tests or permuation tests for clustered binary data, treating the observed proportion in each cluster as the outcome. Chen (1994) also discusses trend tests for clustered binary outcomes.

Lefkopoulou and Ryan (1993) proposed a simple test for multiple binary outcomes based on generalized estimating equation concepts (Liang and Zeger 1986). Like the Rao–Scott test, the one proposed by Lefkopoulou and Ryan can be computed with a handheld calculator and is thus accessible to statisticians and practitioners alike. The Lefkopoulou and Ryan approach also has the advantage of generalizing easily to multiple outcomes. Furthermore, the test can be viewed as a natural extension of the familiar Cochran–Armitage trend test. The purpose of this chapter is to address some technical issues that arise in construction of the Lefkoupoulou and Ryan test.

There are several ways to construct quasi-likelihood, or more generally, GEE score tests. One can derive model-based tests assuming that the variance of the outcome is scaled by a constant overdispersion factor (see, for example, Scott and Rao 1981; Wilson 1989). Alternatively, empirical tests are available that yield valid inferences even when the assumed covariance structure of the data is not correct. The idea of using empirical or robust variance estimators has been discussed by a number of authors (see, for example, White 1982), but has been popularized in the GEE context by Liang and Zeger (1986) and Zeger and Liang (1986). Breslow (1990) compares the deviance test to both model-based and empirical versions of the Wald and score tests. He focuses particularly on the Poisson model, and finds that while the empirical tests perform well in large samples, model-based tests are preferable in smaller samples. In this chapter, we address similar issues, with particular emphasis on models for overdispersed binomial data.

In addition to the question of model-based versus empirical variance calculations, we also address the issue of how one should estimate nuisance parameters in the context of a composite null hypothesis. This is a familiar issue in the standard likelihood context. For example, Cox and Reid (1987) address this issue very generally, and discuss the use of transformations to make the nuisance parameters orthogonal to the parameters of interest. Eberhart and Fligner (1977) discuss the related but more focused issue of whether one should estimate the variance of a binomial score test under the null or alternative hypothesis. Similar issues arise in the context of GEE testing, with the added complication that some of the parameters characterizing the covariance of the data are nuisance parameters, and yet they are not obtained by maximizing a likelihood.

In Section 12.2 we provide background theory for quasi-likelihood models and define the associated Wald and score tests, both model-based and empirical. We also discuss several different ways to estimate unknown nuisance parameters in each of the test statistics. We present asymptotic comparisons of the various tests in Section 12.3. To confirm these results and to assess the performance of various tests in small samples, we performed simulations, the results of which we present in Section 12.4. We apply the various tests to several developmental toxicity data sets in Section 12.5 and conclude in Section 12.6 with some general discussion and recommendations.

12.2 Quasi-likelihood: model definitions and fitting

Consider a study involving K groups, each of which has an associated quantitative covariate (x_i for group i) representing, for example, dose or exposure level.

Suppose group i contains N_i clusters, the jth of which includes n_{ij} individuals whose outcomes sum to y_{ij}. Suppose that the random variables y_{ij} are independent and that y_{ij} has mean $n_{ij}\mu_i$, where μ_i exists and depends linearly on x_i through some link function g:

$$\mu_i = g^{-1}(\beta_1 + \beta_2 x_i), \tag{12.1}$$

where β_1 and β_2 are unknown regression coefficients. Extensions to arbitrary covariates are straightforward, but we consider only a single covariate since our goal is to derive tests for trend. The variance of y_{ij} is assumed to satisfy

$$\text{Var}(y_{ij}) = \sigma_{ij}^2 = \phi n_{ij} v(\mu_i), \tag{12.2}$$

where ϕ is an unknown proportionality constant and $v(\mu_i)$ is defined by the relationship

$$\partial\mu/\partial\beta_1 = v(\mu_i) \qquad \text{and} \qquad \partial\mu/\partial\beta_2 = x_i v(\mu_i). \tag{12.3}$$

Many familiar modelling situations can be expressed in this way. If, for example, y_{ij} represents the number of successes or positive responses among the n_{ij} individuals, then relationship (12.3) is satisfied by the moments of the familiar scaled binomial (McCullagh and Nelder 1989). In general, if $\phi = 1$, the above moment assumptions correspond to those from some regular exponential family in natural form.

Assuming the mean relationship (12.1), consistent estimators of the unknown regression coefficients $\boldsymbol{\beta} = (\beta_1, \beta_2)^{\mathrm{T}}$ may be obtained by solving $\mathbf{S}_N(\boldsymbol{\beta}) = 0$, where

$$\mathbf{S}_N(\boldsymbol{\beta}) = \sum_{i=1}^{K} \sum_{i=1}^{N_i} \mathbf{d}_i [v(\mu_i)]^{-1} (y_{ij} - n_{ij}\mu_i) \tag{12.4}$$

with $N = \sum N_i$ and $\mathbf{d}_i = (\partial\mu_i/\partial\beta_1, \partial\mu_i/\partial\beta_2)^{\mathrm{T}}$, the vector of partial derivatives of the means with respect to the regression parameters. We call the expression $\mathbf{S}_N(\boldsymbol{\beta})$ the quasi-likelihood score. For the natural parametrization (12.1)–(12.3), the term $\mathbf{d}_i[v(\mu_i)]^{-1}$ reduces simply to $(1, x_i)^{\mathrm{T}}$. When $\phi = 1$, the equations (12.1)–(12.3) usually define an exponential family and the resulting estimators are the maximum likelihood estimators. The variance of eqn. (12.4) is

$$\boldsymbol{\Sigma}_N(\boldsymbol{\beta}) = \sum_{i=1}^{K} \sum_{j=1}^{N_i} \mathbf{d}_i \mathbf{d}_i^{\mathrm{T}} [v(\mu_i)]^{-2} \sigma_{ij}^2. \tag{12.5}$$

Much of the popularity of quasi-likelihood methods derives from the 'likelihood-like' property that, when the variance relationships (12.2) and (12.3) are correctly specified, $\sigma_{ij}^2 = n_{ij}\phi v_i$ and the variance of the quasi-likelihood score (12.4) is given by $\phi\mathbf{W}_N(\boldsymbol{\beta})$, where $\mathbf{W}_N(\boldsymbol{\beta})$ is the expected value of the matrix of second derivatives with respect to β_1 and β_2:

$$\mathbf{W}_N(\boldsymbol{\beta}) = \sum_{i=1}^{K} \sum_{j=1}^{N_i} \mathbf{d}_i \mathbf{d}_i^{\mathrm{T}} [v(\mu_i)]^{-1} n_{ij}.$$

By the central limit theorem, $\mathbf{S}_N(\boldsymbol{\beta})$ has an asymptotic normal distribution, so that for N sufficiently large,

$$\frac{1}{\sqrt{N}}\mathbf{S}_N(\boldsymbol{\beta}) \sim \mathcal{N}\left(\mathbf{0}, \frac{1}{N}\boldsymbol{\Sigma}_N(\boldsymbol{\beta})\right). \tag{12.6}$$

If the variance is correctly specified by (12.2) and (12.3), (12.6) becomes

$$\frac{1}{\sqrt{N}}\mathbf{S}_N(\boldsymbol{\beta}) \sim \mathcal{N}\left(\mathbf{0}, \frac{1}{N}\phi\mathbf{W}_N(\boldsymbol{\beta})\right). \tag{12.7}$$

It follows on standard expansions of $\mathbf{S}_N(\boldsymbol{\beta})$ that the quasi-likelihood estimators are also approximately normally distributed. In the next section, we describe how these distributional properties can be used to derive tests for the null hypothesis (12.8) given below.

12.3 Hypothesis testing for quasi-likelihood models

In contrast to parameter estimation, the theory of hypothesis testing for quasi-likelihood models has received relatively little attention. In this section we review several approaches that extend standard likelihood based procedures to the quasi-likelihood context. Suppose we wish to test the null hypothesis that the regression coefficient in eqn. (12.1) equals zero:

$$\mathrm{H}_0\colon \beta_2 = 0. \tag{12.8}$$

The deviance test, extensively discussed by McCullagh and Nelder (1989), provides the most commonly used approach to hypothesis testing in the quasi-likelihood context and can be viewed as an analogy to the likelihood ratio test. Analogies to the Wald and score tests are also readily available for the quasi-likelihood context (see, for example, Breslow 1990; Rotnitzky and Jewell 1990). Let $\tilde{\boldsymbol{\beta}}$ and $\hat{\boldsymbol{\beta}}$ denote estimates of $\boldsymbol{\beta}$ calculated under the null and alternative hypotheses: that is, $\hat{\boldsymbol{\beta}}$ denotes the solution to $\mathbf{S}_N(\boldsymbol{\beta}) = (S_{N1}, S_{N2})^{\mathrm{T}} = \mathbf{0}$ and $\tilde{\boldsymbol{\beta}} = (\tilde{\beta}_1, 0)^{\mathrm{T}}$, where $\tilde{\beta}_1$ is the solution to $S_{N1} = 0$ subject to $\beta_2 = 0$. Then, the Wald test involves comparing $\hat{\beta}_2$ to zero, its hypothesized value under H_0, and the score test involves comparing $S_{N2}(\tilde{\boldsymbol{\beta}})$ to 0. Based on the asymptotic normality of $\mathbf{S}_N(\beta)$ at the true $\boldsymbol{\beta}$, one can use appropriate Taylor series expansions to express both the quasi-likelihood Wald and score tests as quadratic forms that converge to χ^2 distributions.

12.3.1 *Quasi-likelihood score tests*

For the model (12.1)–(12.3) defined in Section 12.2, the quasi-likelihood score equations (12.4) take the form:

$$S_{N1}(\boldsymbol{\beta}) = \sum_{i=1}^{K}\sum_{j=1}^{N_i}(y_{ij} - n_{ij}\mu_i) = 0, \qquad S_{N2}(\boldsymbol{\beta}) = \sum_{i=1}^{K}\sum_{j=1}^{N_i}x_i(y_{ij} - n_{ij}\mu_i) = 0. \tag{12.9, 12.10}$$

The score test for H_0: $\beta_2 = 0$ is based on S_{N2} with μ_i estimated under the null hypothesis,

$$S_{N2} = \sum_{i=1}^{K} \sum_{j=1}^{N_i} x_i(y_{ij} - n_{ij}\tilde{\mu}),$$

where $\tilde{\mu} = \Sigma_{ij} y_{ij}/\Sigma_{ij} n_{ij}$. This statistic can be rewritten as

$$S_{N2} = \sum_{i=1}^{K} \sum_{j=1}^{N_i} y_{ij}(x_i - \tilde{x}),$$

where $\tilde{x} = \Sigma_{ij}\, n_{ij} x_i/\Sigma_{ij}\, n_{ij}$, and it then follows that the statistic

$$\frac{\left[\sum_{i=1}^{K} \sum_{j=1}^{N_i} y_{ij}(x_i - \tilde{x})\right]^2}{\sum_{i=1}^{K} \sum_{j=1}^{N_i} (x_i - \tilde{x})^2 \sigma_{ij}^2} \tag{12.11}$$

has an approximate χ_1^2 distribution.

Different choices for the estimation of the denominator of eqn. (12.11) will lead to different versions of the quasi-likelihood score test. We will consider empirical estimates based on replacing σ_{ij}^2 with

$$(y_{ij} - n_{ij}\,\mu_i)^2$$

and model-based estimates that replace σ_{ij}^2 with

$$\sigma_{ijM}^2 = n_{ij}\phi v(\mu_i).$$

Both estimates require estimating μ_i and we will consider estimating it under the null hypothesis as well as in the unrestricted space ('under the alternative'). The parameter ϕ will also need to be estimated for the model-based approach. The estimate of μ_i under the null is the same for all i and equal to $\tilde{\mu}$, while the estimate of μ_i under the alternative is $\hat{\mu}_i = \mu_i(\hat{\boldsymbol{\beta}})$. Thus the estimate under the alternative requires solving the score equations for $\boldsymbol{\beta}$. We also consider a non-parametric estimate of μ_i, given by $\check{\mu}_i = \Sigma_j\, y_{ij}/\Sigma_j\, n_{ij}$. These estimates of the mean yield three corresponding estimates of ϕ, given by

$$\tilde{\phi} = \frac{1}{N-1} \sum_{i=1}^{K} \sum_{j=1}^{N_i} \frac{(y_{ij} - n_{ij}\tilde{\mu})^2}{n_{ij}v(\tilde{\mu})}, \qquad \hat{\phi} = \frac{1}{N-2} \sum_{i=1}^{K} \sum_{j=1}^{N_i} \frac{(y_{ij} - n_{ij}\hat{\mu}_i)^2}{n_{ij}v(\hat{\mu}_i)}, \tag{12.12, 12.13}$$

and

$$\check{\phi} = \frac{1}{N-K} \sum_{i=1}^{K} \sum_{j=1}^{N_i} \frac{(y_{ij} - n_{ij}\check{\mu}_i)^2}{n_{ij}v(\check{\mu}_i)}. \tag{12.14}$$

We have thus the following six choices for replacing σ_{ij}^2 in eqn. 12.11:

Test	Method	σ_{ij}^2 replacement
EMP_0	Empirical, null	$(y_{ij} - n_{ij}\tilde{\mu})^2$
EMP_A	Empirical, alternative	$(y_{ij} - n_{ij}\hat{\mu}_i)^2$
EMP_{NP}	Empirical, non parametric	$(y_{ij} - n_{ij}\check{\mu}_i)^2$
MOD_0	Model-based, null	$n_{ij}\tilde{\phi}v(\tilde{\mu})$
MOD_A	Model-based, alternative	$n_{ij}\hat{\phi}v(\hat{\mu}_i)$
MOD_{NP}	Model-based, non-parametric	$n_{ij}\check{\phi}v(\check{\mu}_i)$

For clustered binary data where the outcome y_{ij} for the ijth cluster corresponds to the number of responses out of a total of n_{ij} trials, the natural link parametrization implies that the covariate x_i is related to μ_i through a logistic relationship,

$$\mu_i = \frac{\exp[\beta_1 + \beta_2 x_i]}{1 + \exp[\beta_1 + \beta_2 x_i]}, \tag{12.15}$$

and the variance of y_{ij} satisfies

$$\sigma_{ij}^2 = \phi n_{ij}\mu_i(1 - \mu_i).$$

In this case, $v(\mu_i) = \mu_i(1 - \mu_i)$. When ϕ equals one, MOD_0 coincides exactly with the Cochran–Armitage test:

$$\frac{\sum_{i=1}^{K}\sum_{j=1}^{N_i} x_i(y_{ij} - n_{ij}\tilde{\mu})^2}{\tilde{\mu}(1-\tilde{\mu})\sum_{i=1}^{K}\sum_{j=1}^{N_i}(x_i - \bar{x})^2 n_{ij}}.$$

Both MOD_0 and EMP_0 have the strong appeal of not requiring the fitting of the full model. This advantage is certainly lost when EMP_A or MOD_A are used in eqn. (12.11). To address this issue, we considered the non-parametric replacements EMP_{NP} and MOD_{NP}. These replacements mimic the behaviour of EMP_A and MOD_A without requiring the fitting of a model, and result in simple tests available in closed form. They are non-parametric in the sense that they do not assume any functional form on the relationship between the covariate and the response probability.

Presently, we will discuss the properties of these different formulations of the score test. For comparison, we will also consider Wald and scaled deviance tests.

The Wald test compares $\hat{\beta}_2$ to 0, its asymptotic mean under H_0. The asymptotic variance of $\sqrt{N}(\hat{\beta}_2 - \beta_2)$ is approximated by

$$N\frac{\sum_{i=1}^{K}\sum_{j=1}^{N_i}(x_i - \tilde{x}_v)^2\sigma_{ij}^2}{\left[\sum_{i=1}^{K}\sum_{j=1}^{N_i}(x_i - \tilde{x}_v)^2 n_{ij}v(\hat{\mu}_i)\right]^2}, \tag{12.16}$$

where

$$\tilde{x}_v = \frac{\sum_{i=1}^{K}\sum_{j=1}^{N_i} x_i n_{ij} v(\hat{\mu}_i)}{\sum_{i=1}^{K}\sum_{j=1}^{N_i} n_{ij} v(\hat{\mu}_i)}. \tag{12.17}$$

We define the empirical Wald test, based on the quadratic form

$$WALD_{EMP} = \hat{\boldsymbol{\beta}}_2^2 \frac{\left[\sum_{i=1}^{K}\sum_{j=1}^{N_i}(x_i - \tilde{x}_v)^2 n_{ij}v(\hat{\mu}_i)\right]^2}{\sum_{i=1}^{K}\sum_{j=1}^{N_i}(x_i - \tilde{x}_v)^2(y_{ij} - n_{ij}\hat{\mu}_i)^2}. \tag{12.18}$$

Under H_0 this statistic has an asymptotic χ_1^2 distribution. When relationship (12.3) holds then eqn. (12.16) reduces to

$$\frac{N\phi}{\sum_{i=1}^{K}\sum_{j=1}^{N_i}(x_i - \tilde{x}_v)^2 n_{ij}v(\hat{\mu}_i)}, \tag{12.19}$$

so that under H_0 the usual Wald statistic

$$WALD_{MOD} = \hat{\beta}_2^2 \frac{1}{\hat{\phi}} \sum_{i=1}^{K}\sum_{j=1}^{N_i}(x_i - \tilde{x}_v)^2 n_{ij}v(\hat{\mu}_i) \tag{12.20}$$

has an asymptotic χ_1^2 distribution. Here $\hat{\phi}$ is defined as in eqn. (12.13). We will call eqn. (12.20) the model-based Wald test.

The scaled deviance test in the case of the logit link (12.15) has the form

$$DEV = (2/\hat{\phi})\left[\sum_{i=1}^{K}\sum_{j=1}^{N_i} y_{ij}\left(\log\frac{\hat{\mu}_i}{1-\hat{\mu}_i} - \log\frac{\tilde{\mu}}{1-\tilde{\mu}}\right) + \sum_{i=1}^{K}\sum_{j=1}^{N_i} n_{ij}[\log(1-\hat{\mu}_i) - \log(1-\tilde{\mu})]\right].$$

Both the scaled deviance test and the Wald test require estimation of all unknown parameters under the alternative hypothesis.

12.4 Efficiency

It is well known that, in general, score and Wald tests have a Pitman asymptotic relative efficiency (ARE) of one with respect to the deviance or likelihood ratio test. However, the Pitman ARE only compares the power of tests at local alternatives, i.e. at alternatives very close to the null. Hence, it is possible for two tests to have the same local power, and yet for one test to perform better under alternatives that are away from the null. The Bahadur ARE (Serfling 1980) offers a comparison of the performance of tests at fixed alternatives: it compares the rates of convergence of the p-value as $N \to \infty$. Accordingly, we will examine the Bahadur ARE of the various tests discussed in the previous section.

12.4.1 *Bahadur efficiency*

Serfling (1980, theorem 10.4.3, p. 337) provides the following definition of Bahadur efficiency. Consider a test statistic Z_N for some null hypothesis $H_0: \boldsymbol{\beta} \in \Omega_0$ and suppose that the following two conditions hold:

A. Under some alternative hypothesis, $\boldsymbol{\beta} = \boldsymbol{\gamma}$,

$$N^{-1/2} Z_N \to b(\gamma),$$

where $b(\boldsymbol{\gamma})$ is a real function and '$\to$' denotes convergence almost surely.

B.

$$\lim_{N \to \infty} -2N^{-1} \log \sup_{\boldsymbol{\beta} \in \Omega_0} \left[1 - G_{\boldsymbol{\beta}_N}(N^{-1/2} t)\right] = g(t),$$

where $G_{\boldsymbol{\beta}_N}(t)$ is the distribution function of Z_N at a parameter value $\boldsymbol{\beta}$.

Then, the Bahadur non-centrality parameter (Bahadur coefficient) of Z_N is $g(b(\boldsymbol{\gamma}))$. The Bahadur relative efficiency of two test statistics is the ratio of their non-centrality parameters.

When the test statistic Z_N is based on binomial data, this definition is non-informative, because the quantity in square brackets in condition B will always be 1. Heuristically, this means that no matter how large the χ^2 test statistic is, there always exists a baseline probability (i.e. a value of β_1) under which it will have a large exact p-value. Instead, one can calculate the Bahadur coefficients and efficiency for a fixed value of the nuisance parameter: that is, by using $g^*(b(\boldsymbol{\gamma}))$, where

$$\lim_{N \to \infty} -2N^{-1} \log\left[1 - G^*_{\beta N}(N^{1/2} t)\right] = g^*(t),$$

where $G^*_{\beta N}$ is the distribution function of Z_N at parameter value $\boldsymbol{\beta}^{\mathrm{T}} = (\beta, 0)$.

Table 12.1. Non-centrality parameters

EMP_0:	$n^2\left[\sum_i (x_i-\bar{x})\mu_i\right]^2 \Big/ \left[\sum_i (x_i-\bar{x})^2\left(n\phi v(\mu_i)+(n^2+\tau^2)(\mu_i-\bar{\mu})^2\right)\right]$
EMP_A:	$n\left[\sum_i (x_i-\bar{x})\mu_i\right]^2 \Big/ \left[\phi\sum_i (x_i-\bar{x})^2 v(\mu_i)\right]$
EMP_{NP}:	$n\left[\sum_i (x_i-\bar{x})\mu_i\right]^2 \Big/ \left[\phi\sum_i (x_i-\bar{x})^2 v(\mu_i)\right]$
MOD_0:	$Kn\left[\sum_i (x_i-\bar{x})\mu_i\right]^2 \Big/ \left[\sum_i (x_i-\bar{x})^2\left(\phi\sum_i v(\mu_i)+n\sum_i (\mu_i-\bar{\mu})^2\right)\right]$
MOD_A:	$n\left[\sum_i (x_i-\bar{x})\mu_i\right]^2 \Big/ \left[\phi\sum_i (x_i-\bar{x})^2 v(\mu_i)\right]$
MOD_{NP}:	$n\left[\sum_i (x_i-\bar{x})\mu_i\right]^2 \Big/ \left[\phi\sum_i (x_i-\bar{x})^2 v(\mu_i)\right]$
$WALD_{EMP}$:	$\beta_2^2 n\sum_i (x_i-\bar{x}_v)^2 v(\mu_i)/(\phi)$
$WALD_{MOD}$:	$\beta_2^2 n\sum_i (x_i-\bar{x}_v)^2 v(\mu_i)/(\phi)$
DEV:	$\frac{2}{\phi}\sum_i\left[n\mu_i\left(\beta_1+\beta_2 x_i-\log\frac{\bar{\mu}}{1-\bar{\mu}}\right)+n\log\frac{1-\mu_i}{1-\bar{\mu}}\right]$

In the above formulas, $\bar{\mu}=(1/K)\Sigma_i\,\mu_i$, $\bar{x}=(1/K)\Sigma_i\,x_i$, and $\bar{x}_v=[\Sigma_i\,x_i v(\mu_i)]/[\Sigma_i\,v(\mu_i)]$

Even in this case $G^*_{\beta N}$ is not known, since we are using quasi-likelihood, so that exact distributions cannot be calculated. We will use its limiting distribution instead and obtain *approximate* coefficients and efficiencies.

The score, Wald, and deviance tests defined in Section 12.3.1 all converge in law to a χ_1^2 distribution under the null. In the Appendix we show that if $T_N \xrightarrow{\mathscr{L}} \chi_1^2$, then the Bahadur non-centrality parameter of T_N is $\lim_P T_N/N$, where $\lim_P$ denotes limit in probability. The non-centrality parameters of all the statistics considered are given in Table 12.1. These non-centrality parameters were computed assuming equal sample sizes in each of the K groups and iid random cluster sizes with expectation n and variance τ^2.

All the proposed score tests are constructed by squaring S_{N2} and dividing by one of the variance estimates. Thus any differences in the non-centrality parameters of the score tests can be attributed to differences in the limits of the estimates of the variance of S_{N2}. Under the assumptions (12.1)–(12.3) the non-parametric replacements EMP_{NP} and MOD_{NP}, have the same non-centrality parameters as EMP_A and MOD_A. Also, the empirical variance estimate at $\hat{\boldsymbol{\beta}}$ converges to the true variance of S_{N2}, and so does the model-based estimate at $\hat{\boldsymbol{\beta}}$, so that EMP_A and MOD_A have the same non-centrality parameters. For the same reason, the two Wald tests have the same non-centrality parameters and are equally efficient.

From Table 12.1 it is apparent that the non-centrality parameter of EMP_0 is always smaller than the non-centrality parameter of EMP_A, so that EMP_A, the empirical test at the alternative, is always more efficient than EMP_0, the empirical test at the null. A disturbing feature of EMP_0 is that it depends on the variance of the cluster sizes n_{ij}, losing in efficiency as this variance grows. Luckily, this is not the case for the empirical test under the alternative, EMP_A. No clear-cut ordering, valid for all K and all parameter values, exists for the remaining statistics.

We explored the Bahadur efficiency of EMP_0, EMP_A, MOD_0, and the Wald test with respect to the deviance test numerically for the case of four covariate groups at levels 0, 0.25, 0.5, and 1 and for $0.5 \leqslant \phi \leqslant 5$, $\log(0.05/0.95) \leqslant \beta_1 \leqslant \log(0.4/0.6)$ and $0 \leqslant \beta_2 \leqslant \log(3)$. In these computations we assumed a constant cluster size $n = 10$, so that they could be comparable to the subsequent simulation studies.

In this range the Wald test is usually equally efficient to the deviance test, and is more efficient than any of the score tests. The score tests with the nuisance parameters evaluated under the null gain in efficiency as ϕ grows larger. The value of ϕ does not affect the efficiency of EMP_A or the Wald test with respect to the deviance test, as can be seen from the formulas in Table 12.1. The score test with empirical variance under the null (EMP_0) is the least efficient of all, although in the range considered its efficiency with respect to the deviance test does not fall below 80 per cent. The empirical score under the alternative, EMP_A, is less efficient than the model-based score under the null for small values of the control rate ($\mu_1 < 0.2$), but can become more efficient than MOD_0 for $\mu_1 > 0.2$. In fact, the efficiency of EMP_A with respect to the deviance or the Wald test is greater than 95 per cent, even for small values of μ_1.

The Bahadur relative efficiencies of the three score tests EMP_0, EMP_A (or MOD_A or any of the non-parametric tests), and MOD_0, and of the Wald test with respect to the deviance test plotted against β_1, β_2, and ϕ, respectively, are shown in Fig. 12.1. The figure indicates how variable the efficiency of these tests can be.

These asymptotic results seem to favour EMP_A (or, equivalently, EMP_{NP}) among all score tests.

12.5 A simulation study

Simulations were used to evaluate the small-sample performance of the various tests discussed in previous sections. To represent situations typically encountered in many developmental toxicity studies, the dose levels (x_1 to x_4) were set at 0, 0.25, 0.50, and 1, respectively, and the cluster sizes n_{ij} were all equal to 10. Outcomes y_{ij} ($i = 1,\ldots,4$, $j = 1,\ldots,15$) were generated from a beta-binomial

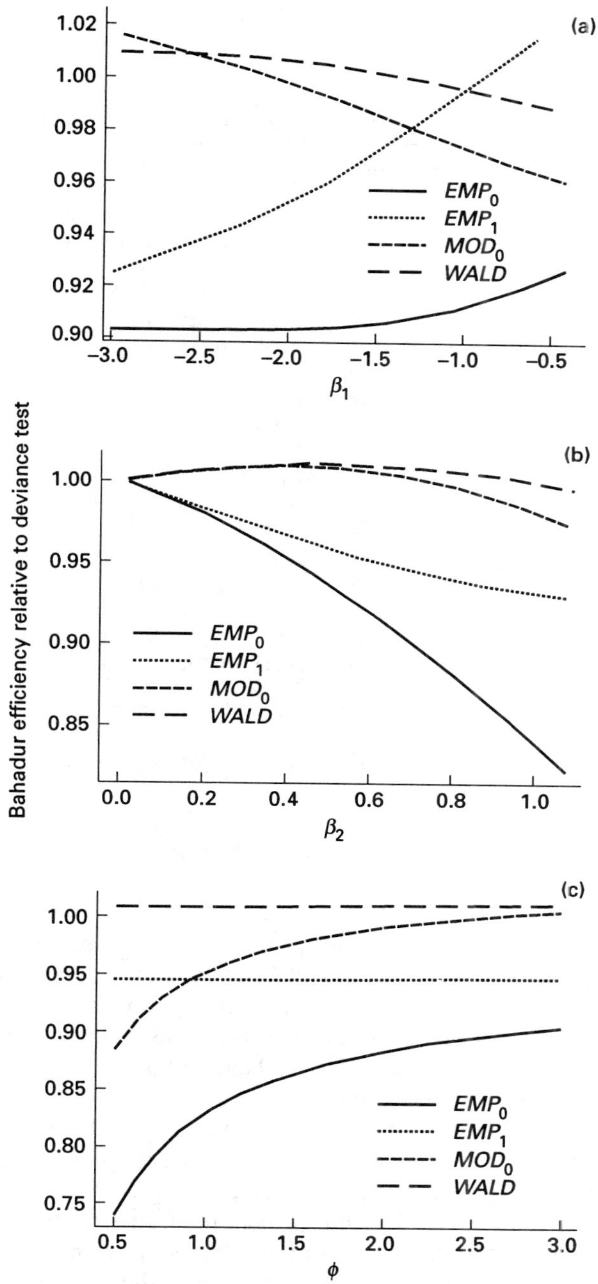

Fig. 12.1. Relative efficiency by (a) baseline, (b) dose effect, and (c) overdispersion.

Table 12.2. Rejection probabilities under H_0

Test/method/model	Baseline	Scale/significance level, $\phi = 1$ 0.01	0.05	0.10	Scale/significance level, $\phi = 3$ 0.01	0.05	0.10
Score/model/null	0.05	0.009	0.040	0.091	0.009	0.045	0.089
	0.15	0.009	0.058	0.103	0.011	0.066	0.111
	0.30	0.006	0.044	0.094	0.011	0.041	0.100
Score/model/non-parametric	0.05	0.009	0.054	0.096	0.020	0.064	0.131
	0.15	0.014	0.062	0.113	0.022	0.083	0.130
	0.30	0.018	0.052	0.104	0.013	0.061	0.114
Score/empirical/null	0.05	0.008	0.047	0.099	0.002	0.035	0.086
	0.15	0.005	0.045	0.106	0.011	0.061	0.121
	0.30	0.006	0.042	0.088	0.008	0.044	0.097
Score/empirical/non-parametric	0.05	0.021	0.062	0.113	0.011	0.058	0.116
	0.15	0.014	0.070	0.118	0.025	0.087	0.133
	0.30	0.014	0.055	0.105	0.015	0.065	0.120
Wald/model/alternative	0.05	0.009	0.044	0.092	0.010	0.049	0.097
	0.15	0.013	0.059	0.107	0.016	0.069	0.110
	0.30	0.013	0.049	0.97	0.012	0.046	0.101
Wald/empirical/non-parametric	0.05	0.013	0.053	0.101	0.017	0.074	0.135
	0.15	0.014	0.069	0.111	0.024	0.083	0.128
	0.30	0.013	0.051	0.051	0.011	0.054	0.103
Deviance/scale/alternative	0.05	0.010	0.052	0.097	0.019	0.060	0.116
	0.15	0.015	0.062	0.113	0.020	0.074	0.116
	0.30	0.013	0.050	0.099	0.013	0.053	0.103

distribution with $E(y_{ij}) = n_{ij}\mu_i$ and $\mathrm{Var}(y_{ij}) = \phi n_{ij}\mu_i(1-\mu_i)$. The μ_i's followed a logistic regression model,

$$\ln[\mu_i/(1-\mu_i)] = \beta_1 + \beta_2 x_i,$$

with β_1 chosen to yield values of μ_1 equal to 0.05, 0.15, and 0.30, respectively, and β_2 equal to 0, log(3), log(4), and log(5). Two overdispersion factors were used, $\phi = 1$ and $\phi = 3$. Each experiment (that is, each choice of ϕ, β_1, and β_2) was replicated 1000 times, and at each replication the test statistics were computed. The proportion of times that the tests rejected among the 1000 replications at the nominal levels of 0.01, 0.05, and 0.10 are the estimates of the rejection probabilities of these tests.

The estimated rejection probabilities of the tests under the null hypothesis are displayed in Table 12.2. In the absence of overdispersion ($\phi = 1$), all tests had actual rejection probabilities that were in agreement with the nominal levels, with the exception of the empirical non-parametric tests that tended to reject at a higher rate than the nominal levels. For moderate amounts of overdispersion, i.e. $\phi = 3$, the non-parametric tests, the empirical Wald test, and the scaled deviance test showed actual significant levels greater than the nominal levels, especially for the smaller baseline probabilities, $\mu_1 = 0.05$ and $\mu_1 = 0.15$. On the other hand, both model-based and empirical score tests under

Table 12.3. Rejection probabilities under the alternative: $\pi_0 = 0.05$

Test/method/model	Odds	Scale/significance level, $\theta = 1$			Scale/significance level, $\theta = 3$		
		0.01	0.05	0.10	0.01	0.05	0.10
Score/model/null	3	0.585	0.806	0.877	0.170	0.391	0.532
	4	0.852	0.958	0.979	0.353	0.598	0.718
	5	0.977	0.993	0.998	0.511	0.752	0.850
Score/model/non-parametric	3	0.576	0.797	0.870	0.166	0.384	0.516
	4	0.852	0.953	0.976	0.343	0.585	0.708
	5	0.974	0.993	0.997	0.504	0.741	0.839
Score/empirical/null	3	0.427	0.747	0.846	0.075	0.305	0.457
	4	0.742	0.935	0.972	0.217	0.510	0.666
	5	0.935	0.989	0.997	0.355	0.685	0.809
Score/empirical/non-parametric	3	0.579	0.792	0.867	0.133	0.362	0.481
	4	0.842	0.948	0.977	0.312	0.576	0.700
	5	0.969	0.993	0.998	0.489	0.735	0.834
Wald/model/alternative	3	0.608	0.812	0.876	0.130	0.383	0.524
	4	0.875	0.957	0.979	0.356	0.591	0.711
	5	0.978	0.994	0.998	0.514	0.749	0.844
Wald/empirical/non-parametric	3	0.624	0.817	0.872	0.210	0.421	0.527
	4	0.873	0.955	0.978	0.383	0.611	0.722
	5	0.980	0.994	0.998	0.537	0.760	0.846
Deviance/scale/alternative	3	0.608	0.809	0.876	0.197	0.386	0.528
	4	0.874	0.956	0.977	0.378	0.599	0.711
	5	0.978	0.993	0.998	0.525	0.752	0.844

the null had acceptable actual levels. The results for $\mu_1 = 0.05$ are in remarkable agreement with those obtained by Breslow (1990) in a simulation study of overdispersed Poisson regression data. This is explained by the similarity between the Poisson and binomial distributions for rare events.

In Table 12.3 are shown the estimated rejection probabilities of the tests at nominal levels 0.01, 0.05, and 0.1, under several alternative models (odds = 3, 4, or 5) and for three values of β_2, when the baseline probability is $\mu_1 = 0.05$. Results for $\mu_1 = 0.15$ and $\mu_1 = 0.30$ were qualitatively similar to those for $\mu_1 = 0.05$, but the discrepancies between the powers of the various tests were smaller, and are not presented here. When nuisance parameters were estimated under the null hypothesis, model-based tests generally had higher power than their empirical counterparts. The increased variability in estimation of the variance of the score statistic probably causes the reduction of the power of the empirical tests. This power reduction is more significant when $\phi = 3$, and for alternatives closer to the null. Furthermore, the relative power loss of empirical with respect to model-based tests seems most pronounced for tests with small nominal rejection probabilities. For tests with nominal level 0.01, the empirical test had about 10 per cent less power than the model-based tests when nuisance parameters were estimated under the null. We found no significant discrepancies between the power of model-based versus empirical tests when nuisance parameters were estimated either non-parametrically or under the alternative hypothesis. The Wald and deviance tests tended to have higher power than all four score tests.

12.6 Examples

To illustrate our findings further, we consider data from two developmental toxicity studies conducted by the Research Triangle Institute under contract to the National Toxicology Program. (The studies investigated the effects of exposing pregnant mice to triethylene glycol dimethyl ether (TGDM) (George *et al.* 1987) or theophylline (THEO) (Lindstrom *et al.* 1990), respectively.)

The standard study design involves exposure of the pregnant animals to the test agent over the period of major organogenesis, beginning just after implantation. The effect on *in utero* development is evaluated just before parturition would normally occur. Each study included a vehicle control group and three or four dosed groups, each including approximately 20–30 pregnant animals. Outcomes included the number of implantation sites in each dam and indications of which sites had resorptions or fetal deaths. Fetuses surviving to the terminal sacrifice were weighed and evaluated for the presence of a variety of different types of malformations. Summary data from the two studies of interest are listed in Table 12.4.

The results of applying various tests discussed in Section 12.3.1 to the malformation and resorption end points are summarized in Table 12.5. For TGDM, dose effects on malformation were strongly significant, and all tests yielded similar conclusions. Exposure had a weaker effect on fetal death, and the various tests all yielded χ^2 values of approximately 2, corresponding to non-significant p-values of around 0.15. For THEO, dose effects were strongest with respect to fetal death, and all tests yielded highly significant χ^2 values. For the malformation end point, there is considerable variability in the χ^2 values, leading to p-values ranging from 0.1 for the Wald tests to around 0.02 for

Table 12.4. Summary statistics

Study/dose	Dams	Implants	Prenatal deaths Number	(%)	Live	Malformed Number	(%)
TGDM							
0	27	342	23	(0.07)	319	1	(0.00)
250	26	296	21	(0.07)	275	0	(0.00)
500	26	296	34	(0.11)	262	2	(0.01)
1000	28	327	41	(0.11)	286	33	(0.12)
THEO							
0	26	324	28	(0.11)	296	1	(0.00)
282	26	327	49	(0.15)	278	2	(0.01)
372	33	394	94	(0.24)	300	7	(0.02)
396	23	258	61	(0.24)	197	5	(0.03)

Table 12.5. Examples

	Score tests											
	Empirical			Model-based						Wald		
	H_0	H_1	H_1^*	$H_0\,\tilde{\rho}$	$H_1\,\tilde{\rho}$	$H_0\,\check{\rho}$	$H_1\,\check{\rho}$	$H_0\,\hat{\rho}$	$H_1\,\hat{\rho}$	Empirical	Model	Deviance
Malformation												
TGDM	9.9	13.2	13.2	22.5	11.6	64.3	33.1	38.3	19.7	22.0	16.4	40.8
THEO	4.1	4.5	4.5	2.9	4.8	3.8	6.2	3.5	5.7	2.7	2.7	4.6
Resorption												
TGDM	2.2	2.2	2.3	2.1	1.9	2.5	2.2	2.4	2.2	3.0	2.3	2.3
THEO	11.7	15.6	15.6	7.0	9.9	7.8	11.0	7.7	11.0	14.1	7.2	8.7

several of the model-based score tests. The empirical score tests and the deviance tests yielded χ^2 values around 4, with corresponding p-values of about 0.04. These examples all suggest that use of the empirical score tests will yield results consistent with tests such as Wald or deviance.

12.7 Discussion and recommendations

The purpose of this chapter was to compare several quasi-likelihood testing procedures for assessing the presence of a trend in K ordered groups where the data within each group are clustered. Quasi-likelihood score tests are appealing in this context because they exist in closed form and are easily explained and presented to non-statisticians. In the absence of clustering, the score tests considered are essentially the same as the familiar Cochran–Armitage test for trend.

The use of empirical variance adjustments has become popular in the context of quasi-likelihood because the resulting inferences are robust to misspecifications of the second moment assumptions. In contrast, model-based tests fail to converge to a χ^2 distribution under such model violations (Rotnitzky and Jewell 1990). A potential drawback to the use of robustified variances is a decrease in small sample efficiency due to the estimation of additional and perhaps unnecessary parameters. To address this, we compared the small sample power of empirical and model-based versions of quasi-likelihood score and Wald tests with the deviance test. These comparisons were made using theoretical considerations (Bahadur efficiency) and simulations. To allow for power comparisons in a context in which all of the considered tests were valid, simulations were conducted assuming the same models as used to derive the model-based tests. Several different approaches were considered for the estimation of nuisance parameters. In analogy to standard likelihood theory, the standard quasi-likelihood score test is constructed by estimating all nuisance parameters under the null hypothesis. We considered several other approaches. One was to estimate nuisance parameters under the alternative model. Another choice was to estimate the nuisance parameters under a non-parametric alternative for which each of the K groups was assumed to have a different response rate.

As expected, the simulations generally confirmed a slightly increased power of the model-based score test over the corresponding empirical test when nuisance parameters were estimated under the null hypothesis. The actual type I error was close to the nominal level for both score tests. This finding was consistent with that discussed by Breslow (1990) in the context of Poisson data. Our findings suggested that empirical adjustments to the variance of the Wald test resulted in minor power loss over the model-based Wald test. However, the model-based and empirical Wald test, along with the deviance test, all tended to have inflated type I error rates. The reported simulations only discuss the case of constant cluster sizes (ten individuals per cluster). Further simulations with variable cluster sizes would be useful.

When nuisance parameters were estimated either non-parametrically or under the alternative model, the empirical score tests were found to have similar power to the model-based tests. However, this advantage was at the cost of a slightly inflated type I error rate. Nevertheless, this inflation was no more extreme than that observed for the Wald and deviance tests.

Our findings suggest that empirical score tests will generally perform quite well and are strongly recommended for assessing dose-related trends in clustered binary data. The decision as to whether or not nuisance parameters should be estimated under the null involves a trade-off between improved power at the cost of an inflated type I error rate. If nuisance parameters are estimated under the null hypothesis, the empirical score test will tend to be slightly less powerful than model-based tests, including score, Wald, or deviance tests. However, the empirical score test with nuisance parameters estimated under the null has a well controlled type I error rate. Non-parametric estimation of nuisance parameters, or estimation under the alternative model, resulted in improved power for the empirical score tests. However, this gain was at the cost of an inflated type I error rate. In general, the inflation of the type I error for the score tests was no worse than that observed for the Wald and deviance tests. The non-parametric empirical score test is particularly appealing, since it has the same simple closed form as the standard empirical score test (with nuisance parameters estimated under the null). The only difference is that the variance of the test is based on group specific means, rather than a pooled mean. An analogy is the choice of whether to use pooled or separate response rates in calculating the variance for a comparison of binomial proportions. The observed inflation of type I error rates suggests that the use of exact inference procedures, such as the permutational distribution, may be useful and certainly worthy of further exploration.

Acknowledgements

The authors wish to thank Dr Bernard Schwetz, formerly of the National Toxicity Program and now at the National Center for Toxicological Research, for assistance in accessing the computerized data base used in the analysis presented in Section 12.6.

References

Altham, P. M. E. (1978). Two generalizations of the binomial distribution. *Applied Statistics*, **27**, 162–7.

Breslow, N. E. (1990). Tests of hypotheses in overdispersed Poisson regression and other quasi-likelihood models. *Journal of the Americal Statistical Association*, **85**, 565–71.

Chen, J. J. (1994). Trend tests for overdispersed proportions. *Biometrical Journal*, in press.

Cox, D. R. and Reid, N. (1987). Parameter orthogonality and approximate conditional inference. *Journal of the Royal Statistical Society, Series B*, **49**, 1–18.

Eberhard, K. R. and Fligner, M. A. (1977). A comparison of two tests for equality of two proportions. *American Statistician*, **31**, 151–5.

Fung, K. Y., Krewski, D., Rao, J. N. K., and Scott, A. J. (1994). Tests for trend in developmental toxicity experiments with correlated binary data. *Risk Analysis*, in press.

George, J. D., Price C. J., Kimmel C. A., and Marr M. C. (1987). The developmental toxicity of triethylene glycol dimethyl ether in mice. *Fundamentals of Applied Toxicology*, **9**, 173–81.

Haseman, J. and Kupper, L. L. (1979). Analysis of dichotomous response data from certain toxicological experiments. *Biometrics*, **35**, 281–93.

Kupper, L. L. and Haseman, J. K. (1978). The use of a correlated binomial model for the analysis of certain toxicological experiments. *Biometrics*, **34** 69–76.

Liang, K. Y. and Zeger, S. L. (1986). Longitudinal data analysis using generalized linear models. *Biometrika*, **73**, 13–22.

Lindstrom, P., Morrissey, R. E., George, J. D., Price, C. J., Marr, M. C., Kimmel, C. A., and Schwetz, B. A. (1990) The developmental toxicity of orally administered theophylline in rats and mice. *Fundamentals of Applied Toxicology*, **14**, 167–78.

Lefkopoulou, M. and Ryan, L. (1993). Global tests for multiple binary outcomes. *Biometrics*, **49**, 975–88.

McCullagh, P. and Nelder, J. A. (1989). *Generalized linear models*. Chapman and Hall, London.

Moore, D. F. (1986). Asymptotic properties of moment estimators for overdispersed counts and proportions. *Biometrika*, **73**, 583–8.

Ochi, Y. and Prentice, R. L. (1984). Likelihood inference in a correlated probit regression model. *Biometrika*, **71**, 531–43.

Piegorsch, W. (1993). Biometrical methods for testing dose effects of environmental stimuli in laboratory studies. *Environmetrics*, **4**, 483–506.

Piegorsch, W. (1994). Environmental biometry: assessing impacts of environmental stimuli via animal and microbial laboratory studies. In *Handbook of statistics*, Vol. 23 (eds. G. P. Patil and C. R. Rao), pp. 535–59. Elsevier Science, Amsterdam.

Rotnitzky, A. and Jewell, N. P. (1990). Hypothesis testing of regression parameters in semiparametric generalized linear models for cluster correlated data. *Biometrika*, **77**, 485–97.

Rao, J. N. K. and Scott, A. J. (1992). A simple method for the analysis of clustered binary data. *Biometrics*, **48**, 577–85.

Scott, A. J. and Rao, J. N. K. (1981). Chi-squared tests for contingency tables with properties estimated from survey data. In *Current Topics in Survey Sampling* (ed. D. Krewski). Academic Press, London.

Serfling, R. J. (1980). *Approximation theorems of mathematical statistics*. John Wiley, New York.

White, H. (1982). Maximum likelihood estimation of misspecified models. *Econometrika*, **50**, 1–26.

Williams, D. A. (1975). The analysis of binary responses from toxicological experiments involving reproduction and teratogenicity. *Biometrics*, **31**, 949–52.

Williams, D. A. (1982). Extra-binomial variation in logistic linear models. *Applied Statistics*, **31**, 144–8.

Wilson, J. R. (1989). Chi-square tests for overdispersion with multiparameter estimates. *Applied Statistics*, **38**, 441–53.

Zeger, S. L. and Liang, K. Y. (1986). Longitudinal data analysis for discrete and continuous outcomes. *Biometrics*, **42**, 121–30.

Appendix: Bahadur efficiencies

Let $T_N \xrightarrow{\mathscr{L}} \chi_1^2$. In order to satisfy the Bahadur condition A, we take $Z_N = \sqrt{T_N}$, so that

$$b(\beta) = \lim_P \sqrt{T_N/N}\,.$$

Now we will compute the quantity $g(t)$ in B, namely:

$$\lim_{N\to\infty} -2N^{-1}\log\left[1-G_{0N}(N^{1/2}t)\right],$$

where $G_{0N}(t)$ is the distribution function of Z_N at the null. Since, under H_0, Z_N^2 has a χ_1^2 distribution, we have

$$\left[1-G_{0N}(N^{1/2}t)\right] = Pr_{\beta=0}(Z_N^2 > Nt^2) = H(Nt^2),$$

where $H(t)$ is the tail probability function of a χ_1^2 distribution. We then need

$$\lim_{N\to\infty} -\frac{2\log H(Nt^2)}{N}.$$

Applying L'Hôpital's rule twice, this quantity is equal to

$$\lim_{N\to\infty}\frac{2h(Nt^2)t^2}{H(Nt^2)} = \lim_{N\to\infty}\frac{-2h'(Nt^2)t^4}{h(Nt^2)t^2} = t^2,$$

since

$$\frac{h'(x)}{h(x)} = \frac{k-2}{2x} - \frac{1}{2}.$$

It follows that the Bahadur non-centrality parameter of T_N is $b(\beta)^2$, which in turn is simply $\lim_P(T_N/N)$.

13 Exploratory and model-based inference in toxicokinetics

W. URFER AND M. BECKA

13.1 Introduction

Risk assessment of potentially harmful chemicals is fundamental in toxicology. Thorough research depends on investigations with animals *in vivo* and *in vitro*.

When animals serve as models of human systems, a critical step is extrapolation from the risk observed in the experimental animals to the risk associated with the human organism. To avoid serious error, the researcher must consider both toxicokinetics in specific experimental animals (including uptake, distribution, elimination, and metabolism of the chemicals), as well as interspecific differences among various animals.

Animals have immensely complicated and interconnected systems and subsystems, all with complex biochemical and physiological functions. Experimental design and evaluation should account for the complexity of the system under study, although such accounting is not always thorough or even possible. The researcher must acknowledge discrepancies between practical experimental design and theoretical accuracy. The development and application of statistical methods offer a means to account for the common discrepancies found in the analysis of toxicokinetic models.

After describing the role of toxicokinetics, the deterministic two-compartment model is further discussed and exemplified by non-invasive toxicokinetic inhalation experiments with rats. The model is characterized by a system of differential equations which results in concentration–time functions for the compartments. Linear and non-linear regression are used to estimate toxicokinetic parameters, and this approach is contrasted to a curve-stripping technique, often used for finding starting values for the non-linear regression approach, or even for estimating the kinetic parameters themselves. Finally, variations within and between individuals are considered, and described by a population model with random parameters. Data following such a model can be analysed by the penalized quasi-likelihood procedure, a method that is equivalent to the non-linear mixed model approach.

13.2 The role of toxicokinetics

Environmental research requires sophisticated tools from all of the well established sciences, and co-operation of experts in these different fields is necessary for success.

One distinguishing mark of much environmental research covering ecological and economical problems is the investigation of global to sub-atomic dynamic systems over time. Using different notations in different sciences, climate changes, disease developments, and chemical interactions are characterized by states and transitions. The human environment is often directly and visibly influenced by chemicals, due to industrial and economic development. Toxicological research is then concerned with the exposure of humans to such substances and their possible adverse effects.

In practical situations, the critical factor of a substance or process is not the intrinsic toxicity but the risk or hazard associated with its use. Risk is the probability that a substance will produce harm under specified conditions. Safety, the reciprocal of risk, is the probability that harm will not occur under specified conditions. Risk assessment is defined as 'the characterisation of the potential adverse health effects of human exposure to environmental hazards' (NAS 1983). The process of risk assessment consists of several elements:

(1) evaluation of the potential adverse health effects of a chemical, mixture of chemicals, or process, based on epidemiological, clinical, toxicological, and environmental research;

(2) extrapolation from those results to predict the type and estimate the extent of health effects in humans under given conditions of exposure;

(3) judgements as to the number and characteristics of persons exposed at various intensities and durations;

(4) summary judgements on the existence and overall magnitude of the public health problem; and

(5) characterization of the uncertainties inherent in the process of inferring risk (NAS 1983).

Risk management, which should be distinct from risk assessment, is the process of weighing policy alternatives and selecting the most appropriate regulatory action, integrating the results of risk assessment with engineering data and with social, economic, and political concerns to reach a decision (NAS 1983).

In the context of environmental research, toxicology is the study of the adverse affects of chemicals or poisons on living organisms. Poison could be defined as any agent capable of producing a deleterious response in a biological system, seriously influencing function or producing death. However, this definition is not useful, because every known chemical has the potential to produce injury or death if present in a sufficient amount.

The toxicologist is trained to examine the nature of the adverse effects, including the cellular, biochemical, and molecular mechanisms of action. They should also be trained to assess the probability of their occurrence. The variety of potential adverse effects and the diversity of chemicals present in our environment combine to make even toxicology, as one environmental science, very broad. The process of risk assessment is commonly divided into four major steps: hazard identification, dose–response assessment, exposure assessment, and risk characterization. The major factors that influence toxicity as it relates to the exposure situation for a specific chemical are the route of administration and the duration and frequency of exposure. The characteristics of exposure and the spectrum of effects come together in a correlative relationship customarily referred to as the dose–response relationship. This relationship is the most fundamental and pervasive concept in toxicology. An understanding of this relationship is essential for the study of toxic materials. From a practical perspective, there are two types of dose–response relationship:

(1) that which describes the response of an individual to varying doses of a chemical, and

(2) that which characterizes the distribution of responses to different doses in a population of individuals.

The toxicity of any substance depends on the dose. The higher the amount of a chemical taken up by an organism and reaching the sites of action, the greater is the toxic response. In general, the observed response to varying doses of a chemical in the whole organism is often complicated by the fact that most toxic substances have multiple sites or mechanisms of toxicity, each with its own dose–response relationship and subsequent adverse effects. Adverse or toxic affects in a biological system are not produced by a chemical unless that agent or its biotransformed products reach appropriate sites in the body at a concentration and for a length of time sufficient to produce the toxic manifestation. The concentration of any chemical at the site of action is proportional to the dose. However, the same dose of two or more chemicals may lead to vastly different concentrations in a particular target organ of toxicity. This differential pattern is due to differences in the disposition of chemicals. Disposition may be conceptualized as consisting of absorption, distribution, biotransformation, and excretion. If dose-dependent absorption, biotransformation, distribution, or excretion occurs, then the relationship between exposed dose and target dose will not be proportional at all doses. The processes of disposition may occur simultaneously. Any or all of the factors may have a minor or major impact on the concentration and thus the toxicity of a chemical in a target organ. If the fraction absorbed or the rate of absorption is low, then a chemical may never attain sufficiently high concentrations at a potential site of action to cause toxicity. The more rapidly a biochemical is eliminated from an organism, the lower will be its concentration and hence its toxicity in target tissues. Biotransformation of a chemical may result in the formation of less or more toxic metabolites at a fast or slow rate, with obvious consequences for the concentration and thus toxicity at the target site. It is known that many chemicals are only carcinogenic after they have been biotransformed. The amount of reactive metabolite formed might not be directly related to dosage because the enzyme that forms the reactive metabolite might become saturated at higher doses, or there may be depletion of cosubstrate. After the reactive metabolite is formed, it is often destroyed by a second enzyme. These enzymes can also be saturated. The reactive metabolites that are not destroyed by these detoxification pathways often bind to DNA. However, the metabolites bound to DNA can be removed by various DNA repair systems. These systems also can be saturated. All of these processes are dynamically interrelated and thus influence each other.

Whether or not a toxic response occurs is dependent, therefore, on the chemical and physical properties of the agent, the exposure situation, and the susceptibility of the biological system or subject. Thus, to characterize fully the potential hazard of a specific chemical agent it is necessary to know not only what type of effect it produces and the dose required to produce the effect, but also to know the characteristics of the agent, the exposure, and the subject.

Toxicokinetics is the modelling and mathematical description of the time course of disposition (absorption, distribution, biotransformation, and excretion) of foreign compounds in the whole organism. The most common way to characterize the kinetics of such xenobiotics is to represent the body as consisting of a number of compartments. In simplifying such a complex biological system to only a few sections, the compartments may have no apparent physiological or anatomical reality. More recently, *p*hysiologically *b*ased *p*harmaco*k*inetic models have been advanced, in which mass balance equations allow the modelling of each organ or tissue based on physiological considerations. The principal intention of this PB-PK modelling is to predict the concentration of carcinogen at the target site, and to describe the relationship between exposed dose and target dose over a range of concentrations. For that purpose, PB-PK models require estimates of the general physiological parameters and the fundamental kinetic microconstants.

Compartment models including the physiologically based pharmacokinetic approach are mechanistic models. The mathematical translation and the handling of such mechanistic models yield a deterministic access to the given problem which makes it possible to estimate the desired parameters by statistical means. For other questions, the deterministic approach may be extended to a stochastic approach. Estimates based on these models allow a species-specific numerical characterization of half-life times, elimination rate constants, tissue concentration profiles, and so on, which are essential for the assessment of the toxicity of a given compound in the special experimental case.

Examination of species differences combined with knowledge of species-specific pathways of action often provide the tools for toxicologists to predict disposition and its role in the toxicity of a compound for human exposure, but the use of mathematical models to extrapolate animal data to estimate human risk is a controversial issue.

Although the need to assess hazards of chemicals is clear, and the value of experimental animals studies in conducting scientifically sound appraisals of risk is widely accepted, the uncertainties and assumptions inherent in quantitative risk assessment are profound. Among the most controversial assumptions are selection of the appropriate mathematical model, the relevance of high doses in experimental testing to low-dose human exposure, and selection of the appropriate means of dose conversion between animals and humans. In addition to a critical evaluation of the design and performance of an experimental chronic bioassay, other available information such as mutagenicity assays, human epidemiology studies, metabolism, mechanistic information, structure–activity relationships, and—last but not least— toxicokinetics have to be considered in the final assessment.

13.3 A kinetic model for two compartments

Compartmental modelling, including PB-PK models, generally suffers from the difficulty of controlling all relevant compartments. In the context of estimating kinetic parameters, multicompartment and PB-PK models are often too complex. They are then decomposed into sub-units in a first step to obtain basic information. The two-compartment model yields an important approach to this problem. It can be widely used for *in vivo* and *in vitro* experiments.

As an example, for volatile chemicals, the 'closed chamber technique', as reviewed by Filser (1992), allows investigation of kinetics of volatile substances *in vivo*. This technique is based on a closed inhalation chamber in which, during the exposure period, the atmospheric concentrations of the substance are measured.

In the inhalation chamber, the experimental animals are exposed to the substance of interest (gas or vapours). The exhaled CO_2 is absorbed by soda lime, and its volume is replaced by pure oxygen. At the beginning of each experiment, the test material (gas or vapour) is injected into the chamber. In the course of time, the change in the atmospheric concentration within the chamber is measured by gas-chromatographic means. The experimental data result from measurements at different time-points. Due to the method of application, the actual concentration in the inhalation chamber at the beginning of each experiment, i.e., at zero time, is not exactly known. In the course of time, the concentration of the test compound declines in the atmosphere. This decline is due to the interaction with the organism, if chemical interactions with the soda lime are ruled out. In the following sections, an approach to the problem of quantitatively describing the underlying kinetic processes is presented.

The two-compartment model used by Filser (1992) for the characterization of exposure to volatile xenobiotics describes uptake, endogenous production, excretion of the unchanged substance, and its metabolic elimination. The model is depicted as follows. A xenobiotic gas enters the body and is exhaled. This is represented by two compartments; one compartment, Cp_1, being the environment outside the body and the other, Cp_2, the body itself. The xenobiotic transits from one compartment to the other through a theoretical interface. During this process, a portion of the volatile xenobiotic present within the organism at any stage is eliminated by metabolic processes, and another portion is exhaled. Special interest is given to the kinetics governing these processes.

Let $y_i(t)$ denote the concentration of a xenobiotic in compartment i at time t. If a process is governed by zero-order kinetics, the elimination rate is constant. In the case of first-order kinetics, the rate of elimination in the compartment is proportional to the concentration present in the compartment; and if second-order kinetics is applicable, it is a quadratic relation. Enzymatic controlled processes are often saturable and modelled by Michaelis–Menten kinetics with parameters $V_{\max}$ and K_m, where $V_{\max}$ denotes the maximal elimination rate, and where K_m is the concentration at which the elimination rate is $\frac{1}{2}V_{\max}$. They are usually described as functions of concentration.

A preliminary assumption is that the compound is metabolized within the body, and that there is no metabolism back to the parent compound, the latter being very likely on toxicological grounds. Furthermore, it is supposed that uptake and exhalation are governed by first-order kinetics. One important assumption is that at low concentrations the metabolic elimination is well approximated by first-order elimination kinetics; which, at low concentrations, also holds for Michaelis–Menten type kinetics.

In the case of overall first-order kinetics, each partial process can be characterized by one rate or velocity constant k; for example, k_{12} for the uptake, k_{21} for the exhalation, and k_{el} for the metabolic elimination. First-order kinetic processes operate as

$$\dot{y}_i(t) = \frac{\mathrm{d}y_i(t)}{\mathrm{d}t} = ky_i(t) \tag{13.1}$$

and, therefore, the first-order elimination kinetics, with $N_{el}(t)$ denoting the amount metabolised up to time t, and V_i denoting the volume of compartment i, this partial process of metabolic turnover is characterized by

$$\dot{N}_{el}(t) = \frac{\mathrm{d}N_{el}(t)}{\mathrm{d}t} = k_{el}V_2y_2(t). \tag{13.2}$$

Assuming merely first-order uptake and exhalation, the two-compartment model then yields a system of linear differential equations with the matched processes in each compartment in the form

$$\begin{aligned} V_1\dot{y}_1(r) &= -k_{12}V_1y_1(t) + k_{21}V_2y_2(t), \\ V_2\dot{y}_2(t) &= +k_{12}V_1y_1(t) - k_{21}V_2y_2(t) - \dot{N}_{el}(t). \end{aligned} \tag{13.3}$$

These yield

$$y_2(t) = \frac{V_1(\dot{y}_1(t) + k_{12}y_1(t))}{k_{21}V_2} \tag{13.4}$$

and

$$\dot{N}_{el}(t) = -(V_1\dot{y}_1(t) + V_2\dot{y}_2(t)). \tag{13.5}$$

Additionally assuming first-order elimination kinetics, the resulting model described by two compartments and three partial processes is represented in Fig. 13.1.

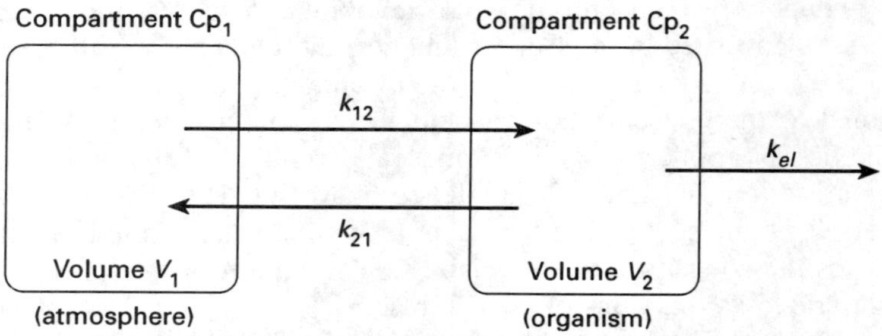

Fig. 13.1. The two-compartment block in the case of metabolic turnover.

The partial processes are then depicted as follows: In the infinitesimal time interval $[t, t + \mathrm{d}t)$ the amount of material $\{k_{12}V_1y_1(t)\mathrm{d}t\}$ passes from compartment 1 into compartment 2, and the amount of material $\{k_{21}V_2y_2(t)\mathrm{d}t\}$ passes from compartment 2 into compartment 1. The amount $\{k_{el}V_2y_2(t)\mathrm{d}t\}$ is eliminated by metabolic processes. The rates of change in the quantity of material in the compartments are given by the system of differential equations

$$\begin{aligned} V_1\frac{\mathrm{d}y_1(t)}{\mathrm{d}t} &= -k_{12}V_1y_1(t) + k_{21}V_2y_2(t), \\ V_2\frac{\mathrm{d}y_2(t)}{\mathrm{d}t} &= +k_{12}V_1y_1(t) - (k_{21} + k_{el})V_2y_2(t), \end{aligned} \tag{13.6}$$

or

$$\begin{pmatrix} \mathrm{d}y_1(t)/\mathrm{d}t \\ \mathrm{d}y_2(t)/\mathrm{d}t \end{pmatrix} =: \dot{y}(t) = \mathbf{A}y(t),$$

with the notation

$$\alpha_1 := V_1V_2, \quad \alpha_2 := V_2/V_1, \qquad \mathbf{y}(t) := [y_1(t), y_2(t)]^{\mathrm{T}},$$

and

$$\mathbf{A} := \begin{pmatrix} -k_{12} & \alpha_2 k_{21} \\ \alpha_1 k_{12} & -(k_{21} + k_{el}) \end{pmatrix}.$$

The matrix **A** is regular (of full rank) and the deterministic solution may be obtained using Laplace transformation or matrix theory.

In some instances, there may be assumed a basic level of compound under question in the second compartment Cp_2 due to an internal production of the substance or a common environmental pollution with the compound that cannot be excluded by the experimental design. If there is an internal production of the chemical, this will also happen during the experiment, and it may be compared with a continuous infusion into the system instead of, or in addition to, a bolus injection.

Let the initial state of any dynamic system modelled by two compartments be given by the vector $(\mathbf{y}0) := [y_1(0), y_2(0)]^{\mathrm{T}}$ and let $\mathbf{B}(t) := [B_1(t), B_2(t)]^{\mathrm{T}}$ be the vector describing a continuous input (production, injection) or output (loss) into or out of the compartments. Furthermore, let the dynamic system be described by the system of differential equations

$$\mathrm{d}y_1(t)/\mathrm{d}t = \alpha(t)y_1(t) + b(t)y_2(t) + B_1(t),$$
$$\mathrm{d}y_2(t)/\mathrm{d}t = c(t)y_1(t) + d(t)y_2(t) + B_2(t),$$

or

$$\dot{\mathbf{y}}(t) := \begin{pmatrix} \mathrm{d}y_1(t)/\mathrm{d}t \\ \mathrm{d}y_2(t)/\mathrm{d}t \end{pmatrix} = \begin{pmatrix} a(t) & b(t) \\ c(t) & d(t) \end{pmatrix} \begin{pmatrix} y_1(t) \\ y_2(t) \end{pmatrix} + \begin{pmatrix} B_1(t) \\ B_2(t) \end{pmatrix} =: \mathbf{A}(t)\cdot\mathbf{y}(t) + \mathbf{B}(t). \tag{13.7}$$

Excluding the problem of validating the chosen model, the basic scientific interest is in the parameters characterizing the special model. In the case of *in vivo* or *in vitro* systems in toxicology, the main levels or dimensions of each parameter are its intra-species or intra-tissue distribution and its inter-species or inter-tissue behaviour. The above is concerned with the intra-species or intra-tissue situation. On this level and in a special species or tissue, the parameters are assumed to be time-invariant but concentration-dependent in terms of orders of reaction. However, concentration may change over time and is therefore time-dependent.

In the case of the two-compartment model, the assumption of time-invariant parameters describing the dynamic model through the order of reaction yields $a(t) = a$, $b(t) = b$, $c(t) = c$, $d(t) = d$, and therefore $\mathbf{A}(t) = \mathbf{A}$, and the solution to

$$\dot{\mathbf{y}}(t) = \mathbf{A}\cdot\mathbf{y}(t) + B(t) \tag{13.8}$$

then becomes

$$\mathbf{y}(t) = \mathrm{e}^{\mathbf{A}t}\cdot\mathbf{y}(0) + \mathrm{e}^{\mathbf{A}t}\cdot\int_0^t (\mathrm{e}^{-\mathbf{A}x}\cdot\mathbf{B}(x))\mathrm{d}x. \tag{13.9}$$

The matrix-integral is calculated by integrating the components of the matrix. Furthermore, the solution contains matrix-exponent forms, which can be evaluated using series expansion of the e-function and spectra decomposition of the matrices.

Let the matrix $\mathbf{A}$ be regular and real, with distinct eigenvalues, and let $c \neq 0$ and $b \neq 0$. The eigenvalues of $\mathbf{A}$ are given by

$$\lambda_1 := \tfrac{1}{2}\left[a + d + \sqrt{(a-d)^2 + 4cb}\right] \quad \text{and} \quad \lambda_2 := \tfrac{1}{2}\left[a + d - \sqrt{(a-d)^2 + 4cb}\right], \tag{13.10}$$

where

$$\lambda_2 \leqslant \lambda_1, \qquad \lambda_1\lambda_2 = ad - cb, \qquad \text{and} \qquad \lambda_1 + \lambda_2 = a + d, \tag{13.11}$$

and **A** can be rewritten as

$$\mathbf{A} = \frac{1}{(\lambda_1 - \lambda_2)cb}\begin{pmatrix} -b & -b \\ (a-\lambda_1) & (a-\lambda_2)\end{pmatrix}\begin{pmatrix} \lambda_1 & 0 \\ 0 & \lambda_2\end{pmatrix}$$
$$\times\begin{pmatrix} -c(\lambda_1 - d) & (a-\lambda_1)(\lambda_1 - d) \\ -c(d-\lambda_2) & (a-\lambda_2)(d-\lambda_2)\end{pmatrix}, \tag{13.12}$$

using the right and left eigenvectors. Noting, that for $i, j = 1, 2$,

$$(a - \lambda_i) = (a + d - d - \lambda_i) = (\lambda_i + \lambda_j - d - \lambda_i) = (\lambda_j - d)$$

and

$$(d - \lambda_i) = (a + d - a - \lambda_i) = (\lambda_i + \lambda_j - a - \lambda_i) = (\lambda_j - a),$$

this yeilds

$$\mathrm{e}^{\mathbf{A}t} = \frac{1}{(\lambda_1 - \lambda_2)cb}\cdot\mathbf{K}, \tag{13.13}$$

with

$$\mathbf{K} = \begin{bmatrix} cb\{(a-\lambda_2)\mathrm{e}^{\lambda_1 t} - (a-\lambda_1)\mathrm{e}^{\lambda_2 t}\} & (\lambda_2 - a)(a-\lambda_1)b\{\mathrm{e}^{\lambda_1 t} - \mathrm{e}^{\lambda_2 t}\} \\ (\lambda_2 - a)(a-\lambda_1)c\{\mathrm{e}^{\lambda_1 t} - \mathrm{e}^{\lambda_2 t}\} & (a-\lambda_1)(a-\lambda_2)\{(a-\lambda_1)\mathrm{e}^{\lambda_1 t} - (a-\lambda_2)\mathrm{e}^{\lambda_2 t}\}\end{bmatrix}.$$

Given this matrix-exponent form, the initial state of the system $\mathbf{y}(0)$, and the input function $\mathbf{B}(t)$ the deterministic solution given by eqn. (13.9) can easily be evaluated.

Returning to the above example, the components of the matrix **A** are given by $a = -k_{12}$, $b = \alpha_2 k_{21}$, $c = \alpha_1 k_{12}$, and $d = -(k_{21} + k_{el})$, whereby the rate parameters are naturally positive. The eigenvalues are then given as

$$\lambda_{1,2} = \tfrac{1}{2}\left\{-(k_{12} + k_{21} + k_{el}) \pm \sqrt{(k_{12} + k_{21} + k_{el})^2 - 4k_{12}k_{el}}\right\} \tag{13.14}$$

with $\lambda_2 < \lambda_1 < 0$, $\lambda_1\lambda_2 = k_{12}k_{el}$, and $\lambda_1 + \lambda_2 = -(k_{12} + k_{21} + k_{el})$.

The assumption of no compound being present in the organism at the beginning of the experiments and the single bolus infusion yield $\mathbf{y}(0) = [y_1(0),\ 0]^{\mathrm{T}}$ as the initial state of the system and $\mathbf{B}(t) = [0,\ 0]^{\mathrm{T}}$ as the input function during the observation phase. The solution is then simply given by $\mathbf{y}(t) = \mathrm{e}^{\mathbf{A}t}\mathbf{y}(0)$, with

$$y_1(t) = \frac{y_1(0)}{(\lambda_1 - \lambda_2)}\{(k_{12} + \lambda_1)\mathrm{e}^{\lambda_2 t} - (k_{12} + \lambda_2)\mathrm{e}^{\lambda_1 t}\} \tag{13.15}$$

and

$$y_2(t) = \frac{y_1(0)(\lambda_2 + k_{12})(k_{12} + \lambda_1)}{(\lambda_1 - \lambda_2)\alpha_2 k_{21}}\{\mathrm{e}^{\lambda_2 t} - \mathrm{e}^{\lambda_1 t}\}. \tag{13.16}$$

The ratio of $y_2(t)$ and $y_1(t)$ yields

$$\frac{y_2(t)}{y_1(t)} = \frac{(\lambda_2 + k_{12})(k_{12} + \lambda_1)\{e^{\lambda_2 t} - e^{\lambda_1 t}\}}{\alpha_2 k_{21}\{(k_{12} + \lambda_1)e^{\lambda_2 t} - (k_{12} + \lambda_2)e^{\lambda_1 t}\}}$$

$$= \frac{(\lambda_2 + k_{12})\{e^{(\lambda_2 - \lambda_1)t} - 1\}}{\alpha_2 k_{21}\left\{e^{(\lambda_2 - \lambda_1)t} - \dfrac{(k_{12} + \lambda_2)}{(k_{12} + \lambda_1)}\right\}}, \tag{13.17}$$

and because $(\lambda_2 - \lambda_1) < 0$ asymptotically,

$$\lim_{t \to \infty}\left\{\frac{y_2(t)}{y_1(t)}\right\} = \frac{(k_{12} + \lambda_1)(k_{12} + \lambda_2)}{\alpha_2 k_{21}(k_{12} + \lambda_2)} = \frac{(k_{12} + \lambda_1)}{\alpha_2 k_{21}}$$

$$= \frac{k_{12}}{\alpha_2(\lambda_1 + k_{21} + k_{el})} = \frac{V_1 k_{12}}{V_2(\lambda_1 + k_{21} + k_{el})}, \tag{13.18}$$

which is known as the steady-state constant K_{st}.

From theoretical considerations (Filser 1992), the parameter k_{12} is inversely proportional to the atmospheric volume V_1, and the product $k_{12}V_1$ is constant. Consequently, referring to an open system, $V_1 \to \infty$ implies $k_{12} \to 0$ and

$$\lim_{V_1 \to \infty}\{K_{st}\} = \frac{V_1 k_{12}}{V_2(k_{21} + k_{el})} < \frac{V_1 k_{12}}{V_2(\lambda_1 + k_{21} + k_{el})}. \tag{13.19}$$

Therefore, the asymptotically defined steady-state constant in the closed exposure system is greater than in the real-life situation.

The most important events happen within the second compartment, and it is therefore useful and necessary to examine the deterministic concentration–time relationship in the second compartment in more detail.

For the given example of Filser's closed chamber technique (Filser 1992) under strict first-order kinetics, with no endogenous production of compound assumed, the deterministic concentration–time function for the organism is given by

$$y_2(t) = \frac{y_1(0)(\lambda_2 + k_{12})(k_{12} + \lambda_1)}{(\lambda_1 - \lambda_2)\alpha_2 k_{21}}\{e^{\lambda_2 t} - e^{\lambda_1 t}\}$$

$$= y_1(0)\left[\frac{V_1(\lambda_2 + k_{12})(k_{12} + \lambda_1)}{V_2(\lambda_1 - \lambda_2)k_{21}}\{e^{\lambda_2 t} - e^{\lambda_1 t}\}\right] =: y_1(0)f(t), \tag{13.20}$$

where $y_1(0)$ denotes the initially administered dose in the experimental atmosphere. The shape of the concentration–time function is completely determined by

$$f(t) = \frac{V_1(\lambda_2 + k_{12})(k_{12} + \lambda_1)}{V_2(\lambda_1 - \lambda_2)k_{21}}\{e^{\lambda_2 t} - e^{\lambda_1 t}\} = \frac{(\lambda_2 - a)(\lambda_1 - a)}{(\lambda_1 - \lambda_2)b}\{e^{\lambda_2 t} - e^{\lambda_1 t}\} \tag{13.21}$$

From $\lambda_2 < \lambda_1 < 0$, it follows that $(\lambda_1 - \lambda_2) > 0$, $e^{\lambda_2 t} < e^{\lambda_1 t}$, and $(e^{\lambda_2 t} - e^{\lambda_1 t}) < 0$. Furthermore, $b > 0$, $f(0) = \lim_{t \to \infty} g(t) = 0$,

$$(\lambda_1 - a) = \left(\tfrac{1}{2}\left[a + d + \sqrt{(a-d)^2 + 4cb}\right] - a\right) = \tfrac{1}{2}\left[(d-a) + \sqrt{(d-a)^2 + 4cb}\right]$$
$$> \tfrac{1}{2}\left[(d-a) + \sqrt{(d-a)^2}\right] = \tfrac{1}{2}[(d-a) + |d-a|] \geqslant 0,$$

and

$$(\lambda_2 - a) = \left(\tfrac{1}{2}\left[a + d - \sqrt{(a-d)^2 + 4cb}\right] - a\right) = \tfrac{1}{2}\left[(d-a) - \sqrt{(d-a)^2 + 4cb}\right]$$
$$< \tfrac{1}{2}\left[(d-a) - \sqrt{(d-a)^2}\right] = \tfrac{1}{2}[(d-a) - |d-a|] \leqslant 0.$$

For determining the time and peak of the maximum, the first derivative of $f(t)$ is given by

$$f'(t) = \frac{(\lambda_2 - a)(\lambda_1 - a)}{(\lambda_1 - \lambda_2)b}\{\lambda_2 e^{\lambda_2 t} - \lambda_1 e^{\lambda_1 t}\}, \tag{13.22}$$

and

$$f'(t) = 0 \Leftrightarrow \{\lambda_2 e^{\lambda_2 t} - \lambda_1 e^{\lambda_1 t}\} = 0 \Leftrightarrow \lambda_2 e^{\lambda_2 t} = \lambda_1 e^{\lambda_1 t}$$
$$\Leftrightarrow \lambda_2 t \ln(\lambda_2) = \lambda_1 t \ln(\lambda_1) \Leftrightarrow t = \ln\left(\frac{\lambda_1}{\lambda_2}\right) \cdot \frac{1}{(\lambda_2 - \lambda_1)} =: t_{\max}.$$

For checking the maximum, the second derivative of $f(t)$ is given by

$$f''(t) = \frac{(\lambda_2 - a)(\lambda_1 - a)}{(\lambda_1 - \lambda_2)b}\{\lambda_2^2 e^{\lambda_2 t} - \lambda_1^2 e^{\lambda_1 t}\}$$

with

$$\{\lambda_2^2 e^{\lambda_2 t_{\max}} - \lambda_1^2 e^{\lambda_1 t_{\max}}\} = \left[\lambda_2^2(\lambda_1/\lambda_2)^{\lambda_2/(\lambda_2 - \lambda_1)} - \lambda_1^2(\lambda_1/\lambda_2)^{\lambda_1/(\lambda_2 - \lambda_1)}\right]$$
$$= (\lambda_1/\lambda_2)^{\lambda_1/(\lambda_2 - \lambda_1)}[\lambda_2 - \lambda_1]\lambda_1 > 0.$$

because $\lambda_2 - \lambda_1 < 0$ and $\lambda_1/\lambda_2 > 0$, so that in summary $f''(t_{\max}) < 0$. The concentration peak in the organism is then given by

$$y_2(t_{\max}) = y_1(0)\left[\frac{(\lambda_2 + k_{12})(k_{12} + \lambda_1)}{\alpha_2 \lambda_2 k_{21}}\left(\frac{\lambda_1}{\lambda_2}\right)^{\lambda_1/(\lambda_2 - \lambda_1)}\right]$$
$$= y_1(0)\left[\frac{-k_{12}V_1}{V_2\lambda_2}\left(\frac{\lambda_1}{\lambda_2}\right)^{\lambda_1/(\lambda_2 - \lambda_1)}\right], \tag{13.23}$$

which corresponds to

$$y_1(t_{\max}) = \frac{y_1(0)}{(\lambda_1 - \lambda_2)}\left(\frac{\lambda_1}{\lambda_2}\right)^{\lambda_1/(\lambda_2-\lambda_1)}\left\{\frac{(k_{12}+\lambda_1)\lambda_1 - \lambda_2(k_{12}+\lambda_2)}{\lambda_2}\right\}$$

$$= y_1(0)\left[\frac{-(k_{21}+k_{el})}{\lambda_2}\left(\frac{\lambda_1}{\lambda_2}\right)^{\lambda_1/(\lambda_2-\lambda_1)}\right] \tag{13.24}$$

in the experimental atmosphere, i.e., the first compartment.

Looking again at the ratio of these two concentrations yields

$$\frac{y_2(t_{\max})}{y_1(t_{\max})} = \frac{k_{12}V_1}{(k_{21}+k_{el})V_2}, \tag{13.25}$$

which is, indeed, the steady-state constant of eqn. (13.19) calculated for the open atmosphere.

13.4 Statistical methods

13.4.1 *Data expression under 'closed chamber' conditions*

The observable concentration–time data in experiments based on 'the closed chamber technique' reflect the totality of kinetic processes in the body. The processes in the body itself depend on the amount of material added to the inhalation chamber at the beginning of the experiments. Once the individual experiment has started, the added amount of material equilibrates with the organism up to the steady state. If there is no metabolism and no loss of material through other pathways, this steady state equals the equilibrium state. After reaching the steady state, the observable decay of concentration is governed by the metabolism or the loss of material within the body. If the kinetic processes in the body are saturable, and if the initial concentration in the inhalation chamber is so high that the kinetic processes within the body are saturated, an obvious linear decay can be seen in the experimental data after the equilibrium phase, until the saturation conditions are decomposed. Because it is a dynamic system, this obvious linear decay may not be justified, as indicated by the deterministic solutions of the compartment models above.

13.4.2 *A statistical strategy for first-order kinetics*

In the present example of experimental design, let the biological system under view be exposed to a variety of n initial concentrations $y_{1m}(0) := y_{0m}$, $m = 1, 2, \ldots, n$. Let the random variable Y_{mj} denote the concentration of propylene in the first compartment Cp_1 in the mth experiment with initial concentration y_{0m} at times t_j, $j = 1, 2, \ldots, d_m$ and $m = 1, 2, \ldots, n$. The n experiments are divided into two subsets E_1 and E_2, where E_1 consists of all those experiments with strict first-order elimination kinetics characterized by low initial concentrations y_{0m}.

The expectation value of Y_{mj} for $m \in E_1$, $j = 1, 2, \ldots, d_m$, is given by $y_1(t_j, k_m)$, where $k_m := (k_{12m}, k_{21m}, k_{elm}, y_{0m})^{\mathrm{T}}$. Thus, the jth measurement in the mth experiment, y_{mj}, is described by the statistical model

$$y_{mj} = y_1(t_j, k_m) + \varepsilon_{mj} \qquad \text{for} \qquad m \in E_1 \quad \text{and} \quad j = 1, 2, \ldots, d_m, \tag{13.26}$$

where the measurement errors ε_{mj} are assumed to be uncorrelated, with $\mathrm{E}(\varepsilon_{mj}) = 0$ and $\mathrm{Var}(\varepsilon_{mj}) = \sigma_m^2$. This model is the basis of the practice in compartmental analysis of estimating the parameter vector k_m by least squares; that is, by minimizing

$$\sum_{j=1}^{d_m} \left\{ y_{mj} - y_1\left(t_j, \hat{k}_m\right) \right\}^2 \qquad \text{for} \qquad m \in E_1, \tag{13.27}$$

where $\hat{k}_m := (\hat{k}_{12m}, \hat{k}_{21m}, \hat{k}_{elm}, \hat{y}_{m0})^{\mathrm{T}}$ and y_{mj} is the observed concentration in Cp_1 at time t_j. If corresponding software is available, the system of differential equations may be solved numerically, and estimates of the rate parameters can be obtained using faster optimization algorithms. Furthermore, model (13.26), with the assumption of constant variances within each experiment, can be extended to the typical case of heterogeneous variances and autocorrelated error structures in biological data.

Let $|E_1|$ denote the number of experiments with first-order kinetics. Then estimates of k_{12} and k_{21} under 'standard' conditions (for a definition of 'standard' conditions, see Filser 1992) may be obtained by calculating the harmonic mean

$$\hat{k}_{12} = \frac{|E_1|}{\sum\limits_{m \in E_1} \left(1/\hat{k}_{12m}\right)} \qquad \text{and} \qquad \hat{k}_{21} = \frac{|E_1|}{\sum\limits_{m \in E_1} \left(1/\hat{k}_{21m}\right)}. \tag{13.28}$$

Adapted to the conditions of the individual experiments, $\hat{k}_{12}$ and $\hat{k}_{21}$ can be used for the analysis of the experiments in E_2, where first-order elimination kinetics may not be assumed.

As an example, in Fig. 13.2 is shown actually measured concentration–time data in Cp_1 (squares) and the fitted curve in a single experiment with low initial concentration (a). The errors of the fit with a sketched error structure (dashed line) and 95 per cent limits are shown in (b). According to the solution of the differential equations, (c) shows the estimated concentration–time curve of propylene in Cp_2 for this experiment. For details, see Becka *et al.* (1992)

13.4.3 *Approach to non-linear elimination kinetics*

Using eqn. (13.4) and substituting the first derivative $\dot{y}_1(t)$ by an appropriate approximation $\hat{\dot{y}}_1(t)$ yields

$$\hat{y}_{2m}(t_j) = \frac{V_{1m}\left(\hat{\dot{y}}_{1m}(t_j) + \hat{k}_{12m} y_{mj}\right)}{\hat{k}_{21m} V_{2m}} \qquad \text{for} \qquad m \in E_2 \quad \text{and} \quad j = 1, 2, \ldots, d_m. \tag{13.29}$$

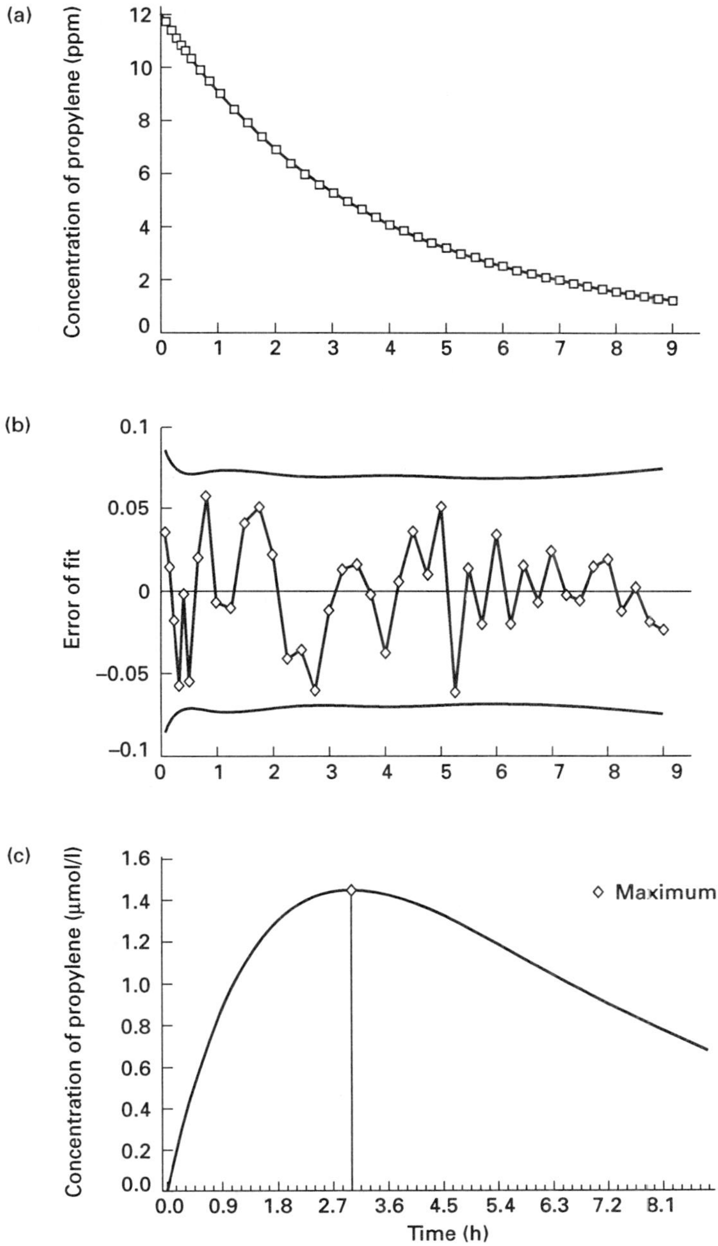

Fig. 13.2. (a) The actually measured concentration–time data in Cp_1 (squares) and the fitted curve for the estimates ($\pm$s.d.) $\hat{k}_{12} = 0.29 \pm 0.004$, $\hat{k}_{21} = 0.052 \pm 0.011$, $\hat{k}_{el} = 0.367 \pm 0.063$, and $\hat{y}_0 = 11.947 \pm 0.021$. (b) Errors of the fit with a sketched error structure (dashed line) and asymptotic 95 per cent limits. (c) The estimated concentration–time curve for propylene in Cp_2, with the marked concentration peak according to Becka *et al.* (1992).

Substituting the first derivative $\dot{y}_2(t)$ in eqn. (13.5) by an approximation using eqn. (13.29) yields an estimate for the metabolic elimination rate $\dot{N}_{el}(t)$ for each time t_j in experiments from E_2 by

$$z_{mj} := -\left(V_{1m}\hat{\dot{y}}_{1m}(t_j) + V_{2m}\dot{y}_{2m}(t_j)\right) \quad \text{for} \quad m \in E_2 \quad \text{and} \quad j = 1, 2, \ldots, d_m. \tag{13.30}$$

For each $m \in E_2$ the maximal value $z_{m,\max}(j^*)$ of the $\{z_{mj}: j = 1, 2, \ldots, d_m\}$ characterizes the maximal elimination rate, since this value corresponds to the theoretical maximal concentration $y_{2m,\max}(j^*)$ in the body, which itself depends on the chosen initial concentration y_{0m}, at the beginning of each individual experiment through the subscript m.

Dropping the time expression j^*, which is not essential here, and looking at the $z_{m,\max}$ alone, these values must be interpreted as individual realizations of random variables $Z_{m,\max}$ with probability density functions Ψ_m. The elimination rate η as a function of concentration can then be modelled, for example, by the Michaelis–Menten equation by using the expected values $\mathrm{E}(Z_{m,\max})$ of the $Z_{m,\max}$ through

$$\eta\{\mathrm{E}(Z_{m,\max})\} = \frac{\nu_{\max}\,\mathrm{E}(Z_{m,\max})}{\kappa_m + \mathrm{E}(Z_{m,\max})}. \tag{13.31}$$

13.4.4 *An approximate approach using the curve-stripping technique*

Given a concentration–time curve of a special compound in a special exposure system, it might be assumed that the kinetic processes are adequately described by an open two-compartment model, in which measurements are only taken from one of the compartments, say from compartment Cp_1. Let the two compartments be mutually connected by two pathways and let there be an outlet to the outside in one of the compartments. An experimental input may be made as a bolus into Cp_1 or as a bolus outside but invading Cp_1. Examples are enzymatic reactions (substrate and product), pharmacokinetics (blood and target tissue), and inhalation experiments. For further discussion, the model shown in Fig. 13.1 will be used.

The deterministic solution for the concentration–time curve in the first compartment is given by eqn. (13.15) and can be defined in the common form as

$$y_1(t) = \frac{y_1(0)}{(\lambda_1 - \lambda_2)}\{(a - \lambda_2)\mathrm{e}^{\lambda_1 t} + (\lambda_1 - a)\mathrm{e}^{\lambda_2 t}\} =: \Psi_1\mathrm{e}^{\lambda_1 t} + \Psi_2\mathrm{e}^{\lambda_2 t}, \tag{13.32}$$

with

$$\Psi_1 := \frac{(a - \lambda_2)y_1(0)}{(\lambda_1 - \lambda_2)} \quad \text{and} \quad \Psi_2 := \frac{(\lambda_1 - a)y_1(0)}{(\lambda_1 - \lambda_2)},$$

and it is obvious that $\Psi_2 + \Psi_1 = y_1(0)$. From this it follows that

$$\Psi_1 = \frac{(a-\lambda_2)y_1(0)}{(\lambda_1-\lambda_2)} \Leftrightarrow a = \frac{\Psi_1(\lambda_1-\lambda_2)}{y_1(0)} + \lambda_2 = \frac{\Psi_1\lambda_1 + \lambda_2\Psi_2}{y_1(0)},$$

and, using $a + d = \lambda_1 + \lambda_2$,

$$d = \lambda_1 + \lambda_2 - a = \lambda_1 - \frac{\Psi_1(\lambda_1-\lambda_2)}{y_1(0)} = \frac{\Psi_1\lambda_2 + \lambda_1\Psi_2}{y_1(0)}.$$

In the given example, and with the additional information that $\lambda_1\lambda_2 = k_{12}k_{el}$, the kinetic parameters can then be written as

$$k_{12} = \frac{-(\Psi_1\lambda_1 + \lambda_2\Psi_2)}{y_1(0)}, \quad k_{el} = \frac{-\lambda_1\lambda_2 y_1(0)}{(\Psi_1\lambda_1 + \lambda_2\Psi_2)}, \quad k_{21} = \frac{-(\lambda_1-\lambda_2)^2\Psi_1\Psi_2}{(\Psi_1\lambda_1 + \lambda_2\Psi_2)y_1(0)}.$$

The special concentration–time curve can be approximately divided into two parts when plotted in semi-logarithmic scale. After the bolus administration of a certain compound into Cp_1, a non-linear phase of fast decay of concentration occurs at the beginning of the experiment, describing the disposition process in the system. This fast decay is followed by an approximately linear phase governed by the elimination process. The whole concentration–time curve is outlined in Fig. 13.3.

The curve-stripping technique, also called the 'method of residuals' or 'back feathering', works as follows. The deterministic concentration–time curve given by eqn. (13.32), also known as the sum of exponentials model, is approximated by its product:

$$y_1(t) = \Psi_1 e^{\lambda_1 t} + \Psi_2 e^{\lambda_2 t} \approx \Psi_1 e^{\lambda_1 t}\Psi_2 e^{\lambda_2 t}. \tag{13.33}$$

From this it follows that

$$\ln\{y_1(t)\} \approx (\ln\{\Psi_1\} + \lambda_1 t) + (\ln\{\Psi_2\} + \lambda_2 t) =: G1 + G2.$$

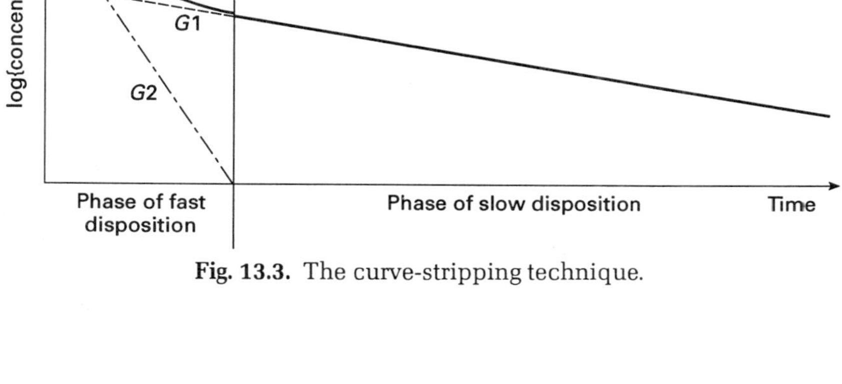

Fig. 13.3. The curve-stripping technique.

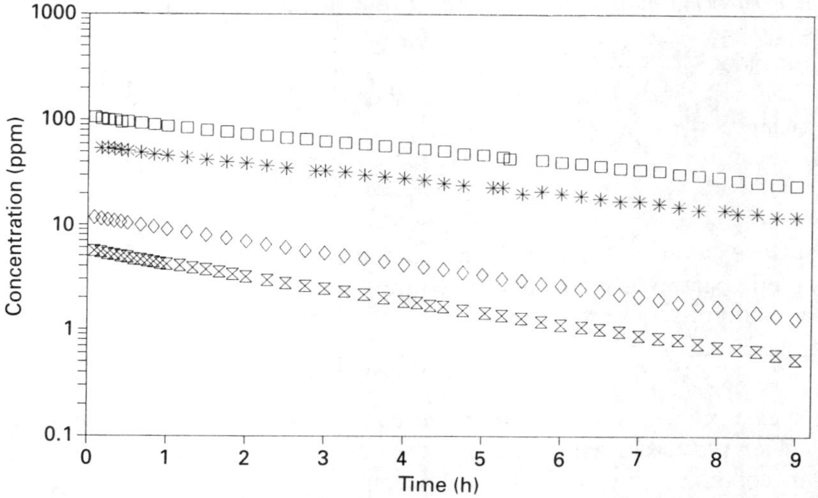

Fig. 13.4. Concentration–time data of propylene in rats from four experiments carried out by Golka *et. al.* (1989). Observations resulting from each experiment are characterized by the same symbol.

Using the experimental data after reaching the phase of slow disposition, the intercept $\ln\{\Psi_1\}$ and slope λ_1 of the straight line $G1$ can be estimated using simple linear regression analysis. The second straight line $G2$, describing the phase of fast disposition in the beginning, is obtained by subtracting the back-extrapolated $G1$-values from the logarithms of the observed data in this phase. The resulting values are then used to estimate the intercept term $\ln\{\Psi_2\}$ and slope λ_2 of the straight line $G2$ using simple linear regression analysis again. These slopes and intercepts allow approximate calculations of the microconstants k_{12}, k_{21}, and k_{el} as described above.

However, the approximation (13.33) might lead to erroneous results. The classification of the experimental data into fast and slow phases of disposition is difficult, as shown in Fig. 13.4, and—even if possible—is always performed at random. The estimated values of the microconstants depend on this classification. Nevertheless, they yield an approximate impression of the order of magnitude and can be used as starting values for more detailed analyses such as non-linear regression. For further discussion, see Becka *et al.* (1993).

13.5 Statistical aspects of population toxicokinetics

13.5.1 *Data structure for considering intra- and inter-individual variation*

Studies and experiments designed for risk assessment are usually based on special collections of individual subjects. One or more interesting response variables are measured at several selected times, leading to so-called time-dependent response curves. The selected individual subjects are assumed to be a representative sample of a population of individuals, all of whose responses are related to time in a basically similar way but with some variation from individual to individual. It is important to consider the measurement process on the individual response curves and also to take into account the variation of these individual response curves around a mean population curve.

The measured data structure is determined by the number k of individuals sampled from the population and the number n_i of observations made on individual i ($i = 1, 2, \ldots, k$). The observed response of the ith individual at time t_{ij} will be denoted by y_{ij} ($i = 1, 2, \ldots, k$; $j = 1, 2, \ldots, n_i$). In the case of no missing observations and if all individuals are observed at comparable times, n_i and t_{ij} will not require the subscript i.

13.5.2 *Population model*

We assume that the relationship between the response y_{ij} and the time of measurement t_{ij} takes the form

$$y_{ij} = f(\theta_i, t_{ij}) + e_{ij}, \qquad i = 1, 2, \ldots, k, \quad j = 1, 2, \ldots, n_i, \tag{13.34}$$

where f describes the expected value of the response at the different times t_{ij} for a given parameter vector θ_i of individual i and e_{ij} is a zero-mean measurement error assumed to be independent from observation to observation and with constant variance.

For a sample of individuals from the same population, the same form of functional relationship f is expected. The parameter vector θ_i which determines the precise shape of the curve for each individual is assumed to vary across the population in the manner of a random sample.

It is reasonable to suppose that $\theta_i = \theta + v_i$, where θ can be interpreted as a mean population parameter vector. The zero-mean random vectors v_i, which are supposed to be independent across individuals, represent the variation of the individual parameter vectors θ_i around the mean population parameter vector θ.

The elements of the covariance matrix $Cov(v_i) = \mathbf{\Sigma}$ describe this variation.

13.5.3 *Outlook*

Several statistical methods have been proposed for the inference of parameters in models that combine individual and population components.

For the special case of a linear growth pattern, Urfer and Thöni (1976) have applied Rao's MINQUE (*m*inimum *n*orm *q*uadratic *u*nbiased *e*stimation) procedure for estimating variance–covariance components in a growth-curve study conducted in a plant physiology experiment. This random coefficient regression approach involves repeated inversion of large matrices, resulting in intensive computations, large storage requirements and numerical instabilities.

The analysis of non-linear individual response curves is described by Racine-Poon and Smith (1990). Technical details of the empirical Bayes approach and its application to simulated and real data are given. All the calculations reported by Racine-Poon and Smith were performed using *PROC GLM* and *PROC NLIN* of SAS (1985).

Particularly in the case of non-linear response curves, population models involve complex covariance structures. They present a challenge for statisticians in terms of both estimation and model validation. Recently, Breslow and Clayton (1993) reviewed approximate inference in generalized linear mixed models, and showed that their penalized quasi-likelihood procedure is equivalent to the non-linear mixed model procedure of Lindstrom and Bates (1990).

Whatever procedure is followed, a substantial amount of diagnostic and cross-validation checking has to be performed to investigate the appropriateness of the choice of response curves, error variance forms, distributional assumptions, and approximations invoked in the inference procedure.

Acknowledgements

The authors would like to thank the editor and the referees for helpful hints and for improving the text.

References

Becka, M., Bolt, H. M., and Urfer, W. (1992). Statistical analysis of toxicokinetic data by nonlinear regression (example: inhalation pharmacokinetics of propylene). *Archives of Toxicology* **66**, 450–3.

Breslow, N. E. and Clayton, D. G. (1993). Approximate inference in generalized linear mixed models. *Journal of the American Statistical Association*, **88** (no. 421) 9–25.

Filser, J. G. (1992). The closed chamber technique—uptake, endogenous production, excretion, steady-state kinetics and rates of metabolism of gases and vapours. *Archives of Toxicology* **66**, 1–10.

Golka, K., Peter, H., Denk, B., and Filser, J. G. (1989). Pharmacokinetics of propylene and its reactive metabolite propylene oxide in Sprague–Dawley rats. *Archives of Toxicology Supplement*, **13**, 240–2.

Lindstrom, M. J. and Bates, D. M. (1990). Nonlinear mixed effects models for repeated measures data. *Biometrics*, **46**, 673–87.

NAS (1983) *Risk assessment in the Federal Government: managing the process*. National Academy of Sciences. National Academy Press, Washington DC.

Racine-Poon, A. and Smith, A. F. M. (1990). Population models. In *Statistical methodology in the pharmaceutical sciences* (ed. D. A. Berry), pp. 139–62. Marcel Dekker, New York.

SAS (1985) *User's guide, version* 6. SAS Institute Inc., Cary, North Carolina, USA.

Urfer, W. and Thöni, H. (1976). Zur Schätzung von Wachstumskurven aufgrund wiederholter Messungen am gleichen Individuum. *EDV in Biologie und Medizin* **6**, 92–5.

Index